Weight Management
-
Challenges and Opportunities

Edited by Hassan M. Heshmati

Published in London, United Kingdom

Weight Management - Challenges and Opportunities
http://dx.doi.org/10.5772/intechopen.95719
Edited by Hassan M. Heshmati

Contributors
Reji Manjunathan, Dharanibalan Kasiviswanathan, Selvaraj Jayaraman, Gwen V. Childs, Angela K. Odle, Melanie C. MacNicol, Melody L. Allensworth-James, Tiffany K. Miles, Noor Akhter, Mohsin M. Syed, Angus M. MacNicol, Shyam Pyari Jaiswar, Apala Priyadarshini, Sunil T. Galatage, Sakshi N. Gurav, Mahadevi R. Moladi, Tejal R. Podjale, Nikita B. Tejam, Arehalli S. Manjappa, Popat S. Kumbhar, Supriya V. Nikade, Swapnil S. Chopade, Sujit A. Desai, Shweta N. Kalebere, Suresh G. Killedar, Indu Saxena, Amar Preet Kaur, Suwarna Suman, Abhilasha, Prasenjit Mitra, Praveen Sharma, Manoj Kumar, Svitlana Drozdovska, Olena Andrieieva, Valeriya Orlenko, Igor Andrieiev, Victoriya Pastukhova, Iuliia Mazur, Olha Hurenko, Anastasiia Nahorna, Wahiba Elhag, Walid El Ansari, Ina Shaw, Travis Triplett, Brandon S. Shaw, Nina Vinot, Emma Baghtchedjian, Clémentine Picolo, Grégory Lambert, Anvi Rana, Kayode Olariike Oyindasola, Folake Funke Adedoyin, Adeoye Adeyemi Adedoyin, Upasana, Danladi Musa, Daniel Iornyior, Andrew Tyoakaa

First published in London, United Kingdom, 2022 by IntechOpen
IntechOpen is the global imprint of INTECHOPEN LIMITED, registered in England and Wales, registration number: 11086078, 5 Princes Gate Court, London, SW7 2QJ, United Kingdom

British Library Cataloguing-in-Publication Data
A catalogue record for this book is available from the British Library

Additional hard and PDF copies can be obtained from orders@intechopen.com

Weight Management - Challenges and Opportunities
Edited by Hassan M. Heshmati
p. cm.
Print ISBN 978-1-80355-186-9
Online ISBN 978-1-80355-187-6
eBook (PDF) ISBN 978-1-80355-188-3

For EU product safety concerns:
IN TECH d.o.o., Prolaz Marije Krucifikse Kozulić 3, 51000 Rijeka, Croatia, info@intechopen.com or visit our website at intechopen.com.

Meet the editor

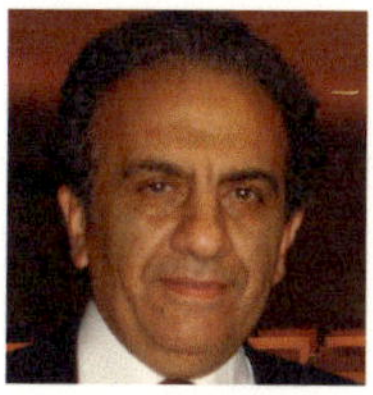

Dr. Hassan Massoud Heshmati is an endocrinologist with 46 years of experience in clinical research in academia (university-affiliated hospitals, Paris, France; Mayo Foundation, Rochester, MN, USA) and pharmaceutical companies (Sanofi, Malvern, PA, USA; Essentialis, Carlsbad, CA, USA; Gelesis, Boston, MA, USA). His research activity focuses on pituitary tumors, hyperthyroidism, thyroid cancers, osteoporosis, diabetes, and obesity. He has extensive knowledge in the development of anti-obesity products. Dr. Heshmati is the author of 309 abstracts, chapters, and articles related to endocrinology and metabolism. He is currently a consultant at Endocrinology Metabolism Consulting, LLC, Anthem, AZ, USA.

Contents

Preface IX

Section 1
Leptin Pathophysiology 1

Chapter 1 3
Biodiversity of the Adipocyte-Derived Hormone, Leptin
by Reji Manjunathan, Dharanibalan Kasiviswanathan and Selvaraj Jayaraman

Chapter 2 25
Leptin: A Metabolic Signal for the Differentiation of Pituitary Cells
by Gwen V. Childs, Angela K. Odle, Melanie C. MacNicol, Melody L. Allensworth-James, Tiffany K. Miles, Noor Akhter, Mohsin M. Syed and Angus M. MacNicol

Chapter 3 45
Leptin and Female Reproductive Health
by Shyam Pyari Jaiswar and Apala Priyadarshini

Chapter 4 59
Role of Leptin in Obesity Management: Current and Herbal Treatment
by Sunil T. Galatage, Sakshi N. Gurav, Mahadevi R. Moladi, Tejal R. Podjale, Nikita B. Tejam, Arehalli S. Manjappa, Popat S. Kumbhar, Supriya V. Nikade, Swapnil S. Chopade, Sujit A. Desai, Shweta N. Kalebere and Suresh G. Killedar

Section 2
Obesity Consequences and Management 73

Chapter 5 75
The Multiple Consequences of Obesity
by Indu Saxena, Amar Preet Kaur, Suwarna Suman, Abhilasha, Prasenjit Mitra, Praveen Sharma and Manoj Kumar

Chapter 6 **109**
Personalized Strategy of Obesity Prevention and Management Based on the Analysis of Pathogenetic, Genetic, and Microbiotic Factors
by Svitlana Drozdovska, Olena Andrieieva, Valeriya Orlenko, Igor Andrieiev, Victoriya Pastukhova, Iuliia Mazur, Olha Hurenko and Anastasiia Nahorna

Chapter 7 **135**
Medical Weight Management: A Multidisciplinary Approach
by Wahiba Elhag and Walid El Ansari

Chapter 8 **161**
Resistance Training and Weight Management: Rationale and Efficacy
by Ina Shaw, Travis Triplett and Brandon S. Shaw

Chapter 9 **173**
The Potential of Precision Probiotic *Hafnia alvei* HA4597 to Support Weight Loss
by Nina Vinot, Emma Baghtchedjian, Clémentine Picolo and Grégory Lambert

Chapter 10 **185**
Inability to Understand the Complexity of Maintaining Weight Loss and the Complications
by Anvi Rana

Section 3
Anorexia Nervosa Treatment **201**

Chapter 11 **203**
Anorexia Nervosa: Opportunities and Challenges in Treatment
by Kayode Olariike Oyindasola, Folake Funke Adedoyin and Adeoye Adeyemi Adedoyin

Section 4
Miscellaneous **213**

Chapter 12 **215**
Mechanism and Impact of Food Components in Burning Calories from White-to-Brown Adipose Tissue
by Upasana

Chapter 13 **225**
Association of Fatness and Leg Power with Blood Pressure in Adolescents
by Danladi Musa, Daniel Iornyior and Andrew Tyoakaa

Preface

Total body weight is the sum of the weight of all body components. Among these components, water, adipose tissue, muscle, and bone are the main contributors. The physiological or pathological variations in the amount or mass of each component can lead to an increase or decrease in total body weight. Some of these changes carry a risk of increased morbidity and mortality. The variations in body weight are increase (retention) or decrease (dehydration) in water amount, increase (hypertrophy, hyperplasia) or decrease (lipodystrophy) in adipose tissue mass, increase (hypertrophy) or decrease (sarcopenia) in muscle mass, and increase (increased bone density) or decrease (osteopenia, osteoporosis) in bone mass. A variety of factors including genes, lifestyle, environment, age, diseases, and medications can promote these conditions. The most common and relevant body weight change is obesity, which is a major health problem worldwide. The prevalence of obesity has doubled in more than 70 countries since 1980. The number of adults with obesity is around 650 million worldwide. This book provides the reader with a comprehensive overview of current knowledge about the pathophysiology, consequences, complications, and treatment of different types of body weight changes, with a special emphasis on obesity.

The book contains thirteen chapters by authors from Dominica, France, India, Nigeria, Qatar, Ukraine, South Africa, the United Kingdom, and the United States. I would like to thank all of them. I would also like to express my appreciation for the great assistance provided by Ms. Ana Javor at IntechOpen who supervised this book project.

Hassan M. Heshmati, MD
Endocrinology Metabolism Consulting, LLC,
Anthem, AZ, USA

Section 1

Leptin Pathophysiology

Chapter 1

Biodiversity of the Adipocyte-Derived Hormone, Leptin

Reji Manjunathan, Dharanibalan Kasiviswanathan and Selvaraj Jayaraman

Abstract

The adipocyte derived hormone leptin is known for its pivotal role in the regulation of a variety of physiological functions mainly associated with metabolism and energy homeostasis. One of the major functions of leptin is pertain with its angiogenic induction in support of organ development as well as under pathological conditions such as atherosclerosis and cancer. Leptin is a well-known pro-angiogenic growth factor which exerts its role through Ob-R receptor present on endothelial cells. The therapeutic application of leptin is based on its potential to maintain various functions at pathological conditions. In this book chapter, the multi-diversity potentials of leptin are discussed in detail.

Keywords: Leptin, obesity, angiogenesis, tumor progression, multi-signaling pathways

1. Introduction

Leptin is a 16 kDa non-glycosylated protein derived from adipose tissue, primarily by adipocytes. Leptin is a well-known mediator for food intake and weight loss [1]. Leptin mediates its functions mainly through the receptor located in the hypothalamus and activates signaling cascades associated with energy intake [2]. It circulates through the bloodstream, engages with normal metabolism, regulates energetic homeostasis, reproductive system, and influences the circadian cycle, lipid inflammation, and carbohydrate mechanisms. Leptin is well known for its pro-angiogenic potential and operates multiple signaling agencies through the receptor located in endothelial cells [3, 4]. Leptin is also secrets by other organs, such as the placenta, bone marrow, ovaries, stomach, and cellular structures, including mammary epithelial cells, P/D1 cells, and gastric chief cells [1]. Research has demonstrated that leptin plays a crucial role in maintaining the normal physiology of various vital systems such as the reproductive system and could balance cell proliferation (**Figure 1**). The pleiotropic hormone also could repair tissue damage and can prevent on-adipocyte lipotoxicity. Though leptin is highly acceptable for its protective mode of action, increased leptin level is often observed in several inflammatory

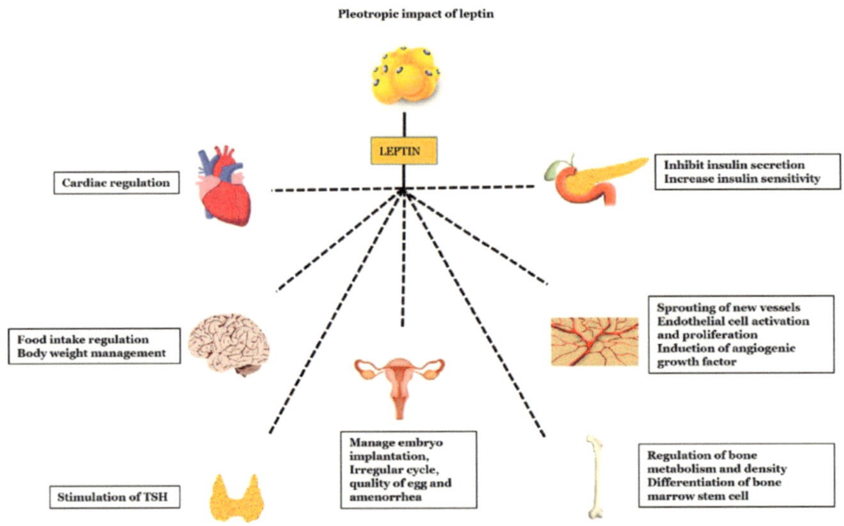

Figure 1.
Leptin exerts its pleiotropic impact on various organs. It maintains muscle tone and regulates cardiac function. Leptin regulates food intake and body weight management through binding with receptor located at brain. In the thyroid gland, leptin stimulates the secretion of TSH. In the female reproductive system, leptin manage menstrual cycle and supports in embryo implantation. Leptin inhibits insulin secretion and maintains blood-glucose level. Leptin induces sprouting of new vessels from existing ones and enhances ECs proliferation and migration and also it regulates bone metabolism and density.

conditions [5]. Hence, a therapeutic approach based on leptin and receptor has become the need of the hour to balance many inflammatory diseases in the human body. The particular book chapter provides an insight into the multi-diversity properties of the pleiotropic hormone leptin.

2. Leptin synthesis and regulation

Leptin derives from adipose tissue's obese gene (OB) transcription product [6]. The OB gene function was first identified in the *ob/ob* obese mice model and is located on chromosome 7 (7q31.3) and has three exons and two introns (18 kb) [7, 8]. Leptin receptors are located on chromosome 1 (1p31) and are noted with 17 introns and 18 exons and encode two proteins of 166 and 1162 amino acids, respectively [9]. Leptin receptors are highly expressed in the hypothalamus, cerebellum, and other tissues associated with the vasculature, stomach, and placental organs [10]. Leptin receptors have five spliced isoforms, the longest form expressed in neuronal tissue and the short forms expressed almost in all tissue types [11]. Leptin receptors (OB-R) are structurally similar to the class I cytokine family receptors. Alternative splicing of leptin receptor RNA results in various isoforms, designated as OB-Ra, OB-Rb, OB-Rc, OB-Rd, OB-Re, and OB-Rf. They all have an extracellular domain of more than 800 amino acids, a transmembrane domain of 34 amino acids, and a variable intracellular domain. The pleiotropic biological effects of leptin are explained based on the wide distribution of leptin receptors in humans [5]. Leptin bind to its hypothalamic receptors (Ob-Rs) in the brain and activates appetite and satiety. The concentration of leptin in plasma depends on the person's dietary behavior, gender, and physical activities. The other hormonal constituents, such as insulin, estrogen, and glucocorticoids, can also influence the regulation mode and the level of leptin in the blood [12, 13]. On the other hand, low energy or fasting, thyroid hormones, androgens, inflammatory cytokines, and adrenergic agonists can inhibit leptin secretion [14].

3. Leptin signaling pathways

Leptin mediates its biological effects by binding to its various alternatively spliced isoforms receptor located at the brain and peripheral tissues. The binding of leptin to its long-form of receptor activates various intracellular signaling pathways, including insulin receptor substrate (IRS)/phosphatidylinositol 3 kinase (PI3K), Janus kinase 2 (JAK2)/Signal transducer, and activator of transcription 3 (STAT3), SH2-containing protein tyrosine phosphatase 2 (SHP2)/Mitogen-activated protein kinase (MAPK), and 5′ adenosine monophosphate-activated protein kinase (AMPK)/acetyl-CoA carboxylase (ACC) [8]. The binding of leptin to its receptor activates JAK2, which in turn phosphorylates the Tyrosine amino acid residues in LepRb and is terminated by a suppressor of cytokine signaling 3 (SOC3) [15].

Leptin input a significant role in energy homeostasis and neuroendocrine function through JAK2/STAT3 signaling pathway. A selective deletion in LepRb or STAT3 in LepRb-expressing neurons ends with obesity and hyperphagia, which further supports the dominant role of the JAK2/STAT3 signaling pathway in the leptin-induced body weight regulation [16]. One interesting fact about leptin and insulin is that both have similar intracellular signaling pathways (PI3K/Akt) in neurons [17]. The ERK, a member of the MAPK family, acts downstream of LepRb and is mediated through

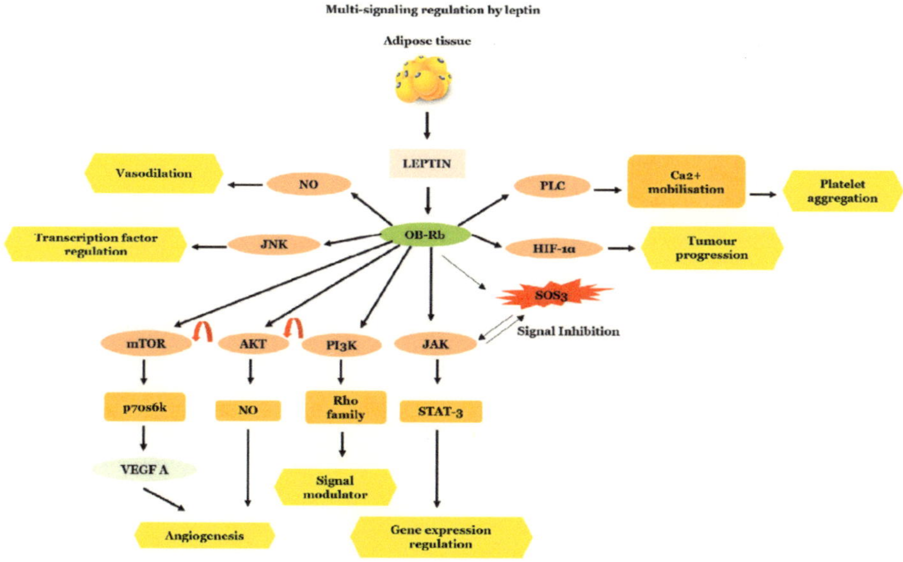

Figure 2.
Leptin regulates many signaling pathways through receptor (Ob-Rb) binding mechanism. It regulates gene expression through JAK/STAT3 pathway, modulates other signals through PI3K/rho family dependent pathway, induces vasodilation through NO-dependent pathway, and accelerates angiogenesis through PI3K/Akt/mTOR/s6 kinase/VEGF a and PI3/Akt/NO-dependent pathways. Promotes tumor progression through HIF-1 alpha pathway and enhances platelet aggregation through the PLC pathway. The SOS3 molecule function as a regulator of leptin induced signaling activations by negative feedback mechanism.

SHP2 or by JAK2. Inhibition of ERK prevents leptin-based sympathetic function in brown adipose, which further supports SHP2/MAPK in leptin energy expenditure and food intake [18]. Leptin's suppressive mode of action on food intake initiates by inhibiting the effect of AMPK in the brain. The inhibition of AMPK regulates feeding through the mTOR (mammalian target of rapamycin)/s6Kinase pathway [19]. In skeletal muscle, leptin directly exists its effect through AMPK signaling and stimulates fatty acid oxidation and glucose uptake [20]. Leptin has a prominent role in the modulation of both innate and adaptive immunity. It stimulates neutrophil chemotaxis and promotes phagocytosis of macrophages through the receptor binding mechanism. It is also known to increase the production of IL-6 and TNF-alpha under pathological conditions [21]. Leptin protective action on neutrophils exerts through PI3K and MAPK depending on signaling and prevents apoptosis of neutrophils. Leptin via STAT3 activation promotes natural killer cell activation [22]. In the adaptive immune response, leptin promotes native T cells proliferation by increasing the expression of interferon-gamma and TNF-alpha in T cells [23].

Apart from the mentioned direct signaling pathways, leptin interacts with many signaling functions as a multifunctional cytokine. Leptin shows a potential functional relationship with Nitric Oxide (NO) and favors NO-mediated lipolysis and vascular tone [24]. The significant other functions of leptin are associated with its predominant role in angiogenesis. It is observed that Endothelial cells (ECs) express OB-R leptin receptors and the binding of leptin to OB-R enables the growth of small blood vessels [3]. Recently, it has been identified that leptin could induce PI3K/Akt/mTOR/s6Kinase signaling pathway and enhance VEGF mRNA's transcription level while inducing angiogenesis [4]. One of the intriguing possibilities of leptin is that it promotes neovascularization through paracrine mode concerning the volume of fat mass [25]. Leptin could promote proliferation in colonic epithelial cells in vitro conditions. Moreover, the presence of OB-R receptor in human colon cancer cell lines and human Colonia tissue thus supports the angiogenic role of leptin under cancer environment through PI3K/AKT, MAPK/ERK, and JAK2/STAT3 pathways [26, 27]. Leptin could induce apoptosis and regulate actin-myosin cytoskeleton associated with Rho family GTPases (**Figure 2**) [28].

4. Leptin as an energy balancer

Leptin acts in the brain and maintains energy homeostasis through a negative feedback mechanism [29]. The process is mediated through the receptors in the hypothalamic area named the paraventricular nucleus, ventromedial hypothalamic nucleus, lateral hypothalamic area (LHA), and arcuate nucleus (ARC). The ARC is the primary site for leptin to integrate peripheral energy balance signals [30]. Recently, it has been observed that leptin could play a significant role in the long-term regulation of energy balance and short-term management of body weight and food intake. The gastric leptin produced because of the actions of the intestinal peptide serves as a local stimulus and plays a vital role in food digestion and absorption [31]. The particular area requires more investigations to prove the role of gastric leptin in food digestion and absorption. Research supported the predominant role of leptin in neuroendocrine mediated starvation through changing sympathetic nervous system activity [32].

Overweight or obesity is characterized by increased fat mass and is proportional to circulating leptin levels in individuals [33]. The elevated levels of leptin in body fluid are explained based on leptin resistance. The hypothesis was proved using rodents fed with a high-fat diet and leptin sensitivity loss in ARC neurons [34]. At the cellular level, the inflammatory signals mediate the process of leptin resistance. The two significant characteristics of obesity connect with hyper-leptinemia and leptin resistance. At the molecular level, the leptin gene is over-expressed in overweight or obese individuals [35]. Apart from these functions, many researchers reported the genetic and epigenetic factors that control leptin action in energy homeostasis and food intake [36–38]. A better understanding of leptin-induced pathogenicity of obesity and obesity-related disorders and the regulation of energy homeostasis will provide an alternative solution in preventing obesity and obesity-related co-morbidities.

5. Leptin as an immune modulator

Despite nutritional regulation, leptin has gained more attention for its pivotal role in inflammation. The innate immune system plays a major role in the regulation of leptin production. Leptin responds to immune cells and its receptors, expressed by most cells, and activates pro-inflammatory features in the host [39]. Leptin plays an essential role in T cell development, and leptin deficiency directly impacts the levels of circulating T cells [40]. Many studies supported the role of leptin in immunity modulation and mentioned the signaling pathways related to the notion [39, 41, 42]. Leptin could accelerate the proliferation process in native $CD4^{+}$T cells and favored by reducing the levels of IFN from T cells [43, 44]. During the wound healing process, leptin activates both inflammatory and proliferative phases in favor of tissue repair [45]. The increased plasma leptin level acts as an indicator of leptin-induced inflammatory response at the injury site. These exciting features of leptin gained attention as a pro-angiogenic molecule in ischemic tissues [46]. Leptin induces monocyte chemoattractant protein1 (MCP1) expression [47].

Leptin plays a vital role in producing GM-CSF and G-CSF and activating hematopoietic cells in humans [48]. In animal models, up-regulation of leptin has been found in acute inflammation states. But, experimental evidence from rodents does not match with human studies [49]. Leptin plays a significant role in basophils and eosinophils functions and acts as a chemoattractant [50]. Leptin is abnormally expressed in autoimmune diseases, particularly in skin disorders [51]. Obesity decorates skin normal physiology such as keratosis pilaris, tags, and striae diseases and increases the levels of pro-inflammatory cytokines and adipokines, including leptin [52, 53]. In the event of inflammation, leptin increases the release of Nitric Oxide and activates the macrophages and neutrophils, and increases natural killer cells' activity (NK) [54]. Leptin up-regulates the cytokines production and phagocytic function in obese conditions [55]. It balances monocytes and activations markers and directly involves in interleukin1 and cyclooxygenase expression [56]. One of the prominent roles of leptin pertains to maintaining the balance between the immune system and metabolism regulation. Under malnutrition state, leptin acts as an immunosuppressive factor [42].

6. Leptin as a pro-angiogenic factor

In 1998, Sierra-Hongmans reported that vascular endothelial cells express leptin receptors, especially the long-form. This discovery leads to an insight into the role of leptin in angiogenesis [57]. The angiogenic impact of leptin was conformed used on in vitro and in vivo models analysis [3, 58]. Jin et al. proved that leptin could induce angiogenesis in the cornea of the Zucker obese rat model through the activation of the Ob-R gene [59]. Leptin exerts a paracrine mode of action in tissues and activates various signaling during the promotion of angiogenesis. This endocrine hormone activates Akt signaling pathway and mediates NO-induced vasodilation [60]. In endothelial cell migration, leptin signals through the ERK pathway and activates the PI3k, Akt, and eNOS molecules. By stimulating the local neovascularization in adipose tissue, leptin promotes its release into the vascular system. This process enhances fatty acid oxidation and supports maintaining a proper balance between adipose tissue's fat deposits and blood supply [61]. Even though the vascular fenestration capacity of leptin is poorly understood, the effect is found similar to VEGF [62]. Leptin plays a crucial role in exchanging nutrients between the fetus and maternal circulation in the placenta via enhancing vascular permeability and could induce angiogenesis in the placenta [61].

7. Leptin and pathogenesis

Leptin does not only imply energy homeostasis but also extends its regulatory function at infectious conditions. But the contagious status regulation mode of leptin is the least explored signaling mechanism. Latest research support that leptin could activate phagocytosis of macrophages and could secure the immune cells from pathogenic infections [63]. In *Klebsiella pneumonia* infection, exogenous administration of leptin shows CD11b dependent phagocytosis [64]. It protects lymphocyte deficient mice from various conditions [65]. Several studies have strongly highlighted the therapeutic application of the molecule to innervate infectious diseases, including AIDS [66].

8. Leptin resistance with disease

However, under certain conditions, like obesity, leptin levels decrease in association with leptin resistance. But it is still unclear how the leptin resistance mechanism is exerted throughout the tissue. So far, studies have suggested leptin resistance with metabolic process and revealed a defect in the Ob-R leptin receptor gene [67]. Up to date, the leptin resistance mechanism has been categorized as follows: gene mutation specific to the leptin structure, defect in the transport of leptin through the blood–brain barrier, and malfunctions of leptin receptors. Among these, mutations are rare in humans, occurring in substitution of guanine by adenine at the donor splice site of exon 16 of the leptin gene [68]. Second, the brain's blood vessels usually express leptin receptors and transport leptin into the cerebrospinal fluid. But excessive levels of leptin in the bloodstream decrease the permeability of BBB, thus develops leptin resistance [69]. Finally, the serum level of leptin significantly affects the transcriptional level of the OB (*ob*) gene and the equilibrium of leptin secretion in adipose tissue. In such cases, these dramatic changes promote leptin resistance until leptin level remains standard in the bloodstream. These changes have been widely observed in obesity [70].

Furthermore, several stimuli affect leptin resistance, including the circadian cycle. Interestingly, leptin also develops its leptin resistance, observed in diet-induced obesity [71]. This leptin resistance also provides an environment for the accumulation of immune response against pathogens, particularly high-fat diet-induced inflammation, which activates inflammatory cytokines [72]. But, in-depth leptin resistance mechanisms need much more attention.

9. Leptin role in disease conditions

9.1 Metabolic syndrome and obesity

Fat tissue is an energy storage tissue that functions as a negative feedback loop in energy homeostasis [73]. Homozygous mutation of leptin causes extreme obesity, diabetes and suppresses glucose metabolism in insulin-deficient diabetes [8]. The ob/ob mice model has relatively higher food intake and observed a larger volume of lipid accumulation in the liver than the control group [74]. It has been assumed that nearly 95% of individuals have resistance against leptin [75]. The type 2 diabetes condition is noted with an increased level of leptin and suggested using leptin as a biomarker to study the effect of obesity in diabetes-related morbidities [76]. Some studies also reported that higher leptin levels are associated with the risk of heart-related problems in obese individuals [76, 77]. In younger adults, elevated leptin levels are positively correlated with HOMA-IR and BMI index [78].

Development of severe early-onset obesity and hyperphagia are common in people with homozygous *LEP* mutation [79]. Replacement of leptin from a therapeutic viewpoint has improved insulin sensitivity and thus proved the role of leptin in metabolic disorders, including T2DM. In humans, serum leptin level is positively correlated with the percentage of body fat, fat mass, size of adipocytes, and BMI [80]. Obesity connected with the enlargement of adipose cells enhances the serum leptin level, which further results in the progression of chronic hyperinsulinemia. The majority of obese patients are hyper leptinaemic which supports the development of hypertension, metabolic syndrome, and cardiovascular diseases [81]. Mutation in the leptin receptor located at the hypothalamus alters the transport of leptin across the blood–brain barrier. This incidence increases the level of serum leptin and hence diet-induced obesity. Obesity connected with the leptin receptor mutation is linked with insulin resistance and in the development of T2DM [82].

9.2 Cardiovascular diseases

The level of leptin could influence the function of the heart. It could lead to the progression of many heart-related problems such as coronary artery disease, stroke, chronic kidney disease (CKD), peripheral artery disease (DAP), carotid plaque instability [83]. It was observed that elevated level of serum leptin in obese patients contributes to the low-grade systemic inflammation in favor to develop cardiovascular disease. Moreover, a high level of leptin is used as a biomarker to measure the progression of heart failure in patients with dilated cardiomyopathy [84]. On the other hand, many studies using rodent, obese and diabetic models highlighted the beneficial impact of leptin on cardiac metabolism through glucose metabolism and fatty acid oxidation. This evidence suggested that leptin compensates for cardiac insults due to ischemia and heart failure [85]. Leptin signaling in the modulation of heart function is studied extensively using animal models. These studies demonstrated that impaired cardiac leptin signaling majorly reflects in metabolic inflexibility for glucose utilization, defects in cardiac contractibility, impaired recovery of cardiac function due to coronary artery ligation [86, 87]. Clinical data cemented that plasma leptin levels are associated with LV hypertrophy and increased myocardial wall thickening [88]. Leptin also increased the blood pressure level in obese individuals with a loss-of-function mutation in leptin or leptin receptor [89]. Thus, a leptin-mediated increase in blood pressure directly increases the heartbeat rate, developing into cardiac hypertrophy through the sympathetic nervous mechanism [90].

Leptin-mediated aldosterone synthesis impairs myocardial relaxation and contributes to cardiovascular diseases through a novel mechanism associated with endothelial dysfunctions [91]. Increased plasma leptin levels positively correlate with the number of stenotic coronary arteries in patients with coronary artery disease [92]. In vitro analysis using HUVEC cells demonstrated that leptin induces chronic oxidative stress in ECs and contributes to vascular pathology development [93]. Also, the cytokine hormone leptin could stimulate vascular smooth muscle cells proliferation and migration, thereby increasing calcification and vascular lesions [94]. Altogether, it was suggested that hypertension, obesity, and endothelial dysfunctions are more frequent in T2DM patients with elevated leptin levels [95].

9.3 Tumor progression

Cancer progression is a complex process that includes the interaction between ECs, fibroblast, insusceptible cells, and adipocytes [96]. Normal epithelial cells do not express leptin and leptin receptors but are overexpressed in a cancerous environment. Leptin enhances the survival rate of cancer cells through the activation of a downstream signaling molecule known as sirtuin-dependent NAD-dependent deacetylase 1 (SIRT 1) [97]. Leptin can activate many signaling pathways in cancer directly by activating TNF alpha, IL-6, ROS, VEGF, MMP2, and MMP9. It can also support tumor growth by activating JAK/STAT, Akt, FGF2, and NO molecules through receptor (Ob-R) binding mechanisms in ECs [98, 99]. The appetite hormone can potentially interact with pre-neoplastic or cancerous breast epithelium in a breast cancer environment. Leptin secreted by the breast cancer surroundings inhibits inflammatory cytokines and thus blocks macrophages' production [100, 101]. The cytokine enhances neovascularization through VEGF in many cancerous conditions [102, 103].

Increased levels of serum leptin and insulin under obese conditions cause colorectal cancer [104]. Leptin supports the proliferation and invasiveness of colonic cells. Leptin receptors are found to express in human colon cell lines and are believed to initiate cancer angiogenesis. Hyperlipidemia and insulin resistance can cause low-grade systemic inflammation that promotes proliferation and angiogenesis and inhibits apoptotic rate in colon cancer [105]. Leptin and its receptors express in papillary thyroid tumors and enhance the pathogenicity through PI3K/Akt pathway [106].

Obesity enhances the concentration of leptin around the pancreatic carcinogenic environment. The enhanced concentration of leptin favors vascularization, migration, and invasiveness of pancreatic tumor cells [105]. Leptin has a crucial role in developing the non-alcoholic fatty liver disease (NAFLD) via insulin resistance. This imbalance ultimately worsens hepatic inflammation and results in the development of liver fibrosis [107]. The receptor Ob-R identified in Kupffer cells (KC), and binding of leptin with receptor enhances the expression of TGF beta, TIMP1 in liver fibrosis scenario [108]. However, the direct role of leptin in liver cancer is controversial, with some reports suggesting its role in liver cancer. In contrast, others offer its inhibitory potential on tumor size in hepatic cancer [109, 110]. The level of leptin was found to decrease in patients with cancer cachexia compared to non-cancer cachexia [111].

10. Leptin therapeutics past and future

The significant need for clinical implications of leptin is to regulate the regular physiological role of leptin in pathological conditions. There is a correlation between body weight loss and serum levels of leptin. As a result, several therapeutic approaches have been implemented for the use of leptin in obesity control. However, increased resistance to leptin is also a significant issue in the treatment of obesity. But, a combination of therapeutic approaches may be helpful to these problems [112, 113].

Among the adipocyte secreted hormones, leptin is the front that has been used for the treatment of hypoleptinemia status clinically. The most important therapeutic benefits of leptin are rely on providing a novel method for treating the conditions connected with mutation of leptin gene and lipodystrophy in humans [114]. Treatment with exogenous leptin in obese patients concluded that leptin can decrease the body weight and fat tissue of the subjects [115]. It was also noted that leptin excerpts a dose-dependent regulating potential as individuals energy intake and appetite [116, 117]. Development of leptin analogous with full biological effect, especially with the potential to cross the blood–brain barrier, can improve the results obtained from leptin therapy focusing on obesity management. The administration of leptin can accelerate wound healing in diabetic ob/ob and wild-type mice in a dose-dependent manner through leptin receptor mediation [118].

Exogenous administration of leptin can regulate fatty acid oxidation in muscles and control triglyceride synthesis in the liver [119, 120]. Even though the mechanisms in humans are not clear, administration of leptin and adiponectin was found to improve insulin resistance in type 2 diabetic conditions [121, 122]. The immune-modulatory impact of exogenous leptin administration in rodents highlighted that the cytokine could activate encephalomyelitis [123]. Various in vitro assays also supported the immune stimulator action of leptin [124, 125]. Identifying high-affinity-binding molecules to control the level of circulating leptin is suggested as an advanced therapy for treating arthritis and inflammatory bowel disease. In addition, replacement with recombinant methionyl human leptin is a brilliant choice for treating pathological conditions associated with relative or absolute leptin deficiency and restoring immune functions [126]. One of the future therapeutic approaches of leptin relies on its use as a natural adjuvant in vaccinations since it can stimulate T helper I responses while down-modulating regulatory T cells [127].

Considering the cancerous conditions, ATLO-ACA, an Ob-R antagonist peptide, finds effective for treating triple-negative breast cancers in experimental models [128]. Also, therapy based on leptin/Ob R axis function inhibition was identified as adjunctive therapy for newly diagnosed and recurrent glioblastoma [129]. The modern therapeutic approaches of leptin are connected with molecular approaches at gene levels are 1) CRISPR-Cas 9 connected with floxed leptin-locus based approaches - to lower the leptin levels, 2) Cre-lox P- generation of one copy of Lep eliminates – to lower the leptin levels, glucose and insulin tolerance, c) administration of neutralizing leptin-specific antibodies –to reduce the circulating levels of leptin to reduce food intake and hepatic stenosis [130]. Administration of human recombinant leptin accelareated dose-dependent sprouting angiogenesis and hypothesized that the application of human recombinant leptin could improve the wound healing process through neovascularization [3]. So far, evidence gathered from previous studies highlights the role of leptin in therapeutic applications. But overcoming leptin resistance is a significant challenge in leptin-based therapy.

11. Conclusion

In conclusion, leptin is considered an essential pleiotropic adipokine with various effects on biological systems. However, leptin's structural and functional characteristics and its receptors are characterized by a unique signaling mechanism. Focusing on leptin could be a therapeutic approach to manage autoimmune inflammation associated with obesity, cancer, and metabolic diseases. But further research is needed to understand the relationship between leptin on biological systems, as it has complex signaling mechanisms.

Acknowledgements

Financial support from the Science and Engineering Research Board (DST-SERB), Government of India (Project file no: EEQ/2019/000568) is greatly acknowledged.

Authors Contribution

DK collected information and prepared the first draft, RM and JS critically evaluated and coordinated with final draft preparation.

Conflicts of interest

The authors declare no conflict of interest.

Author details

Reji Manjunathan[1,2,3*], Dharanibalan Kasiviswanathan[2] and Selvaraj Jayaraman[4*]

1 Department of Genetics, Dr. Alagappa Mudaliyar Post Graduate Institute of Basic Medical Sciences, University of Madras, Tamil Nadu, India

2 Vascular Biology Lab, AU-KBC Research Centre, Anna University, Tamil Nadu, India

3 R CELL Diagnostic and Research Centre, Calicut, Kerala, India

4 Department of Biochemistry, Saveetha Dental College and Hospitals, Saveetha Institute of Medical and Technical Sciences, Tamil Nadu, India

*Address all correspondence to: rejimanjunath@gmail.com
and jselvaendo@gmail.com

References

[1] Ramos-Lobo AM, Donato J Jr. The role of leptin in health and disease. Temperature (Austin). 2017 May 26;**4**(3):258-291. DOI: 10.1080/23328940.2017.1327003. PMID: 28944270; PMCID: PMC5605162

[2] Pralong FP, Gaillard RC. Neuroendocrine effects of leptin. Pituitary. 2001 Jan-Apr;**4**(1-2):25-32. DOI: 10.1023/a:1012930609563. PMID: 11824505

[3] Manjunathan R, Ragunathan M. In ovo administration of human recombinant leptin shows dose-dependent angiogenic effect on chicken chorioallantoic membrane. Biol Res. 2015 Jun 10;**48**(1):29. DOI: 10.1186/s40659-015-0021-z. PMID: 26060038; PMCID: PMC4470073

[4] Manjunathan R, Devarajan N, Ragunathan M. Possible Mechanism of Human Recombinant Leptin-Induced VEGF A Synthesis via PI3K/Akt/mTOR/S6 Kinase Signaling Pathway while Inducing Angiogenesis: An Analysis Using Chicken Chorioallantoic Membrane Model. J Vasc Res. 2021 Jun 24:1-18. DOI: 10.1159/000516498. Epub ahead of print. PMID: 34167108

[5] Lee GH, Proenca R, Montez JM, Carroll KM, Darvishzadeh JG, Lee JI, Friedman JM. Abnormal splicing of the leptin receptor in diabetic mice. Nature. 1996 Feb 15;**379**(6566):632-635. DOI: 10.1038/379632a0. PMID: 8628397

[6] Vázquez-Del Mercado M, Martínez-García EA. Leptin as an open secret in the physiopathology of rheumatic diseases. Clin Rheumatol. 2020 Feb;**39**(2):301-303. DOI: 10.1007/s10067-019-04908-4. Epub 2020 Jan 11. PMID: 31927713

[7] Chan JL, Heist K, DePaoli AM, Veldhuis JD, Mantzoros CS. The role of falling leptin levels in the neuroendocrine and metabolic adaptation to short-term starvation in healthy men. J Clin Invest. 2003 May;**111**(9):1409-21. DOI: 10.1172/JCI17490. PMID: 12727933; PMCID: PMC154448

[8] Zhang Y, Proenca R, Maffei M, Barone M, Leopold L, Friedman JM. Positional cloning of the mouse obese gene and its human homologue. Nature. 1994 Dec 1;**372**(6505):425-32. DOI: 10.1038/372425a0. Erratum in: Nature 1995 Mar 30;**374**(6521):479. PMID: 7984236

[9] Chung WK, Power-Kehoe L, Chua M, Leibel RL. Mapping of the OB receptor to 1p in a region of nonconserved gene order from mouse and rat to human. Genome Res. 1996 May;**6**(5):431-438. DOI: 10.1101/gr.6.5.431. PMID: 8743992

[10] Campfield LA, Smith FJ, Burn P. The OB protein (leptin) pathway--a link between adipose tissue mass and central neural networks. Horm Metab Res. 1996 Dec;**28**(12):619-632. DOI: 10.1055/s-2007-979867. PMID: 9013731

[11] Bjørbaek C, Uotani S, da Silva B, Flier JS. Divergent signaling capacities of the long and short isoforms of the leptin receptor. J Biol Chem. 1997 Dec 19;**272**(51):32686-32695. DOI: 10.1074/jbc.272.51.32686. PMID: 9405487

[12] Levine JA, Eberhardt NL, Jensen MD. Leptin responses to overfeeding: relationship with body fat and nonexercise activity thermogenesis. J Clin Endocrinol Metab. 1999 Aug;**84**(8):2751-2754. DOI: 10.1210/jcem.84.8.5910. PMID: 10443673

[13] stlund Jr, R., Yang, J. W., Klein, S. & Gingerich, R. Relation between plasma

leptin concentration and body fat, gender, diet, age, and metabolic covariates. *The journal of clinical endocrinology & metabolism* **81**, 3909-3913 (1996)

[14] Licinio J, Mantzoros C, Negrão AB, Cizza G, Wong ML, Bongiorno PB, Chrousos GP, Karp B, Allen C, Flier JS, Gold PW. Human leptin levels are pulsatile and inversely related to pituitary-adrenal function. Nat Med. 1997 May;**3**(5):575-579. DOI: 10.1038/nm0597-575. PMID: 9142131

[15] Jiang L, You J, Yu X, Gonzalez L, Yu Y, Wang Q, Yang G, Li W, Li C, Liu Y. Tyrosine-dependent and -independent actions of leptin receptor in control of energy balance and glucose homeostasis. Proc Natl Acad Sci U S A. 2008 Nov 25;**105**(47):18619-24. DOI: 10.1073/pnas.0804589105. Epub 2008 Nov 17. PMID: 19015522; PMCID: PMC2587560

[16] Bates SH, Stearns WH, Dundon TA, Schubert M, Tso AW, Wang Y, Banks AS, Lavery HJ, Haq AK, Maratos-Flier E, Neel BG, Schwartz MW, Myers MG Jr. STAT3 signalling is required for leptin regulation of energy balance but not reproduction. Nature. 2003 Feb 20;**421**(6925):856-859. DOI: 10.1038/nature01388. PMID: 12594516

[17] Varela L, Horvath TL. Leptin and insulin pathways in POMC and AgRP neurons that modulate energy balance and glucose homeostasis. EMBO Rep. 2012 Dec;**13**(12):1079-86. DOI: 10.1038/embor.2012.174. Epub 2012 Nov 13. PMID: 23146889; PMCID: PMC3512417

[18] Rahmouni K, Sigmund CD, Haynes WG, Mark AL. Hypothalamic ERK mediates the anorectic and thermogenic sympathetic effects of leptin. Diabetes. 2009 Mar;**58**(3):536-42. DOI: 10.2337/db08-0822. Epub 2008 Dec 9. PMID: 19066310; PMCID: PMC2646051

[19] Minokoshi Y, Alquier T, Furukawa N, Kim YB, Lee A, Xue B, Mu J, Foufelle F, Ferré P, Birnbaum MJ, Stuck BJ, Kahn BB. AMP-kinase regulates food intake by responding to hormonal and nutrient signals in the hypothalamus. Nature. 2004 Apr 1;**428**(6982):569-574. DOI: 10.1038/nature02440. PMID: 15058305

[20] Minokoshi Y, Kim YB, Peroni OD, Fryer LG, Müller C, Carling D, Kahn BB. Leptin stimulates fatty-acid oxidation by activating AMP-activated protein kinase. Nature. 2002 Jan 17;**415**(6869):339-343. DOI: 10.1038/415339a. PMID: 11797013

[21] Paz-Filho G, Mastronardi C, Franco CB, Wang KB, Wong ML, Licinio J. Leptin: molecular mechanisms, systemic pro-inflammatory effects, and clinical implications. Arq Bras Endocrinol Metabol. 2012 Dec;**56**(9):597-607. DOI: 10.1590/s0004-27302012000900001. PMID: 23329181

[22] Iikuni N, Lam QL, Lu L, Matarese G, La Cava A. Leptin and Inflammation. Curr Immunol Rev. 2008 May 1;**4**(2):70-79. DOI: 10.2174/157339508784325046. PMID: 20198122; PMCID: PMC2829991

[23] Procaccini C, Jirillo E, Matarese G. Leptin as an immunomodulator. Mol Aspects Med. 2012 Feb;**33**(1):35-45. DOI: 10.1016/j.mam.2011.10.012. Epub 2011 Oct 21. PMID: 22040697

[24] Frühbeck G, Gómez-Ambrosi J. Modulation of the leptin-induced white adipose tissue lipolysis by nitric oxide. Cell Signal. 2001 Nov;**13**(11):827-833. DOI: 10.1016/s0898-6568(01)00211-x. PMID: 11583918

[25] Frühbeck G. A heliocentric view of leptin. Proc Nutr Soc. 2001 Aug;**60**(3): 301-318. DOI: 10.1079/pns200196. PMID: 11681805

[26] Hardwick JC, Van Den Brink GR, Offerhaus GJ, Van Deventer SJ,

Peppelenbosch MP. Leptin is a growth factor for colonic epithelial cells. Gastroenterology. 2001 Jul;**121**(1):79-90. DOI: 10.1053/gast.2001.25490. PMID: 11438496

[27] Islam MS, Morton NM, Hansson A, Emilsson V. Rat insulinoma-derived pancreatic beta-cells express a functional leptin receptor that mediates a proliferative response. Biochem Biophys Res Commun. 1997 Sep 29;**238**(3):851-855. DOI: 10.1006/bbrc.1997.7399. PMID: 9325180

[28] Sweeney G. Leptin signalling. Cell Signal. 2002 Aug;**14**(8):655-663. DOI: 10.1016/s0898-6568(02)00006-2. PMID: 12020765

[29] Guyenet SJ, Schwartz MW. Clinical review: Regulation of food intake, energy balance, and body fat mass: implications for the pathogenesis and treatment of obesity. J Clin Endocrinol Metab. 2012 Mar;**97**(3):745-55. DOI: 10.1210/jc.2011-2525. Epub 2012 Jan 11. PMID: 22238401; PMCID: PMC3319208

[30] Morton GJ, Cummings DE, Baskin DG, Barsh GS, Schwartz MW. Central nervous system control of food intake and body weight. Nature. 2006 Sep 21;**443**(7109):289-295. DOI: 10.1038/nature05026. PMID: 16988703

[31] Picó C, Oliver P, Sánchez J, Palou A. Gastric leptin: a putative role in the short-term regulation of food intake. Br J Nutr. 2003 Oct;**90**(4):735-741. DOI: 10.1079/bjn2003945. PMID: 13129441

[32] Chan JL, Heist K, DePaoli AM, Veldhuis JD, Mantzoros CS. The role of falling leptin levels in the neuroendocrine and metabolic adaptation to short-term starvation in healthy men. J Clin Invest. 2003 May;**111**(9):1409-21. DOI: 10.1172/JCI17490. PMID: 12727933; PMCID: PMC154448

[33] Maffei M, Halaas J, Ravussin E, Pratley RE, Lee GH, Zhang Y, Fei H, Kim S, Lallone R, Ranganathan S, et al. Leptin levels in human and rodent: measurement of plasma leptin and ob RNA in obese and weight-reduced subjects. Nat Med. 1995 Nov;**1**(11): 1155-1161. DOI: 10.1038/nm1195-1155. PMID: 7584987

[34] Münzberg H, Flier JS, Bjørbaek C. Region-specific leptin resistance within the hypothalamus of diet-induced obese mice. Endocrinology. 2004 Nov;**145**(11): 4880-4889. DOI: 10.1210/en.2004-0726. Epub 2004 Jul 22. PMID: 15271881

[35] Igel M, Becker W, Herberg L, Joost HG. Hyperleptinemia, leptin resistance, and polymorphic leptin receptor in the New Zealand obese mouse. Endocrinology. 1997 Oct;**138**(10):4234-4239. DOI: 10.1210/endo.138.10.5428. PMID: 9322935

[36] Zhang Y, Dallner OS, Nakadai T, Fayzikhodjaeva G, Lu YH, Lazar MA, Roeder RG, Friedman JM. A noncanonical PPARγ/RXRα-binding sequence regulates leptin expression in response to changes in adipose tissue mass. Proc Natl Acad Sci U S A. 2018 Jun 26;**115**(26):E6039-E6047. DOI: 10.1073/pnas.1806366115. Epub 2018 Jun 11. PMID: 29891714; PMCID: PMC6042069

[37] Dallner OS, Marinis JM, Lu YH, Birsoy K, Werner E, Fayzikhodjaeva G, Dill BD, Molina H, Moscati A, Kutalik Z, Marques-Vidal P, Kilpeläinen TO, Grarup N, Linneberg A, Zhang Y, Vaughan R, Loos RJF, Lazar MA, Friedman JM. Dysregulation of a long noncoding RNA reduces leptin leading to a leptin-responsive form of obesity. Nat Med. 2019 Mar;**25**(3):507-516. DOI: 10.1038/s41591-019-0370-1. Epub 2019 Mar 6. PMID: 30842678

[38] Derghal A, Djelloul M, Azzarelli M, Degonon S, Tourniaire F, Landrier JF,

Mounien L. MicroRNAs are involved in the hypothalamic leptin sensitivity. Epigenetics. 2018;**13**(10-11):1127-1140. DOI: 10.1080/15592294.2018.1543507. Epub 2018 Nov 11. PMID: 30395773; PMCID: PMC6342074

[39] Kiernan K, MacIver NJ. The Role of the Adipokine Leptin in Immune Cell Function in Health and Disease. Front Immunol. 2021 Jan 29;**11**:622468. DOI: 10.3389/fimmu.2020.622468. PMID: 33584724; PMCID: PMC7878386

[40] Gerriets VA, Danzaki K, Kishton RJ, Eisner W, Nichols AG, Saucillo DC, Shinohara ML, MacIver NJ. Leptin directly promotes T-cell glycolytic metabolism to drive effector T-cell differentiation in a mouse model of autoimmunity. Eur J Immunol. 2016 Aug;**46**(8):1970-83. DOI: 10.1002/eji.201545861. Epub 2016 Jun 13. PMID: 27222115; PMCID: PMC5154618

[41] Busso N, So A, Chobaz-Péclat V, Morard C, Martinez-Soria E, Talabot-Ayer D, Gabay C. Leptin signaling deficiency impairs humoral and cellular immune responses and attenuates experimental arthritis. J Immunol. 2002 Jan 15;**168**(2):875-882. DOI: 10.4049/jimmunol.168.2.875. PMID: 11777985

[42] Pérez-Pérez A, Vilariño-García T, Fernández-Riejos P, Martín-González J, Segura-Egea JJ, Sánchez-Margalet V. Role of leptin as a link between metabolism and the immune system. Cytokine Growth Factor Rev. 2017 Jun;**35**:71-84. DOI: 10.1016/j.cytogfr.2017.03.001. Epub 2017 Mar 4. PMID: 28285098

[43] Lord GM, Matarese G, Howard JK, Baker RJ, Bloom SR, Lechler RI. Leptin modulates the T-cell immune response and reverses starvation-induced immunosuppression. Nature. 1998 Aug 27;**394**(6696):897-901. DOI: 10.1038/29795. PMID: 9732873

[44] Saucillo DC, Gerriets VA, Sheng J, Rathmell JC, Maciver NJ. Leptin metabolically licenses T cells for activation to link nutrition and immunity. J Immunol. 2014 Jan 1;**192**(1):136-44. DOI: 10.4049/jimmunol.1301158. Epub 2013 Nov 22. PMID: 24273001; PMCID: PMC3872216

[45] Su X, Cheng Y, Chang D. The Important Role of Leptin in Modulating the Risk of Dermatological Diseases. Front Immunol. 2021 Feb 1;**11**:593564. DOI: 10.3389/fimmu.2020.593564. PMID: 33597945; PMCID: PMC7882601

[46] Grosfeld A, Turban S, André J, Cauzac M, Challier JC, Hauguel-de Mouzon S, Guerre-Millo M. Transcriptional effect of hypoxia on placental leptin. FEBS Lett. 2001 Aug 3;**502**(3):122-126. DOI: 10.1016/s0014-5793(01)02673-4. PMID: 11583112

[47] Bouloumie A, Marumo T, Lafontan M, Busse R. Leptin induces oxidative stress in human endothelial cells. FASEB J. 1999 Jul;**13**(10):1231-1238. PMID: 10385613

[48] Gainsford T, Willson TA, Metcalf D, Handman E, McFarlane C, Ng A, Nicola NA, Alexander WS, Hilton DJ. Leptin can induce proliferation, differentiation, and functional activation of hemopoietic cells. Proc Natl Acad Sci U S A. 1996 Dec 10;**93**(25):14564-8. DOI: 10.1073/pnas.93.25.14564. PMID: 8962092; PMCID: PMC26173

[49] Janik JE, Curti BD, Considine RV, Rager HC, Powers GC, Alvord WG, Smith JW 2nd, Gause BL, Kopp WC. Interleukin 1 alpha increases serum leptin concentrations in humans. J Clin Endocrinol Metab. 1997 Sep;**82**(9):3084-3086. DOI: 10.1210/jcem.82.9.4214. PMID: 9284748

[50] Conus S, Bruno A, Simon HU. Leptin is an eosinophil survival factor. J Allergy

Clin Immunol. 2005 Dec;**116**(6):1228-1234. DOI: 10.1016/j.jaci.2005.09.003. Epub 2005 Oct 24. PMID: 16337450

[51] Ünlü B, Türsen Ü. Autoimmune skin diseases and the metabolic syndrome. Clin Dermatol. 2018 Jan-Feb;**36**(1):67-71. DOI: 10.1016/j.clindermatol.2017.09.012. Epub 2017 Sep 8. PMID: 29241755

[52] Deng T, Lyon CJ, Bergin S, Caligiuri MA, Hsueh WA. Obesity, Inflammation, and Cancer. Annu Rev Pathol. 2016 May 23;**11**:421-449. DOI: 10.1146/annurev-pathol-012615-044359. PMID: 27193454

[53] Hirt PA, Castillo DE, Yosipovitch G, Keri JE. Skin changes in the obese patient. J Am Acad Dermatol. 2019 Nov;**81**(5):1037-1057. DOI: 10.1016/j.jaad.2018.12.070. PMID: 31610857

[54] Buttgereit F, Burmester GR, Brand MD. Bioenergetics of immune functions: fundamental and therapeutic aspects. Immunol Today. 2000 Apr;**21**(4):192-199. DOI: 10.1016/s0167-5699(00)01593-0. PMID: 10740243

[55] Lee FY, Li Y, Yang EK, Yang SQ, Lin HZ, Trush MA, Dannenberg AJ, Diehl AM. Phenotypic abnormalities in macrophages from leptin-deficient, obese mice. Am J Physiol. 1999 Feb;**276**(2):C386-C394. DOI: 10.1152/ajpcell.1999.276.2.C386. PMID: 9950766

[56] Zarkesh-Esfahani H, Pockley G, Metcalfe RA, Bidlingmaier M, Wu Z, Ajami A, Weetman AP, Strasburger CJ, Ross RJ. High-dose leptin activates human leukocytes via receptor expression on monocytes. J Immunol. 2001 Oct 15;**167**(8):4593-4599. DOI: 10.4049/jimmunol.167.8.4593. PMID: 11591788

[57] Sierra-Honigmann MR, Nath AK, Murakami C, García-Cardeña G, Papapetropoulos A, Sessa WC, Madge LA, Schechner JS, Schwabb MB, Polverini PJ, Flores-Riveros JR. Biological action of leptin as an angiogenic factor. Science. 1998 Sep 11;**281**(5383):1683-1686. DOI: 10.1126/science.281.5383.1683. PMID: 9733517

[58] Bouloumié A, Drexler HC, Lafontan M, Busse R. Leptin, the product of Ob gene, promotes angiogenesis. Circ Res. 1998 Nov 16;**83**(10):1059-1066. DOI: 10.1161/01.res.83.10.1059. PMID: 9815153

[59] Jin X, Fukuda N, Su J, Takagi H, Lai Y, Lin Z, Kanmatsuse K, Wang ZW, Unger RH. Effects of leptin on endothelial function with OB-Rb gene transfer in Zucker fatty rats. Atherosclerosis. 2003 Aug;**169**(2):225-233. DOI: 10.1016/s0021-9150(03)00159-x. PMID: 12921973

[60] Vecchione C, Maffei A, Colella S, Aretini A, Poulet R, Frati G, Gentile MT, Fratta L, Trimarco V, Trimarco B, Lembo G. Leptin effect on endothelial nitric oxide is mediated through Akt-endothelial nitric oxide synthase phosphorylation pathway. Diabetes. 2002 Jan;**51**(1):168-173. DOI: 10.2337/diabetes.51.1.168. PMID: 11756337

[61] Cao R, Brakenhielm E, Wahlestedt C, Thyberg J, Cao Y. Leptin induces vascular permeability and synergistically stimulates angiogenesis with FGF-2 and VEGF. Proc Natl Acad Sci U S A. 2001 May 22;**98**(11):6390-5. DOI: 10.1073/pnas.101564798. Epub 2001 May 8. PMID: 11344271; PMCID: PMC33478

[62] Senger DR, Galli SJ, Dvorak AM, Perruzzi CA, Harvey VS, Dvorak HF. Tumor cells secrete a vascular permeability factor that promotes accumulation of ascites fluid. Science. 1983 Feb 25;**219**(4587):983-985. DOI: 10.1126/science.6823562. PMID: 6823562

[63] Bruno A, Conus S, Schmid I, Simon HU. Apoptotic pathways are

inhibited by leptin receptor activation in neutrophils. J Immunol. 2005 Jun 15;**174**(12):8090-8096. DOI: 10.4049/jimmunol.174.12.8090. PMID: 15944317

[64] Moore SI, Huffnagle GB, Chen GH, White ES, Mancuso P. Leptin modulates neutrophil phagocytosis of Klebsiella pneumoniae. Infect Immun. 2003 Jul;**71**(7):4182-5. DOI: 10.1128/IAI.71.7.4182-4185.2003. PMID: 12819114; PMCID: PMC161963

[65] Merrick JC, Edelson BT, Bhardwaj V, Swanson PE, Unanue ER. Lymphocyte apoptosis during early phase of Listeria infection in mice. Am J Pathol. 1997 Sep;**151**(3):785-92. PMID: 9284827; PMCID: PMC1857845

[66] Coffey MJ, Phare SM, Kazanjian PH, Peters-Golden M. 5-Lipoxygenase metabolism in alveolar macrophages from subjects infected with the human immunodeficiency virus. J Immunol. 1996 Jul 1;**157**(1): 393-399. PMID: 8683143

[67] Malli F, Papaioannou AI, Gourgoulianis KI, Daniil Z. The role of leptin in the respiratory system: an overview. Respir Res. 2010 Oct 31;**11**(1):152. DOI: 10.1186/1465-9921-11-152. PMID: 21040518; PMCID: PMC2988727

[68] Wabitsch M, Funcke JB, Lennerz B, Kuhnle-Krahl U, Lahr G, Debatin KM, Vatter P, Gierschik P, Moepps B, Fischer-Posovszky P. Biologically inactive leptin and early-onset extreme obesity. N Engl J Med. 2015 Jan 1;**372**(1):48-54. DOI: 10.1056/NEJMoa1406653. PMID: 25551525

[69] Mantzoros CS. The role of leptin in human obesity and disease: a review of current evidence. Ann Intern Med. 1999 Apr 20;**130**(8):671-680. DOI: 10.7326/0003-4819-130-8-199904200-00014. PMID: 10215564.

[70] Mainardi M, Pizzorusso T, Maffei M. Environment, leptin sensitivity, and hypothalamic plasticity. Neural Plast. 2013;**2013**:438072. DOI: 10.1155/2013/438072. Epub 2013 Jul 18. PMID: 23970977; PMCID: PMC3732608

[71] Gonzalez-Carter D, Goode AE, Fiammengo R, Dunlop IE, Dexter DT, Porter AE. Inhibition of Leptin-ObR Interaction Does not Prevent Leptin Translocation Across a Human Blood-Brain Barrier Model. J Neuroendocrinol. 2016 Jun;**28**(6). DOI: 10.1111/jne.12392. PMID: 27037668

[72] Mattace Raso G, Simeoli R, Russo R, Iacono A, Santoro A, Paciello O, Ferrante MC, Canani RB, Calignano A, Meli R. Effects of sodium butyrate and its synthetic amide derivative on liver inflammation and glucose tolerance in an animal model of steatosis induced by high fat diet. PLoS One. 2013 Jul 5;**8**(7):e68626. DOI: 10.1371/journal.pone.0068626. PMID: 23861927; PMCID: PMC3702592

[73] Kelesidis T, Kelesidis I, Chou S, Mantzoros CS. Narrative review: the role of leptin in human physiology: emerging clinical applications. Ann Intern Med. 2010 Jan 19;**152**(2):93-100. DOI: 10.7326/0003-4819-152-2-201001190-00008. PMID: 20083828; PMCID: PMC2829242

[74] Minokoshi Y, Toda C, Okamoto S. Regulatory role of leptin in glucose and lipid metabolism in skeletal muscle. Indian J Endocrinol Metab. 2012 Dec;**16**(Suppl 3):S562-8. DOI: 10.4103/2230-8210.105573. PMID: 23565491; PMCID: PMC3602985

[75] Maffei M, Halaas J, Ravussin E, Pratley RE, Lee GH, Zhang Y, Fei H, Kim S, Lallone R, Ranganathan S, et al. Leptin levels in human and rodent: measurement of plasma leptin and ob RNA in obese and weight-reduced

subjects. Nat Med. 1995 Nov;**1**(11): 1155-1161. DOI: 10.1038/nm1195-1155. PMID: 7584987

[76] Ahima RS. Central actions of adipocyte hormones. Trends Endocrinol Metab. 2005 Sep;**16**(7):307-313. DOI: 10.1016/j.tem.2005.07.010. PMID: 16098759

[77] igneshwaran B, Wahal A, Aggarwal S, Priyadarshini P, Bhattacharjee H, Khadgawat R, Yadav R. Impact of Sleeve Gastrectomy on Type 2 Diabetes Mellitus, Gastric Emptying Time, Glucagon-Like Peptide 1 (GLP-1), Ghrelin and Leptin in Non-morbidly Obese Subjects with BMI 30-35.0 kg/m^2: a Prospective Study. Obes Surg. 2016 Dec;**26**(12):2817-2823. DOI: 10.1007/s11695-016-2226-9. PMID: 27185177

[78] Belhayara MI, Mellouk Z, Hamdaoui MS, Bachaoui M, Kheroua O, Malaisse WJ. Relationship between the insulin resistance and circulating predictive biochemical markers in metabolic syndrome among young adults in western Algeria. Diabetes Metab Syndr. 2019 Jan-Feb;**13**(1):504-509. DOI: 10.1016/j.dsx.2018.11.019. Epub 2018 Nov 3. PMID: 30641755

[79] Dodd GT, Worth AA, Nunn N, Korpal AK, Bechtold DA, Allison MB, Myers MG Jr, Statnick MA, Luckman SM. The thermogenic effect of leptin is dependent on a distinct population of prolactin-releasing peptide neurons in the dorsomedial hypothalamus. Cell Metab. 2014 Oct 7;**20**(4):639-49. DOI: 10.1016/j.cmet.2014.07.022. Epub 2014 Aug 28. PMID: 25176149; PMCID: PMC4192552

[80] Elmquist JK, Ahima RS, Maratos-Flier E, Flier JS, Saper CB. Leptin activates neurons in ventrobasal hypothalamus and brainstem. Endocrinology. 1997 Feb;**138**(2):839-842. DOI: 10.1210/endo.138.2.5033. PMID: 9003024

[81] Fischer AW, Hoefig CS, Abreu-Vieira G, de Jong JMA, Petrovic N, Mittag J, Cannon B, Nedergaard J. Leptin Raises Defended Body Temperature without Activating Thermogenesis. Cell Rep. 2016 Feb 23;**14**(7):1621-1631. DOI: 10.1016/j.celrep.2016.01.041. Epub 2016 Feb 11. PMID: 26876182

[82] Garfield AS, Li C, Madara JC, Shah BP, Webber E, Steger JS, Campbell JN, Gavrilova O, Lee CE, Olson DP, Elmquist JK, Tannous BA, Krashes MJ, Lowell BB. A neural basis for melanocortin-4 receptor-regulated appetite. Nat Neurosci. 2015 Jun;**18**(6):863-71. DOI: 10.1038/nn.4011. Epub 2015 Apr 27. PMID: 25915476; PMCID: PMC4446192

[83] Athyros VG, Katsiki N, Karagiannis A, Mikhailidis DP. Editorial: should chronic kidney disease be considered as a coronary heart disease equivalent? Curr Vasc Pharmacol. 2012 May;**10**(3):374-377. DOI: 10.2174/157016112799959422. PMID: 22272896

[84] Levine JA, Eberhardt NL, Jensen MD. Role of nonexercise activity thermogenesis in resistance to fat gain in humans. Science. 1999 Jan 8; 283(5399):212-214. DOI: 10.1126/science.283.5399.212. PMID: 9880251

[85] Lute B, Jou W, Lateef DM, Goldgof M, Xiao C, Piñol RA, Kravitz AV, Miller NR, Huang YG, Girardet C, Butler AA, Gavrilova O, Reitman ML. Biphasic effect of melanocortin agonists on metabolic rate and body temperature. Cell Metab. 2014 Aug 5;**20**(2):333-45. DOI: 10.1016/j.cmet.2014.05.021. Epub 2014 Jun 26. PMID: 24981835; PMCID: PMC4126889

[86] Monda M, Sullo A, De Luca B. Lesions of the ventromedial hypothalamus reduce postingestional thermogenesis. Physiol

Behav. 1997 May;**61**(5):687-691. DOI: 10.1016/s0031-9384(96)00520-3. PMID: 9145938

[87] Monge-Roffarello B, Labbe SM, Lenglos C, Caron A, Lanfray D, Samson P, Richard D. The medial preoptic nucleus as a site of the thermogenic and metabolic actions of melanotan II in male rats. Am J Physiol Regul Integr Comp Physiol. 2014 Jul 15;**307**(2):R158-R166. DOI: 10.1152/ajpregu.00059.2014. PMID: 24808495

[88] Rosenbaum M, Murphy EM, Heymsfield SB, Matthews DE, Leibel RL. Low dose leptin administration reverses effects of sustained weight-reduction on energy expenditure and circulating concentrations of thyroid hormones. J Clin Endocrinol Metab. 2002 May;**87**(5):2391-2394. DOI: 10.1210/jcem.87.5.8628. PMID: 11994393

[89] usyniak DE, Zaretskaia MV, Zaretsky DV, DiMicco JA. Microinjection of muscimol into the dorsomedial hypothalamus suppresses MDMA-evoked sympathetic and behavioral responses. Brain Res. 2008 Aug 21;**1226**:116-23. DOI: 10.1016/j.brainres.2008.06.011. Epub 2008 Jun 14. PMID: 18586013; PMCID: PMC2600867

[90] te Marie L, Miura GI, Marsh DJ, Yagaloff K, Palmiter RD. A metabolic defect promotes obesity in mice lacking melanocortin-4 receptors. Proc Natl Acad Sci U S A. 2000 Oct 24;**97**(22):12339-44. DOI: 10.1073/pnas.220409497. PMID: 11027312; PMCID: PMC17343

[91] Tam CS, Lecoultre V, Ravussin E. Brown adipose tissue: mechanisms and potential therapeutic targets. Circulation. 2012 Jun 5;**125**(22):2782-2791. DOI: 10.1161/CIRCULATIONAHA.111.042929. PMID: 22665886.

[92] van Marken Lichtenbelt W. Brown adipose tissue and the regulation of nonshivering thermogenesis. Curr Opin Clin Nutr Metab Care. 2012 Nov;**15**(6): 547-552. DOI: 10.1097/MCO.0b013e3283599184. PMID: 23037904

[93] Vaughan CH, Shrestha YB, Bartness TJ. Characterization of a novel melanocortin receptor-containing node in the SNS outflow circuitry to brown adipose tissue involved in thermogenesis. Brain Res. 2011 Sep 9;**1411**:17-27. DOI: 10.1016/j.brainres.2011.07.003. Epub 2011 Jul 13. PMID: 21802070; PMCID: PMC3426614

[94] Welle S, Schwartz RG, Statt M. Reduced metabolic rate during beta-adrenergic blockade in humans. Metabolism. 1991 Jun;**40**(6):619-622. DOI: 10.1016/0026-0495(91)90053-y. PMID: 1650879

[95] Zhou X, Gomez-Smith M, Qin Z, Duquette PM, Cardenas-Blanco A, Rai PS, Harper ME, Tsai EC, Anisman H, Chen HH. Ablation of LMO4 in glutamatergic neurons impairs leptin control of fat metabolism. Cell Mol Life Sci. 2012 Mar;**69**(5):819-28. DOI: 10.1007/s00018-011-0794-3. Epub 2011 Aug 27. PMID: 21874351; PMCID: PMC3276759

[96] Jiang L, You J, Yu X, Gonzalez L, Yu Y, Wang Q, Yang G, Li W, Li C, Liu Y. Tyrosine-dependent and -independent actions of leptin receptor in control of energy balance and glucose homeostasis. Proc Natl Acad Sci U S A. 2008 Nov 25;**105**(47):18619-24. DOI: 10.1073/pnas.0804589105. Epub 2008 Nov 17. PMID: 19015522; PMCID: PMC2587560

[97] Varela L, Horvath TL. Leptin and insulin pathways in POMC and AgRP neurons that modulate energy balance and glucose homeostasis. EMBO Rep. 2012 Dec;**13**(12):1079-86. DOI: 10.1038/embor.2012.174. Epub 2012 Nov 13. PMID: 23146889; PMCID: PMC3512417

[98] Paz-Filho G, Mastronardi C, Franco CB, Wang KB, Wong ML, Licinio J. Leptin: molecular mechanisms, systemic pro-inflammatory effects, and clinical implications. Arq Bras Endocrinol Metabol. 2012 Dec;**56**(9):597-607. DOI: 10.1590/s0004-27302012000900001. PMID: 23329181

[99] Carbone F, La Rocca C, Matarese G. Immunological functions of leptin and adiponectin. Biochimie. 2012 Oct;**94**(10):2082-2088. DOI: 10.1016/j.biochi.2012.05.018. Epub 2012 Jun 26. PMID: 22750129

[100] Iikuni N, Lam QL, Lu L, Matarese G, La Cava A. Leptin and Inflammation. Curr Immunol Rev. 2008 May 1;**4**(2):70-79. DOI: 10.2174/157339508784325046. PMID: 20198122; PMCID: PMC2829991

[101] Procaccini C, Jirillo E, Matarese G. Leptin as an immunomodulator. Mol Aspects Med. 2012 Feb;**33**(1):35-45. DOI: 10.1016/j.mam.2011.10.012. Epub 2011 Oct 21. PMID: 22040697

[102] Sharma V, Mustafa S, Patel N, Wambolt R, Allard MF, McNeill JH. Stimulation of cardiac fatty acid oxidation by leptin is mediated by a nitric oxide-p38 MAPK-dependent mechanism. Eur J Pharmacol. 2009 Sep 1;**617**(1-3):113-117. DOI: 10.1016/j.ejphar.2009.06.037. Epub 2009 Jun 30. PMID: 19573526

[103] German JP, Thaler JP, Wisse BE, Oh-I S, Sarruf DA, Matsen ME, Fischer JD, Taborsky GJ Jr, Schwartz MW, Morton GJ. Leptin activates a novel CNS mechanism for insulin-independent normalization of severe diabetic hyperglycemia. Endocrinology. 2011 Feb;**152**(2):394-404. DOI: 10.1210/en.2010-0890. Epub 2010 Dec 15. PMID: 21159853; PMCID: PMC3037161

[104] Hill JW, Williams KW, Ye C, Luo J, Balthasar N, Coppari R, Cowley MA, Cantley LC, Lowell BB, Elmquist JK. Acute effects of leptin require PI3K signaling in hypothalamic proopio-melanocortin neurons in mice. J Clin Invest. 2008 May;**118**(5):1796-805. DOI: 10.1172/JCI32964. PMID: 18382766; PMCID: PMC2276395

[105] Agrawal S, Gollapudi S, Su H, Gupta S. Leptin activates human B cells to secrete TNF-α, IL-6, and IL-10 via JAK2/STAT3 and p38MAPK/ERK1/2 signaling pathway. J Clin Immunol. 2011 Jun;**31**(3):472-8. DOI: 10.1007/s10875-010-9507-1. Epub 2011 Jan 18. PMID: 21243519; PMCID: PMC3132280

[106] Paz-Filho G, Mastronardi C, Franco CB, Wang KB, Wong ML, Licinio J. Leptin: molecular mechanisms, systemic pro-inflammatory effects, and clinical implications. Arq Bras Endocrinol Metabol. 2012 Dec;**56**(9):597-607. DOI: 10.1590/s0004-27302012000900001. PMID: 23329181

[107] Burguera B, Couce ME, Long J, Lamsam J, Laakso K, Jensen MD, Parisi JE, Lloyd RV. The long form of the leptin receptor (OB-Rb) is widely expressed in the human brain. Neuroendocrinology. 2000 Mar;**71**(3):187-195. DOI: 10.1159/000054536. PMID: 10729790

[108] Weigle DS, Duell PB, Connor WE, Steiner RA, Soules MR, Kuijper JL. Effect of fasting, refeeding, and dietary fat restriction on plasma leptin levels. J Clin Endocrinol Metab. 1997 Feb;**82**(2):561-565. DOI: 10.1210/jcem.82.2.3757. PMID: 9024254

[109] Pelleymounter MA, Cullen MJ, Baker MB, Hecht R, Winters D, Boone T, Collins F. Effects of the obese gene product on body weight regulation in ob/ob mice. Science. 1995 Jul 28;**269**(5223):540-543.

DOI: 10.1126/science.7624776. PMID: 7624776

[110] Halaas JL, Gajiwala KS, Maffei M, Cohen SL, Chait BT, Rabinowitz D, Lallone RL, Burley SK, Friedman JM. Weight-reducing effects of the plasma protein encoded by the obese gene. Science. 1995 Jul 28;**269**(5223):543-546. DOI: 10.1126/science.7624777. PMID: 7624777

[111] Satoh N, Ogawa Y, Katsuura G, Tsuji T, Masuzaki H, Hiraoka J, Okazaki T, Tamaki M, Hayase M, Yoshimasa Y, Nishi S, Hosoda K, Nakao K. Pathophysiological significance of the obese gene product, leptin, in ventromedial hypothalamus (VMH)-lesioned rats: evidence for loss of its satiety effect in VMH-lesioned rats. Endocrinology. 1997 Mar;**138**(3):947-954. DOI: 10.1210/endo.138.3.4989. PMID: 9048594

[112] Roujeau C, Jockers R, Dam J. New pharmacological perspectives for the leptin receptor in the treatment of obesity. Front Endocrinol (Lausanne). 2014 Oct 13;**5**:167. DOI: 10.3389/fendo.2014.00167. PMID: 25352831; PMCID: PMC4195360

[113] Obradovic M, Sudar-Milovanovic E, Soskic S, Essack M, Arya S, Stewart AJ, Gojobori T, Isenovic ER. Leptin and Obesity: Role and Clinical Implication. Front Endocrinol (Lausanne). 2021 May 18;**12**:585887. DOI: 10.3389/fendo.2021.585887. PMID: 34084149; PMCID: PMC8167040

[114] Gorden P, Gavrilova O. The clinical uses of leptin. Curr Opin Pharmacol. 2003 Dec;**3**(6):655-659. DOI: 10.1016/j.coph.2003.06.006. PMID: 14644019

[115] Salvador J, Gomez-Ambrosi J, Frühbeck G. Perspectives in the therapeutic use of leptin. Expert Opin Pharmacother. 2001 Oct;**2**(10):1615-1622. DOI: 10.1517/14656566.2.10.1615. PMID: 11825304

[116] Hukshorn CJ, Saris WH, Westerterp-Plantenga MS, Farid AR, Smith FJ, Campfield LA. Weekly subcutaneous pegylated recombinant native human leptin (PEG-OB) administration in obese men. J Clin Endocrinol Metab. 2000 Nov;**85**(11): 4003-4009. DOI: 10.1210/jcem.85.11.6955. PMID: 11095423

[117] Heymsfield SB, Greenberg AS, Fujioka K, Dixon RM, Kushner R, Hunt T, Lubina JA, Patane J, Self B, Hunt P, McCamish M. Recombinant leptin for weight loss in obese and lean adults: a randomized, controlled, dose-escalation trial. JAMA. 1999 Oct 27;**282**(16):1568-1575. DOI: 10.1001/jama.282.16.1568. PMID: 10546697

[118] Ring BD, Scully S, Davis CR, Baker MB, Cullen MJ, Pelleymounter MA, Danilenko DM. Systemically and topically administered leptin both accelerate wound healing in diabetic ob/ob mice. Endocrinology. 2000 Jan;**141**(1):446-449. DOI: 10.1210/endo.141.1.7373. PMID: 10614668

[119] Yamauchi T, Waki H, Kamon J, Murakami K, Motojima K, Komeda K, Miki H, Kubota N, Terauchi Y, Tsuchida A, Tsuboyama-Kasaoka N, Yamauchi N, Ide T, Hori W, Kato S, Fukayama M, Akanuma Y, Ezaki O, Itai A, Nagai R, Kimura S, Tobe K, Kagechika H, Shudo K, Kadowaki T. Inhibition of RXR and PPARgamma ameliorates diet-induced obesity and type 2 diabetes. J Clin Invest. 2001 Oct;**108**(7):1001-13. DOI: 10.1172/JCI12864. PMID: 11581301; PMCID: PMC200951

[120] Cohen P, Miyazaki M, Socci ND, Hagge-Greenberg A, Liedtke W,

Soukas AA, Sharma R, Hudgins LC, Ntambi JM, Friedman JM. Role for stearoyl-CoA desaturase-1 in leptin-mediated weight loss. Science. 2002 Jul 12;**297**(5579):240-243. DOI: 10.1126/science.1071527. PMID: 12114623

[121] Lindsay RS, Funahashi T, Hanson RL, Matsuzawa Y, Tanaka S, Tataranni PA, Knowler WC, Krakoff J. Adiponectin and development of type 2 diabetes in the Pima Indian population. Lancet. 2002 Jul 6;**360**(9326):57-58. DOI: 10.1016/S0140-6736(02)09335-2. PMID: 12114044

[122] Spranger J, Kroke A, Möhlig M, Bergmann MM, Ristow M, Boeing H, Pfeiffer AF. Adiponectin and protection against type 2 diabetes mellitus. Lancet. 2003 Jan 18;**361**(9353):226-8. DOI: 10.1016/S0140-6736(03)12255-6. Erratum in: Lancet. 2002 Mar 22;**361**(9362):1060. PMID: 12547549

[123] Sanna V, Di Giacomo A, La Cava A, Lechler RI, Fontana S, Zappacosta S, Matarese G. Leptin surge precedes onset of autoimmune encephalomyelitis and correlates with development of pathogenic T cell responses. J Clin Invest. 2003 Jan;**111**(2):241-50. DOI: 10.1172/JCI16721. PMID: 12531880; PMCID: PMC151876

[124] Farooqi IS, Matarese G, Lord GM, Keogh JM, Lawrence E, Agwu C, Sanna V, Jebb SA, Perna F, Fontana S, Lechler RI, DePaoli AM, O'Rahilly S. Beneficial effects of leptin on obesity, T cell hyporesponsiveness, and neuroendocrine/metabolic dysfunction of human congenital leptin deficiency. J Clin Invest. 2002 Oct;**110**(8):1093-103. DOI: 10.1172/JCI15693. PMID: 12393845; PMCID: PMC150795

[125] Moran S, Young J, Ruiz E, Sebring N, Premkumar A, Depaoli A, Oral E, Skarulis M, Gorden P: Changes in body composition in patients with lipodystrophic diabetes after leptin replacement therapy. Diabetes 2003, 52:A76

[126] Frühbeck G. Intracellular signalling pathways activated by leptin. Biochem J. 2006 Jan 1;**393**(Pt 1):7-20. DOI: 10.1042/BJ20051578. PMID: 16336196; PMCID: PMC1383660

[127] Hileman SM, Tornøe J, Flier JS, Bjørbaek C. Transcellular transport of leptin by the short leptin receptor isoform ObRa in Madin-Darby Canine Kidney cells. Endocrinology. 2000 Jun;**141**(6):1955-1961. DOI: 10.1210/endo.141.6.7450. PMID: 10830277

[128] Arvaniti K, Huang Q, Richard D. Effects of leptin and corticosterone on the expression of corticotropin-releasing hormone, agouti-related protein, and proopiomelanocortin in the brain of ob/ob mouse. Neuroendocrinology. 2001 Apr;**73**(4):227-236. DOI: 10.1159/000054639. PMID: 11340336

[129] Pandit R, Beerens S, Adan RAH. Role of leptin in energy expenditure: the hypothalamic perspective. Am J Physiol Regul Integr Comp Physiol. 2017 Jun 1;**312**(6):R938-R947. DOI: 10.1152/ajpregu.00045.2016. Epub 2017 Mar 29. PMID: 28356295

[130] hao S, Zhu Y, Schultz RD, Li N, He Z, Zhang Z, Caron A, Zhu Q, Sun K, Xiong W, Deng H, Sun J, Deng Y, Kim M, Lee CE, Gordillo R, Liu T, Odle AK, Childs GV, Zhang N, Kusminski CM, Elmquist JK, Williams KW, An Z, Scherer PE. Partial Leptin Reduction as an Insulin Sensitization and Weight Loss Strategy. Cell Metab. 2019 Oct 1;**30**(4):706-719.e6. DOI: 10.1016/j.cmet.2019.08.005. Epub 2019 Sep 5. PMID: 31495688; PMCID: PMC6774814

Chapter 2

Leptin: A Metabolic Signal for the Differentiation of Pituitary Cells

Gwen V. Childs, Angela K. Odle, Melanie C. MacNicol, Melody L. Allensworth-James, Tiffany K. Miles, Noor Akhter, Mohsin M. Syed and Angus M. MacNicol

Abstract

Pituitary cell function is impacted by metabolic states and therefore must receive signals that inform them about nutritional status or adiposity. A primary signal from adipocytes is leptin, which recent studies have shown regulates most pituitary cell types. Subsets of all pituitary cell types express leptin receptors and leptin has been shown to exert transcriptional control through classical JAK/STAT pathways. Recent studies show that leptin also signals through post-transcriptional pathways that involve the translational regulatory protein Musashi. Mechanistically, post-transcriptional control would permit rapid cellular regulation of critical pre-existing pituitary transcripts as energy states change. The chapter will review evidence for transcriptional and/or post-transcriptional regulation of leptin targets (including *Gnrh*r, activin, *Fshb, Gh, Ghrhr,* and *Pou1f1*) and the consequences of the loss of leptin signaling to gonadotrope and somatotrope functions.

Keywords: Leptin, somatotropes, gonadotropes, Musashi, post-transcriptional, *Pou1f1*, *Ghrhr*, *Gnrhr*, *Fshb*

1. Introduction

To perform their vital functions, anterior pituitary cells must respond appropriately to their unique hypothalamic releasing hormones, while also responding to extrinsic signals informing them of the body's nutritional and metabolic state. Leptin is one of the most important of these extrinsic signals. However, recent studies show that leptin does more than simply signal levels of fat stores [1–11]. Leptin plays a trophic role that optimizes and maintains differentiation of at least two of these cell types, somatotropes and gonadotropes.

Anterior pituitary somatotropes produce growth hormone (GH) to support growth in muscles and bones before puberty and build muscle, bone, and reduce fat to optimize body composition in the adult [12, 13]. Gonadotropes produce the gonadotropins, luteinizing hormone (LH) and follicle stimulating hormone (FSH), which differentially regulate gonadal functions, ovulation and reproductive cyclicity [14]. Both somatotrope and gonadotrope functions are impacted by the nutritional state and therefore it is not surprising that they exhibit a dependency on leptin. Early studies showed significant reductions in numbers of gonadotropes in leptin-deficient animals [6, 15–19]. Similarly, rodents that lack leptin or leptin receptors (LEPR) had reduced numbers of somatotropes [20, 21]. Our studies on the distribution of pituitary LEPR showed expression in nearly all cells [1, 22].

A dependency on normal levels of serum leptin was seen in our studies of 24 h fasted rats, when we correlated the reduction in serum leptin with reduced numbers of immunolabeled somatotropes and gonadotropes, along with reduced receptivity for gonadotropin releasing hormone (GnRH) and growth hormone releasing hormone (GHRH) [23]. As these findings pointed to potential trophic actions by leptin, we continued *in vitro* studies to determine if leptin would rescue either cell population, restoring hormone stores lost during the acute fast. We cultured pituitary cells from fasted rats overnight and then incubated them with 10-100 pg./ml leptin for 1 h. This brief treatment rapidly restored stores as detected by increases in numbers of immunolabeled somatotropes and gonadotropes [23], confirming direct effects of leptin on these cell populations.

These findings agree with recent *in vivo* studies of rodents by Luque et al. [24], which showed that both GH secretion and *Ghrhr* mRNA levels were restored by leptin in leptin-deficient *ob/ob* mice. Furthermore, studies of non-human primates by this same group confirmed both somatotropes and gonadotropes as leptin targets in primates [25, 26], reporting that leptin stimulated release of GH and follicle stimulating hormone (FSH) *in vitro* [25].

Leptin's restorative or stimulatory effects directly on somatotropes and gonadotropes have since led to studies that explored the significance of this regulatory influence as well as basic mechanisms of action, including the identification of signaling pathways and transcription factors. This chapter will review the studies which have identified critical leptin target molecules that are vital to the differentiated function of gonadotropes and somatotropes. We will also review signaling pathways used by leptin to stimulate production of these targets. Finally, we will show how leptin may contribute to plasticity of the pituitary by supporting multihormonal cell populations.

2. Leptin regulation of reproduction

The overall importance of leptin to reproduction was established soon after its discovery [5]. Leptin alone will restore fertility in leptin-deficient animals and humans [4, 15, 16, 27–36]. There are distinct sex differences in serum leptin levels in the adult. After puberty, adult males have relatively low leptin levels, when compared with females [37–41]. This sex difference may reflect the differential regulation of leptin by gonadal steroids. Androgens inhibit leptin secretion to prevent leptin inhibition of testicular function (reviewed in [5]). In females by contrast, estrogens stimulate leptin secretion. The rise in estrogen early in the cycle may contribute to the 2-3-fold increase in leptin levels known as the midcycle leptin surge [37, 39].

With respect to gonadotrope function, studies have also reported a synchrony between nocturnal leptin and LH pulses in normal cycling women [36, 37]. Indeed, a comprehensive study of 259 cycling women reported that the highest levels of leptin were correlated with the timing of the LH surge [37]. In contrast, anovulatory cycles were associated with overall low leptin levels.

3. Leptin regulation of gonadotropes

Shortly after leptin was discovered, pioneering studies by Yu et al. [10] demonstrated that leptin stimulated LH and FSH release, *in vitro*, from hemi-anterior pituitaries. They reported a dose dependent increase in LH after 3 h in 10^{-11}-10^{-9} M leptin. Higher concentrations, however, were not stimulatory suggesting the development of leptin resistance. It is interesting to note that the relatively narrow concentration range that stimulates gonadotropin release matches that of the normal cyclic rise in leptin [36, 39]. Yu et al. reported that leptin alone stimulated LH release, *in vitro* and it did not add to the stimulatory effect of GnRH [11]. Their studies also identified nitric oxide as a signaling pathway for leptin regulation of gonadotropes. They showed that a competitive inhibitor of nitric oxide synthase (NOS), N6-monomethyl-L-arginine (NMMA), inhibited the leptin stimulation of LH release *in vitro* [11] suggesting that leptin may use the NOS pathway to stimulate gonadotropes directly.

Our studies on the importance of leptin to gonadotropes began with the detection of leptin receptors (LEPR) in dispersed pituitary cells from male and cycling female rats and mice [1]. The expression of LEPR varied with the stage of the cycle and was seen in 40-50% of anterior pituitary cells from males and females in metestrus or diestrus. LEPR expression increased to 60-80% of AP cells in proestrous and estrous females, which coincided with the midcycle rise in serum leptin [1].

To determine if the increase reflected changes in gonadotrope receptivity, dual labeling was performed for LEPR and gonadotropins. The results showed that 90% of gonadotropes identified by the stores of luteinizing hormone (LH) or follicle stimulating hormone (FSH) expressed LEPR in males and throughout all stages of the cycle in females [1]. Some of the increase in LEPR in proestrous females was due to an increase in cells expressing LH and LEPR, which occurs just before the LH surge.

The findings showing an overall increase in LEPR early in the estrous cycle stimulated studies to determine potential regulators for this expression. We treated one day cultures of anterior pituitary cells from diestrous female mice with estradiol overnight and then treated a subset of these cultures with 10 or 100 pg./ml neuropeptide Y (NPY) for 3 h. **Figure 1** shows that estradiol or NPY alone (100 pg./ml) stimulated a

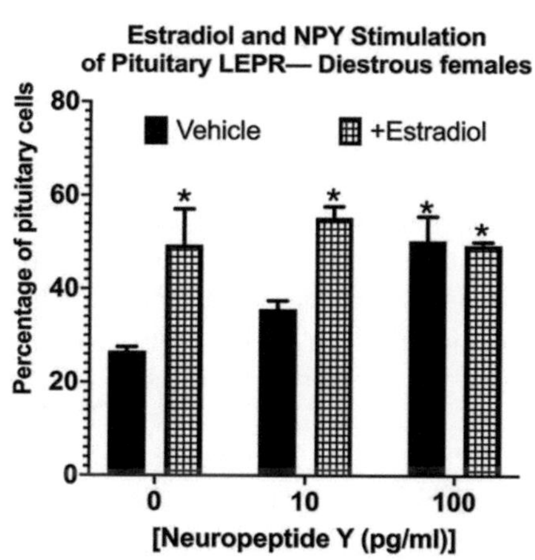

Figure 1.
*Estradiol and NPY stimulate LEPR expression in 1-day cultures of anterior pituitary cells. * = significantly higher values than all other values; ANOVA + Bonferroni's post hoc test. Note: These are original data, not published elsewhere.*

significant 2--fold increase in LEPR-bearing cells and that the effects of the two were not additive. In contrast, NPY did not stimulate LEPR expression in anterior pituitary cells from male mice (data not shown). Collectively, these data support the hypothesis that rising estradiol early in the cycle may stimulate an increase in pituitary receptivity to leptin which may serve as a gateway for leptin's permissive actions [7].

Having established the presence of the receptor population in gonadotropes, we determined if leptin acted on gonadotropes through the Janus Kinase-Signal Transducer and Activator of Transcription (JAK–STAT) pathway. Following leptin stimulation for 10-60 min *in vitro*, pituitary cells from diestrous females were dual immunolabeled for phosphorylated STAT3 and LH or FSH [1]. In 30-60 min, leptin stimulation increased the overall percentage of LH or FSH-bearing gonadotropes and the percentages of gonadotropes bearing pSTAT3 [1]. Thus, leptin acts through both NOS [11] and the JAK–STAT [1] pathways to increase LH or FSH stores in gonadotropes.

4. The importance of leptin to gonadotrope function

The next series of studies investigated leptin's importance to gonadotrope function by selectively ablating LEPR in gonadotropes with Cre-LoxP technology. This work fills a critical knowledge gap, because, as summarized in our recent review [5], much of the research surrounding leptin's role in reproduction has been focused in the hypothalamus. There was a growing body of evidence showing that leptin's regulatory actions were mediated through its stimulation of Kisspeptin neuronal pathways that regulate GnRH neurons (reviewed in [5]).

Our first set of studies used Cre-recombinase driven by the *rLhb* promoter to delete either the JAK binding site (floxed LEPR exon 17) [1] or the signaling peptide of the LEPR (floxed LEPR exon 1). Deletion of LEPR exon 17 resulted in a non-signaling receptor. Deletion of exon 1 resulted in ablation of all isoforms of LEPR. because the deletion removed the signal peptide thereby preventing the protein from entering the rough endoplasmic reticulum. Ongoing studies are using Cre-recombinase driven by the *Gnrhr* promoter to delete LEPR exon 1.

The first question to be addressed related to the impact of loss of LEPR in gonadotropes on pubertal development, growth, and fertility of the mice [1]. When LEPR exon 17 was deleted in gonadotropes with the Cre-*Lhb* driver, mice showed no evidence of delayed puberty or growth. Mutant males showed no evidence of impaired fertility. However, mutant females exhibited a 36% increase in time to first pregnancy and the litters contained significantly fewer pups. Pup survival was 98% from either parent and there was no evidence of growth defects in weanlings from mutant females. Therefore, mutant females appeared to lactate normally.

We analyzed hormone levels in mice lacking LEPR exon 17 and reported that loss of LEPR resulted in several deficits [1]. In mutant diestrous females, serum levels of LH, FSH, and GH were reduced. In contrast, mutant males showed reductions in GH, prolactin (Prl), and thyroid stimulating hormone (TSH), but no reductions in gonadotropins. The loss of LEPR resulted in reduced *Fshb* mRNA levels in both males and females but no reductions in *Lhb, Cga* (in females) or *Gnrhr* mRNA levels. In addition, there was a reduction in inhibin/activin beta subunit mRNA (*Actßa* and *Actßb*) in females. The most striking reduction, however, was in GnRHR proteins, as detected by immunolabeling or binding to a biotinylated analog of GnRH [1]. The reduced binding was most severe in diestrous females, a stage where GnRHR expression is normally at the highest levels.

However, during this phase of the study, we detected Cre-recombinase in the testes and therefore continued these studies focusing only on mutant females [7] bearing Cre-*Lhb* and floxed LEPR exon 1. The deletion of this exon was impactful because it results in loss of all isoforms of the receptor. Tests of fertility showed normal litter numbers from three breeding cages of F2 generation heterozygous females (bearing only one deleted allele of LEPR exon 1). However, the study showed severe subfertility/infertility in F3 generation mutant homozygous and heterozygous females [7]. Out of the five F3 generation homozygous females, only two were fertile, producing litters more slowly than control females (one every 30-45 days). One of the litters did not survive. In addition, three F3 homozygous females and two F3 heterozygous females were completely infertile in breeding tests that lasted from 65 to 281 days with a fertile male [7].

We were able to study cyclicity in the progeny from the two F3 fertile females. These mutant F4 female progeny cycled irregularly. Two of them remained in diestrus and the remaining females spent more time in diestrus than normal females. Collectively, these breeding studies showed that ablation of all isoforms of LEPR in gonadotropes had a profound impact on a subset of females; less than half could cycle and were fertile [7]. This highlighted the importance of leptin to gonadotrope functions. However, because of the infertility issues in the line expressing Cre-LH X LEPR exon 1, our ongoing studies have now switched to mice bearing Cre-recombinase driven by the *Gnrhr* promoter. Whereas the mutant females in this line are still subfertile, they produce sufficient progeny for our ongoing and continuing studies of this line.

5. Leptin regulates target genes through different pathways

After we characterized the deletion mutants lacking LEPR in gonadotropes, we hypothesized that rising leptin early in the cycle may have a permissive effect on the rise in pituitary GnRHR levels [7], which could serve as a gateway that permitted full receptivity to GnRH and facilitates the LH surge. We treated pituitary cells from normal diestrous female mice with 10 nM leptin and showed a significant increase in GnRHR proteins [7]. We also detected leptin-stimulated increases in pituitary activin (but not inhibin) mRNA (*Actβa* and *Actβb*) in the same sets of experiments. However, leptin did not stimulate increases in *Gnrhr* mRNA levels [7], which correlated well with the lack of change in mRNA levels evident in the LEPR-null gonadotropes. Thus, we identified three targets of leptin in our animal model, and proposed that leptin may activate these by different pathways.

5.1 Transcriptional regulation of FSH and activin by leptin

We have demonstrated that expression of *Fshb* and activin transcripts are dependent on a normal leptin signal [1, 7]. Other workers have shown that activin and FSH may be dependent on the timing of this leptin signal during postnatal development, which is characterized by a rapid rise in serum leptin. Wen et al. [42] studied the link between the postnatal rise in leptin and FSH and reported that full co-expression of GnRHR and FSH is seen by postnatal day 7, which coincides with the peak leptin surge. A parallel rise in *Fshb* and *Actβa* and *Actβb* mRNA levels during the postnatal leptin rise has also been reported [43–46]. Researchers investigating the impact of altering the neonatal leptin surge on the reproductive system reported that blockade or alteration of the leptin surge decreased testicular or ovarian growth, delayed puberty, and reduced FSH in rat pups [47]. In addition, females showed reduced numbers of ovarian primordial follicles [48].

Another link between leptin and FSH was reported by studies that restored LEPR in gonadotropes from mice that were genetically engineered to be globally deficient in LEPR [49]. As expected, fertility was not restored, because the mice were morbidly obese, and kisspeptin and GnRH neuronal function was still deficient. However, they did report elevated FSH levels in these mice. It was not determined whether restoration of the leptin signal influenced GnRHR expression.

The reduced *Fshb* mRNA detected in our gonadotrope LEPR-null mutants correlates well with the reduced activin (*Actßa* and *Actßb*) mRNA [1], which is a critical regulator of *Fshb* transcription [50, 51]. Our studies show that leptin stimulates activin mRNA [7], which could thus serve as a pathway for FSH stimulation. Leptin regulation of FSH also agrees with studies of rats [10, 11] and non-human primates [25] in which leptin directly stimulated FSH secretion, *in vitro*. Collectively, these findings suggest that leptin may be an important transcriptional regulator of FSH production both postnatally and early in the cycle, either directly or indirectly. Additional studies are needed to determine if this pathway is mediated through JAK–STAT activation or NOS [10, 11].

Figure 2 illustrates how the ovary and adipocytes may partner in the remodeling of gonadotropes to support the development of the follicles with key cellular regulatory pathways and outputs indicated. This cartoon focuses mainly on leptin, FSH and estrogen. We propose that normal levels of leptin permit a rise in FSH early in the cycle regulating FSH directly or through activin. This could be an important checkpoint if leptin levels drop due to fasting, for example [23] as this may signal poor nutrition and reduce FSH production. The cartoon then shows that FSH stimulates

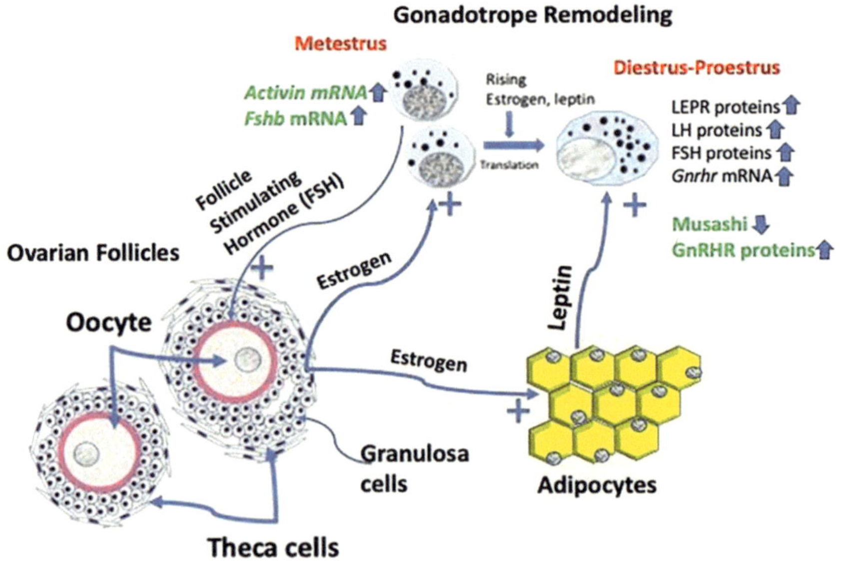

Figure 2.
Gonadotropes are remodeled early in the cycle by estrogens, GnRH, and leptin to support the ovary. We postulate that normal levels of leptin permit FSH release directly or through activin. FSH stimulates the growing population of follicles, which produce more estrogen. This rise in estrogen may stimulate leptin release from adipocytes and the expression of LEPR in gonadotropes. Estrogen also exerts positive feedback on the neuronal circuit that regulates GnRH, which produce more rapid GnRH pulses, which also stimulate Gnrhr *mRNA. As* Gnrhr *mRNA rises, leptin works post-transcriptionally to permit translation of GnRHR proteins by de-repressing the actions of the translational regulator Musashi (MSI). Leptin also causes a reduction in expression of MSI. This is an original figure drawn by the corresponding author and not published elsewhere.*

ovarian follicles to produce and secrete estrogen, which stimulates a rise in serum leptin. The growth in ovarian follicles and subsequent rise in estrogen also has positive feedback actions on GnRH neurons (shown in ref. [5]) and the gonadotropes. Estrogen may also stimulate a rise in pituitary LEPR (**Figure 1**), which renders the gonadotropes more responsive to leptin.

Not shown in this cartoon is GnRH, which is secreted in response to estradiol positive feedback to stimulate gonadotrope production of gonadotropins and GnRHR (pathway shown in ref. [5]). GnRH and estradiol both stimulate *Gnrhr* mRNA during this time (reviewed in [9]). Leptin's role is to de-repress Musashi's actions on *Gnrhr* mRNA and permit translation. Leptin also reduces Musashi expression [7, 8]. Thus, our studies show that, whereas leptin does not regulate *Gnrhr* mRNA directly, it works in partnership with estradiol and GnRH to permit its translation by regulating MSI. This is another checkpoint in reproductive cycles [7, 9]. Reduced leptin, due to fasting for example, may signal poor nutrition and thus reduce translation of GnRHR [7–9] and GnRH binding sites [23]. Ultimately, leptin reduction of ablation slows or prevents reproduction. Our animal models lacking LEPR in gonadotropes support this hypothesis [1, 5, 7].

5.2 Post-transcriptional regulation of GnRHR by leptin

Figure 2 also shows the pathway that regulates the third target for leptin, GnRHR. This receptor appears to be regulated post-transcriptionally by leptin, because *Gnrhr* mRNA is unchanged when diestrous female or male gonadotrope LEPR-null mutants were compared with control males or diestrous females. Additionally, stimulation of control diestrous female pituitary cultures by leptin increases GnRHR, but not *Gnrhr* mRNA levels [7, 8]. We investigated post-transcriptional mediators of leptin action and determined that a putative miRNA repressor of *Gnrhr* mRNA translation, *miR-581/669d,* was increased in LEPR-null gonadotropes [7]. The most promising regulation, however, came from the translational regulatory protein, Musashi (MSI), as we identified 3 consensus binding elements for Musashi (MBEs) in the 3' UTR of murine *Gnrhr* mRNA [8]. The evolutionarily conserved Musashi family of sequence-specific RNA binding proteins (Musashi1 and Musashi2) have long been known to be expressed in stem and progenitor cell populations, where they act to oppose differentiation and promote stem cell self-renewal [52]. Although originally identified as a repressor of target mRNA translation, Musashi was subsequently shown capable of directing translational activation of target mRNAs in a context-dependent manner [53].

Our studies of leptin stimulation of GnRHR proteins showed a dose response relationship between leptin and expression of GnRHR (detected by enzyme assays) or Biotinylated GnRH binding to living pituitary cells (detected cytochemically) [8] After we confirmed that leptin stimulated GnRHR proteins, but not mRNA, we determined by electrophoretic mobility shift assays that Musashi1 interacted directly with the *Gnrhr* 3' UTR [8] . This pituitary association was confirmed by immunoprecipitation with anti-Musashi antibody and the detection of an enrichment of the endogenous *Gnrhr* mRNA (17-fold over control immunoprecipitates). Moreover, the use of luciferase mRNA reporter assays showed that Musashi1 repressed translation of the *Gnrhr* 3' UTR. Tests of leptin actions on Musashi showed that leptin stimulation caused a reduction in Musashi protein levels in gonadotropes, suggesting that leptin may inhibit Musashi expression [8].

To summarize, our studies of leptin actions on gonadotropes have shown severe functional deficiencies in gonadotropes lacking exon 1 of LEPR. The total absence of the LEPR caused infertility in a subset of females [7]. Collectively, studies of these animal models point to key gene products that are affected by loss of leptin signals. Leptin may be important in the transcription of *Fshb* mRNA either directly and/or through the transcription of activin. In addition, leptin's actions may serve to regulate the translation of GnRHR protein [7–9]. Our studies suggest that leptin opposes Musashi-dependent repression of target mRNAs and/or reduces expression of Musashi directly in gonadotropes, leading to enhanced translation of the *Gnrhr* mRNA. This may provide a pathway which permits full expression of GnRHR early in the cycle to reach peak levels in diestrus and proestrus. Estradiol may also stimulate the expression of LEPR, which peaks on proestrus (**Figure 1**). Rising leptin may then partner with estradiol to promote the production of GnRHR (**Figure 2**). We hypothesize that leptin's permissive actions on GnRHR may be to de-repress actions of the translational regulatory protein Musashi and promote full receptivity of the gonadotrope to GnRH [7–9].

6. Impact of ablation of LEPR in gonadotropes on other pituitary cell types

The loss of leptin receptors in gonadotropes also had a broader impact on pituitary function. We reported a profound reduction in serum GH, in both mutant males and females (**Figure 3**) [1]. This reduction would expect to result in growth hormone deficiency, which, in our other models has resulted in significant changes in body weight (adult-onset obesity) [22]. However, when mice were weighed regularly for nearly a year, these deletion mutant animals grew normally and did not gain more weight than normal mice during their first year of life [1]. In addition, male mutants show reduced levels of serum TSH and prolactin [1]. There were also sex-specific differences in mRNA levels. As stated earlier, in deletion mutant females, *Fshb* and activin were reduced. In contrast, male deletion mutants showed reduced mRNA levels of *Fshb, Cga, Gh,* and *Ghrhr.* This phenotype may be the result of deficits in the production of paracrine factors from gonadotropes, which are needed to regulate the function of these cell types. Alternatively, we hypothesized that this phenotype may simply result from of the loss of multihormonal function in subsets of gonadotropes themselves. Evidence for the presence of multihormonal gonadotropes is reviewed in the next few paragraphs.

The presence of multihormonal gonadotropes in the rodent pituitary cell population is not unexpected since our group previously reported cells that stored gonadotropins

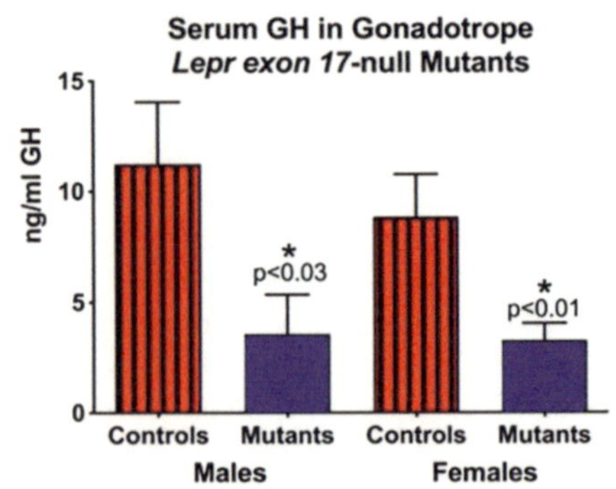

Figure 3.
Mutants lacking Lepr exon 17 in gonadotropes show significantly reduced levels of serum GH. This colored figure has not been published elsewhere. However, the data were published as separate figures (separating sexes) in ref. [1] in a completely different, black and white graph.

and either ACTH [54–56] or GH [57, 58]. Early studies of gonadotropes purified by centrifugal elutriation reported a fraction that contained 91-93% immunolabeled LH-FSH cells (a 9-fold enrichment). This group of cells were enriched based on their response to GnRH. The stimulated secretion caused them to enlarge. Which allowed them to be separated and enriched in a fraction containing larger cells. The fraction also contained gonadotropes that immunolabeled for other hormones. In the female gonadotrope fraction, we detected: 29.2% GH cells, 4% prolactin cells, 6.8% adrenocorticotropin (ACTH) cells, and 2.8% thyroid stimulating hormone cells (TSH [59]).

More recently we bred a Cre-reporter gene into our Cre-LH line to purify gonadotropes by fluorescence activated cell sorting mice [60]. Floxed tdTomato (red fluorescence) was expressed in all pituitary cells. However, in cells bearing Cre-recombinase (Cre-Lhb), the tdTomato was ablated promoting the expression of eGFP (green fluorescence). Thus, all non-gonadotropes (not producing Cre-*Lhb*) fluoresced red and all gonadotropes bearing LH expressed the green eGFP fluorescence. The red and green fractions were then separated by Fluorescence Activated Cell Sorting (FACS).

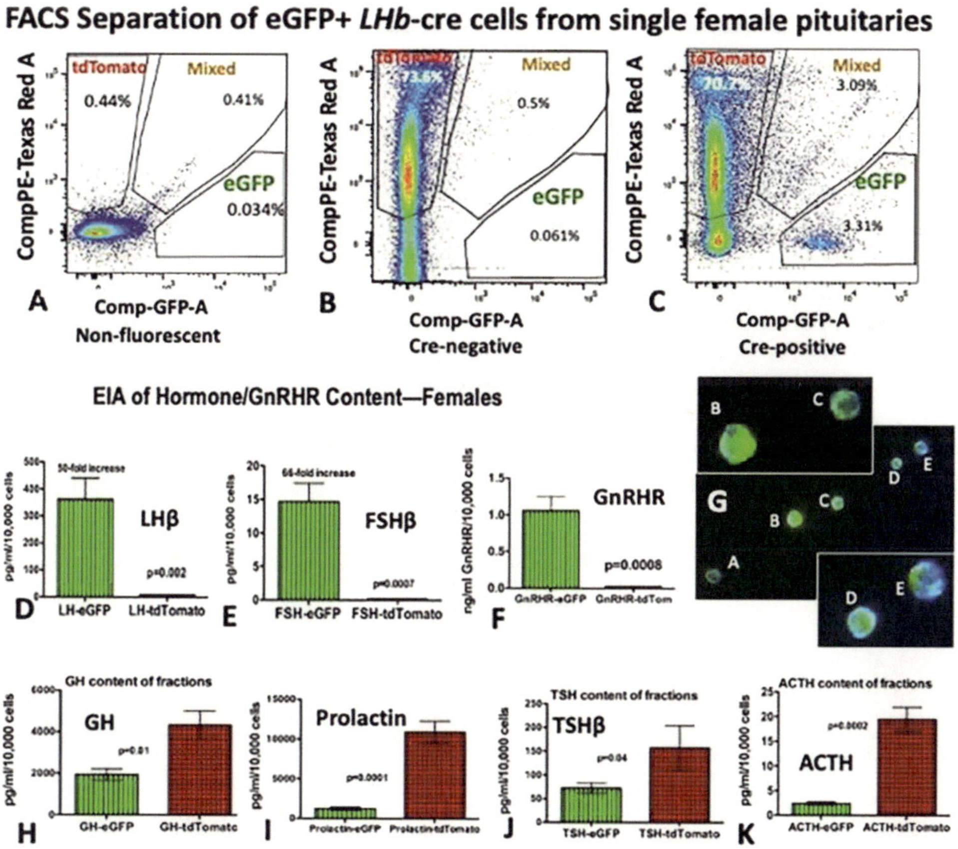

Figure 4.
FACS experiment comparing non-fluorescent cells (4A) with those bearing tdTomato-eGFP, but no Cre-recombinase (4B) and those bearing Cre-recombinase, which ablates the tdTomato, allowing expression of eGFP (4C). Only the profile in 4C shows the presence of eGFP cells. (D–F) show that >90% of LH, FSH, and GnRHR is assayed in the eGFP fraction and barely detectable in the tdTomato fraction. Immunolabeling in (G) shows that >90% of the eGFP cells are labeled for LH (cyan shows blue label over eGFP green). (H–K) detect 70-90% of other pituitary hormones in the tdTomato fraction, but 10-30% of these hormones are found in the pure gonadotrope fraction. These data have never been published elsewhere and are original to this chapter.

The FACS and assay methods are identical to those used for the Cre-GH line, as described by Odle et al. [60].

Figure 4 shows the FACS separation profiles for non-fluorescent pituitary cells (**Figure 4A**); fluorescent Cre-negative populations bearing only tdTomato (**Figure 4B**) and Cre-positive populations, which contain the eGFP cells (**Figure 4C**). Assays for content of gonadotropins and GnRH receptors show that over 95% of the total content is in the eGFP fraction (**Figure 4D–F**). Over 90% of eGFP cells were immunolabeled for LH (**Figure 4G**). However, multihormonal expression is evident as shown in **Figure 4H–K**. The eGFP fraction contains 30% of the GH and TSH content and 10% of the ACTH and prolactin content. In contrast, the non-gonadotrope, tdTomato fraction (red bars) contain over 70% of the content of GH and TSH and 90% of the content of ACTH and prolactin.

When mRNA levels were assayed by qPCR, similar results were seen. **Figure 5A** shows the 72-88% enrichment in gonadotropin and *Gnrhr* mRNAs in the eGFP fractions, with little evidence for expression in the tdTomato fraction. **Figure 5B** shows that 10-20% of the levels of *Gh, Tsh*, and *Pomc* mRNA were also found in the gonadotrope fraction with the remaining tdTomato fraction containing the bulk of these RNAs (80%). It is also interesting to note that *Pou1f1* (also known as *Pit1*) mRNA, a transcription factor important in the production of *Gh, Tshb* and *Prl* is also found in the eGFP-gonadotrope fraction at about the same levels as that of *Gh* and *Tshb*. This expression would be important as Pou1f1 would be available to support the transcription of *Gh, Tsh*, and *Prl.*

FACS fractions from male mice from this line were also analyzed for mRNA content and similar enrichment of gonadotropins and *Gnrhr* mRNA levels was evident as well as similar levels of *Gh*, *Prl* and *Tshb* mRNAs in the eGFP-gonadotrope fractions (data not shown). Also, it is interesting to compare the expression profile of these purified gonadotrope fractions with that of the purified fractions produced in mice bearing Cre-GH. As previously reported, the Cre-GH/eGFP fraction contains most of the GH but very little LH, FSH or ACTH (see Figure 5 in [60]). The pure somatotropes contain significant amounts of Pou1f1, prolactin and TSH proteins and mRNA. Thus, somatotropes also include a multihormonal subset, but the expression profile is different.

More recently, multihormonal pituitary cell populations have been detected by single cell RNA-sequencing, especially in the study by Ho et al. [61], which investigated

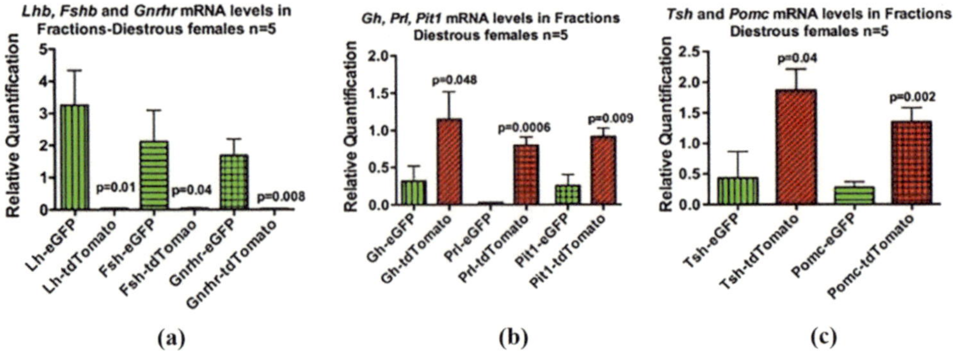

Figure 5.
(A) qPCR assays show enrichment in Lhb, Fshb, and Gnrhr mRNA in eGFP fraction. These data have not been published elsewhere and are original. (B) Shows enrichment of Gh, Prl, and Pit1 mRNA levels in tdTomato fractions, but expression of about 20% of the total in the gonadotrope fraction. (C) Shows Tshb and Pomc mRNA levels and about 20% are in the gonadotrope fraction and 80% in the tdTomato fraction. These data have not been published elsewhere and are original to this chapter.

changes in multihormonal cell transcriptome patterns in mice subjected to different physiological stresses. As we have outlined in a recent review [62], these pools of multihormonal cells may serve to support pituitary plasticity and add to the functions of pituitary populations as physiological needs arise. We hypothesize that these cells may include progenitor cells. Our data showing that gonadotrope LEPR-null mice have deficiencies in other hormones suggest that leptin may regulate multihormonal expression from this group of cells. The fact that secretion of a particular hormone is reduced in animals with LEPR-null gonadotropes highlights the importance of leptin to multihormonal function and suggests a role for leptin in the regulation of pituitary plasticity.

7. Leptin regulation of somatotropes

Somatotropes are vital metabolic sensors because they directly regulate stores of fat as they build muscle, bone, and regulate optimal body composition [63]. Most somatotropes bear leptin receptors [64, 65] and leptin deficiency results in reduced somatotrope functions [4, 20, 66–68]. As stated in the introduction, leptin treatment of leptin deficient *ob/ob* mice restores pituitary GH secretion and *Ghrhr* mRNA levels, but not hypothalamic production or secretion of GHRH [24].

Our studies of leptin's regulation of somatotropes began with the ablation of LEPR exon 17 or exon 1 with Cre-recombinase driven by the rat GH promoter [22, 69]. Both models showed GH deficiency, adult-onset obesity and metabolic dysfunction. At the level of the pituitary, this deficiency was seen as a reduction in GH and GHRHR.

We also reported sex-specific deficiencies during postnatal development with the discovery that leptin may target two transcription factors important in the production of GH, GHRHR, PRL, and TSH. These included Prophet of Pit1 (Prop1) and Pou1f1 [70]. Ablation of LEPR exon 1 in somatotropes reduced Pou1f1 in neonatal females along with serum prolactin. GH stores detected by immunolabeling were also reduced in both neonatal males and females. Interestingly, the lack of LEPR promoted an increase in Prop1 in neonatal males.

The studies of the impact of loss of LEPR were continued on FACS purified somatotropes [60]. Purified somatotropes showed reductions in GH, as expected, however they also contained a subset of multihormonal cells storing TSH and/or prolactin. In somatotrope LEPR-null females, TSH and prolactin stores were reduced in the pure somatotrope fraction [60]. Taken together, our analysis of somatotropes that lack LEPR shows that this multihormonal subset is significantly reduced, suggesting once more that leptin may play a role in maintaining multihormonal expression and promoting pituitary cell plasticity. Finally, these studies also demonstrated that Pou1f1 was reduced in pure somatotropes, which may explain the reduction in any or all hormones dependent on this transcription factor (GH, GHRHR, TSH and prolactin) [60].

We continued the investigation of leptin signaling pathways in somatotropes and reported that they included both transcriptional and posttranscriptional regulators [3]. Our tests of pathway inhibitors showed that full GH expression may be maintained by leptin through the JAK/STAT3 pathway but not nitric oxide. This contrasts with leptin pathways that regulate gonadotropins, which include NOS. Leptin regulation is likely to be transcriptional as loss of LEPR in somatotropes reduced *Gh* and *Ghrhr* mRNA and proteins [3]. In addition, leptin regulation of the *Pou1f1* transcription factor may also serve as a pathway for the transcriptional regulation of *Gh* and *Ghrhr* [2, 3, 60].

However, regulation of POU1F1 by leptin appears to be via post-transcriptional mechanisms as loss of LEPR in somatotropes causes reduction in mRNA levels of the Pou1f1 protein, but not the *Pou1f1* mRNA [2, 60]. Conversely, leptin stimulation results in increased expression of Pou1f1 proteins, but not mRNA [60].

An *in silico* analysis detected eight Musashi binding elements in the 3'UTR of the *Pou1f1* mRNA and tests of Musashi binding showed direct interaction of Musashi with this region and repression of translation, which was reversed by leptin [2]. Furthermore, Musashi immunoprecipitation of whole pituitary extract showed co-association of Musashi and the endogenous *Pou1f1* mRNA. Our analyses of transcripts by scRNA-sequencing studies of normal pituitary cells showed that *Msi1* mRNA was expressed in somatotropes. This was confirmed in pure somatotrope populations [2].

8. Leptin regulation of pituitary musashi

Our studies of animal models in which LEPR was ablated in gonadotropes or somatotropes opened the door to the discovery that leptin may regulate some of its target gene products by post-transcriptional pathways. The post-transcriptional targets included *Gnrhr* mRNA in gonadotropes [1, 7, 8] and the mRNA encoding the POU1F1 transcription factor in somatotropes [2, 60, 70].

The concept that Musashi would be involved in the translational regulation of either *Gnrhr* or *Pou1f*1 mRNA was novel, as both transcripts are important in the function and differentiation of somatotropes and gonadotropes. The expression and involvement of Musashi in differentiated hormone-producing cell lineages was surprising as Musahsi is typically implicated in stem and progenitor cell self-renewal. Nonetheless, while *Msi1* and *Msi2* are expressed in pituitary stem cells as expected, our scRNA sequencing clearly demonstrated that *Msi1* and *Msi2* mRNAs were also expressed in all hormone-producing cell lineages of the anterior pituitary [2].

Since our findings indicated that Musashi was involved in the repression of translation of *Gnrhr* or *Pou1f*1 mRNAs, we hypothesized that normal signals from leptin were needed to reverse this repression [2, 7]. This was based on the fact that the loss of leptin signals resulted in a reduction in the proteins (but not the mRNA). We were able to demonstrate a role for leptin in regulating the actions of Musashi s in reporter assays, where leptin mediated the reversal of Musashi-dependent repression [2].

Our studies also showed that leptin may directly reduce expression of Musashi in its target cells. In pituitaries from proestrous female mice lacking LEPR in gonadotropes, *Msi* mRNA expression is higher. Furthermore, leptin treatment of normal pituitaries from proestrous females resulted in reduced levels of *Msi1* mRNA [8]. More specifically, leptin treatment of normal pituitaries reduced Musashi1 immunolabeling in gonadotropes, identified by their expression of binding to biotinylated GnRH [8].

Similarly, Musashi1 protein and *Msi1* mRNA levels were increased in pure somatotropes lacking LEPR [2]. Furthermore, leptin treatment of pure somatotropes significantly reduced their expression of Musashi1 proteins. Collectively these findings point to a post-transcriptional pathway for leptin, which would reverse repression of translation of key target molecules in somatotropes or gonadotropes by regulating the function and expression of the Musashi family of translational regulatory proteins.

Our *in silico* analyses have identified other potential Musashi targets in the anterior pituitary, which may be regulated by leptin as well. Notably, there are MBEs in the *Fshb, Tshb, Prl* and *Pomc* mRNAs. However, no MBEs are found in *Lhb, Gh, or Ghrhr* mRNAs. It is interesting to speculate that this differential targeting may reflect specific roles for Musashi in regulating differentiated pituitary cells. Musashi could act in multihormonal cells by repressing translation of one set of hormones but not another.

Furthermore, our studies of leptin regulation of Musashi, GnRHR, and Pou1f1 protein levels suggest that leptin may use this Musashi pathway to promote selective differentiation of a given cell type depending on the body's needs.

9. Conclusions

Pituitary gonadotropes and somatotropes were initially shown to be most vulnerable to the global loss in leptin signals as demonstrated by their reduction in numbers in the population, even following acute fasting. As little as 10-100 pg./ml leptin directly restored hormone levels in these populations, so they could once more be detected by immunolabeling. We now have much more information about the impact of loss of leptin signaling to model animals including infertility when they carried LEPR-null gonadotropes and adult-onset obesity and GH deficiency when they carried LEPR-null somatotropes. We have identified specific leptin targets in each of these cell types and determined that leptin regulation may involve both transcriptional and post-transcriptional pathways. The target molecules are vital to the differentiated function of these cells, which highlights a role for leptin in maintaining their differentiated state. Regarding post-transcriptional pathways, we have shown that leptin also regulates expression of the translational regulatory protein, Musashi. Our studies have led to the discovery of novel roles for Musashi, implicating this regulator in the repression of targets in specific pituitary cell types. This broadens the scope of Musashi's regulatory role beyond that of regulation of stem cells. Finally, our studies of purified somatotropes and gonadotropes have confirmed the presence of multihormonal expression in a subpopulation of cells and have led to the discovery that leptin signaling is needed to maintain this subset. The presence of these multihormonal pituitary cells is also evident in single cell RNA-sequencing studies. Future studies are needed that focus on the role leptin plays in maintaining this cell population, which supports pituitary plasticity. Future investigation will elucidate the role Musashi may play in the selective regulation of specific hormones or their transcription factors.

Acknowledgements

The authors are grateful for the outstanding technical assistance of Anessa Haney, Linda Hardy, and Alex Lagasse. The authors acknowledge funding from the following sources; National Institute of Health (NIH) R01 HD059056 (GVC); NIH R01 HD-087057 (GVC, AMM); NIH R01 HD-093461 (AMM, GVC, and MCM); NIH R01 DK113776 (GVC, AMM, and MCM); and NIH R01 DK 127723 (GVC, AMM, and MCM). We also acknowledge pilot studies grants from the Sturgis Foundation (AMM, GVC) and Development Enhancement Awards (GVC, AO) from UAMS. We also acknowledge support for core facilities from Center grants- NIGMS P20 GM103425 and P30 GM11070 (Dr. Edgar Garcia-Rill PI).

Conflict of interest

The authors declare no conflict of interest.

Author details

Gwen V. Childs*, Angela K. Odle, Melanie C. MacNicol,
Melody L. Allensworth-James, Tiffany K. Miles, Noor Akhter, Mohsin M. Syed
and Angus M. MacNicol
Department of Neurobiology and Developmental Sciences, College of Medicine,
University of Arkansas for Medical Sciences, Little Rock, AR, USA

*Address all correspondence to: childsgwenv@uams.edu

References

[1] Akhter N, CarlLee T, Syed MM, Odle AK, Cozart MA, Haney AC, et al. Selective deletion of leptin receptors in gonadotropes reveals activin and GnRH-binding sites as leptin targets in support of fertility. Endocrinology. 2014;**155**(10):4027-4042. DOI: 10.1210/en.2014-1132

[2] Allensworth-James M, Banik J, Odle A, Hardy L, Lagasse A, Moreira ARS, et al. Control of the Anterior Pituitary Cell Lineage Regulator POU1F1 by the Stem Cell Determinant Musashi. Endocrinology. 2021;**162**(3). DOI: 10.1210/endocr/bqaa245

[3] Allensworth-James ML, Odle AK, Lim J, LaGasse AN, Miles TK, Hardy LL, et al. Metabolic signalling to somatotrophs: Transcriptional and post-transcriptional mediators. J Neuroendocrinol. 2020;**32**(11):e12883. DOI: 10.1111/jne.12883

[4] Carro E, Pinilla L, Seoane LM, Considine RV, Aguilar E, Casanueva FF, et al. Influence of endogenous leptin tone on the estrous cycle and luteinizing hormone pulsatility in female rats. Neuroendocrinology. 1997;**66**(6): 375-377. DOI: 10.1159/000127262

[5] Childs GV, Odle AK, MacNicol MC, MacNicol AM. The Importance of Leptin to Reproduction. Endocrinology. 2021;**162**(2). DOI: 10.1210/endocr/bqaa204

[6] Lloyd RV, Jin L, Tsumanuma I, Vidal S, Kovacs K, Horvath E, et al. Leptin and leptin receptor in anterior pituitary function. Pituitary. 2001;**4**(1-2): 33-47. DOI: 10.1023/a:1012982626401

[7] Odle AK, Akhter N, Syed MM, Allensworth-James ML, Benes H, Melgar Castillo AI, et al. Leptin Regulation of Gonadotrope Gonadotropin-Releasing Hormone Receptors As a Metabolic Checkpoint and Gateway to Reproductive Competence. Front Endocrinol (Lausanne). 2017;**8**:367. DOI: 10.3389/fendo.2017.00367

[8] Odle AK, Benes H, Melgar Castillo A, Akhter N, Syed M, Haney A, et al. Association of Gnrhr mRNA With the Stem Cell Determinant Musashi: A Mechanism for Leptin-Mediated Modulation of GnRHR Expression. Endocrinology. 2018;**159**(2):883-894. DOI: 10.1210/en.2017-00586

[9] Odle AK, MacNicol MC, Childs GV, MacNicol AM. Post-Transcriptional Regulation of Gnrhr: A Checkpoint for Metabolic Control of Female Reproduction. International Journal of Molecular Sciences. 2021;**22**(7):3312. DOI: 10.3390/ijms22073312

[10] Yu WH, Kimura M, Walczewska A, Karanth S, McCann SM. Role of leptin in hypothalamic-pituitary function. Proc Natl Acad Sci USA. 1997;**94**(3): 1023-1028. DOI: 10.1073/pnas.94.3.1023

[11] Yu WH, Walczewska A, Karanth S, McCann SM. Nitric oxide mediates leptin-induced luteinizing hormone-releasing hormone (LHRH) and LHRH and leptin-induced LH release from the pituitary gland. Endocrinology. 1997;**138**(11):5055-5058. DOI: 10.1210/endo.138.11.5649

[12] Veldhuis JD, Roemmich JN, Richmond EJ, Bowers CY. Somatotropic and gonadotropic axes linkages in infancy, childhood, and the puberty-adult transition. Endocr Rev. 2006;**27**(2):101-140. DOI: 10.1210/er.2005-0006

[13] Veldhuis JD, Roemmich JN, Richmond EJ, Rogol AD, Lovejoy JC, Sheffield-Moore M, et al. Endocrine control of body composition in infancy, childhood, and puberty. Endocr Rev. 2005;**26**(1):114-146. DOI: 10.1210/er.2003-0038

[14] Childs GV. Gonadotropes and Lactotropes. In Physiology of Reproduction; J Neill and E Knobil, Eds, Elsevier Press, NY. 2006:1483-579

[15] Casanueva FF, Dieguez C. Neuroendocrine regulation and actions of leptin. Frontiers in Neuro endocrinology. 1999;**20**(4):317-363. DOI: 10.1006/frne.1999.0187

[16] Chan JL, Mantzoros CS. Leptin and the hypothalamic-pituitary regulation of the gonadotropin-gonadal axis. Pituitary. 2001;**4**(1-2):87-92. DOI: 10.1023/a:1012947113197

[17] Montague CT, Farooqi IS, Whitehead JP, Soos MA, Rau H, Wareham NJ, et al. Congenital leptin deficiency is associated with severe early-onset obesity in humans. Nature. 1997;**387**(6636):903-908. DOI: 10.1038/43185

[18] Welt CK. Will leptin become the treatment of choice for functional hypothalamic amenorrhea? Nat Clin Pract Endocrinol Metab. 2007;**3**(8): 556-557. DOI: 10.1038/ncpendmet0561

[19] Welt CK, Chan JL, Bullen J, Murphy R, Smith P, DePaoli AM, et al. Recombinant human leptin in women with hypothalamic amenorrhea. N Engl J Med. 2004;**351**(10):987-997. DOI: 10.1056/NEJMoa040388

[20] Isozaki O, Tsushima T, Miyakawa M, Demura H, Seki H. Interaction between leptin and growth hormone (GH)/IGF-I axis. Endocr J. 1999;**46** Suppl:S17-S24. DOI: 10.1507/endocrj.46.suppl_s17

[21] Popovic V, Damjanovic S, Dieguez C, Casanueva FF. Leptin and the pituitary. Pituitary. 2001;**4**(1-2):7-14. DOI: 10.1023/a:1012938308654

[22] Childs GV, Akhter N, Haney A, Syed M, Odle A, Cozart M, et al. The somatotrope as a metabolic sensor: deletion of leptin receptors causes obesity. Endocrinology. 2011;**152**(1): 69-81. DOI: 10.1210/en.2010-0498

[23] Crane C, Akhter N, Johnson BW, Iruthayanathan M, Syed F, Kudo A, et al. Fasting and glucose effects on pituitary leptin expression: is leptin a local signal for nutrient status? J Histochem Cytochem. 2007;**55**(10):1059-1074. DOI:10.1369/jhc.7A7214.2007

[24] Luque RM, Huang ZH, Shah B, Mazzone T, Kineman RD. Effects of leptin replacement on hypothalamic-pituitary growth hormone axis function and circulating ghrelin levels in ob/ob mice. Am J Physiol Endocrinol Metab. 2007;**292**(3):E891-E899. DOI: 10.1152/ajpendo.00258.2006

[25] Sarmento-Cabral A, Peinado JR, Halliday LC, Malagon MM, Castano JP, Kineman RD, et al. Adipokines (Leptin, Adiponectin, Resistin) Differentially Regulate All Hormonal Cell Types in Primary Anterior Pituitary Cell Cultures from Two Primate Species. Sci Rep. 2017;**7**:43537. DOI: 10.1038/srep43537

[26] Vazquez-Borrego MC, Gahete MD, Martinez-Fuentes AJ, Fuentes-Fayos AC, Castano JP, Kineman RD, et al. Multiple signaling pathways convey central and peripheral signals to regulate pituitary function: Lessons from human and non-human primate models. Mol Cell Endocrinol. 2018;**463**:4-22. DOI: 10.1016/j.mce.2017.12.007

[27] Caprio M, Fabbrini E, Isidori AM, Aversa A, Fabbri A. Leptin in

reproduction. Trends Endocrinol Metab. 2001;**12**(2):65-72. DOI: 10.1016/s1043-2760(00)00352-0

[28] De Biasi SN, Apfelbaum LI, Apfelbaum ME. In vitro effect of leptin on LH release by anterior pituitary glands from female rats at the time of spontaneous and steroid-induced LH surge. Eur J Endocrinol. 2001;**145**(5): 659-665. DOI: 10.1530/eje.0.1450659

[29] Jin L, Burguera BG, Couce ME, Scheithauer BW, Lamsan J, Eberhardt NL, et al. Leptin and leptin receptor expression in normal and neoplastic human pituitary: evidence of a regulatory role for leptin on pituitary cell proliferation. J Clin Endocrinol Metab. 1999;**84**(8):2903-2911. DOI: 10.1210/jcem.84.8.5908

[30] Jin L, Zhang S, Burguera BG, Couce ME, Osamura RY, Kulig E, et al. Leptin and leptin receptor expression in rat and mouse pituitary cells. Endocrinology. 2000;**141**(1):333-339. DOI: 10.1210/endo.141.1.7260

[31] Ogura K, Irahara M, Kiyokawa M, Tezuka M, Matsuzaki T, Yasui T, et al. Effects of leptin on secretion of LH and FSH from primary cultured female rat pituitary cells. Eur J Endocrinol. 2001;**144**(6):653-658. DOI: 10.1530/eje.0.1440653

[32] Schneider JE, Blum RM, Wade GN. Metabolic control of food intake and estrous cycles in syrian hamsters. I. Plasma insulin and leptin. Am J Physiol Regul Integr Comp Physiol. 2000; 278(2):R476-R485. DOI: 10.1152/ajpregu.2000.278.2.R476

[33] Schneider JE, Buckley CA, Blum RM, Zhou D, Szymanski L, Day DE, et al. Metabolic signals, hormones and neuropeptides involved in control of energy balance and reproductive success in hamsters. Eur J Neurosci. 2002;**16**(3):377-379. DOI: 10.1046/j.1460-9568.2002.02118.x

[34] Schneider JE, Wade GN. Availability of metabolic fuels controls estrous cyclicity of Syrian hamsters. Science. 1989;**244**(4910):1326-1328. DOI: 10.1126/science.2734610

[35] Schneider JE, Zhou D. Interactive effects of central leptin and peripheral fuel oxidation on estrous cyclicity. Am J Physiol. 1999;**277**(4 Pt 2):R1020-R1024. DOI: 10.1152/ajpregu.1999.277.4.R1020

[36] Schoeller DA, Cella LK, Sinha MK, Caro JF. Entrainment of the diurnal rhythm of plasma leptin to meal timing. J Clin Invest. 1997;**100**(7):1882-7. DOI: 10.1172/JCI119717 [doi]

[37] Licinio J, Negrao AB, Mantzoros C, Kaklamani V, Wong ML, Bongiorno PB, et al. Synchronicity of frequently sampled, 24-h concentrations of circulating leptin, luteinizing hormone, and estradiol in healthy women. Proc Natl Acad Sci USA. 1998;**95**(5):2541-2546. DOI: 10.1073/pnas.95.5.2541

[38] Luukkaa V, Pesonen U, Huhtaniemi I, Lehtonen A, Tilvis R, Tuomilehto J, et al. Inverse correlation between serum testosterone and leptin in men. J Clin Endocrinol Metab. 1998;**83**(9):3243-3246. DOI: 10.1210/jcem.83.9.5134

[39] Riad-Gabriel MG, Jinagouda SD, Sharma A, Boyadjian R, Saad MF. Changes in plasma leptin during the menstrual cycle. Eur J Endocrinol. 1998;**139**(5):528-531. DOI: 10.1038/srep43537

[40] Wabitsch M, Blum WF, Muche R, Braun M, Hube F, Rascher W, et al. Contribution of androgens to the gender difference in leptin production in obese

children and adolescents. J Clin Invest. 1997;**100**(4):808-813. DOI: 10.1172/JCI119595

[41] Wauters M, Considine RV, Van Gaal LF. Human leptin: from an adipocyte hormone to an endocrine mediator. Eur J Endocrinol. 2000;**143**(3):293-311. DOI: 10.1530/eje.0.1430293

[42] Wen S, Ai W, Alim Z, Boehm U. Embryonic gonadotropin-releasing hormone signaling is necessary for maturation of the male reproductive axis. Proc Natl Acad Sci U S A. 2010; **107**(37):16372-16377. DOI: 10.1073/pnas.1000423107

[43] Bjelobaba I, Janjic MM, Kucka M, Stojilkovic SS. Cell Type-Specific Sexual Dimorphism in Rat Pituitary Gene Expression During Maturation. Biol Reprod. 2015;**93**(1):21. DOI: 10.1095/biolreprod.115.129320

[44] Dohler KD, Wuttke W. Changes with age in levels of serum gonadotropins, prolactin and gonadal steroids in prepubertal male and female rats. Endocrinology. 1975;**97**(4):898-907. DOI: 10.1210/endo-97-4-898

[45] Wilson ME, Handa RJ. Ontogeny of gene expression in the gonadotroph of the developing female rat. Biol Reprod. 1997;**56**(2):563-568. DOI: 10.1095/biolreprod56.2.563

[46] Wilson ME, Handa RJ. Activin subunit, follistatin, and activin receptor gene expression in the prepubertal female rat pituitary. Biol Reprod. 1998;**59**(2):278-283. DOI: 10.1095/biolreprod59.2.278

[47] Leonhardt M, Lesage J, Croix D, Dutriez-Casteloot I, Beauvillain JC, Dupouy JP. Effects of perinatal maternal food restriction on pituitary-gonadal axis and plasma leptin level in rat pup at birth and weaning and on timing of puberty. Biol Reprod. 2003;**68**(2):390-400. DOI: 10.1095/biolreprod.102.003269

[48] Attig L, Larcher T, Gertler A, Abdennebi-Najar L, Djiane J. Postnatal leptin is necessary for maturation of numerous organs in newborn rats. Organogenesis. 2011;**7**(2):88-94. DOI: 10.4161/org.7.2.14871

[49] Allen SJ, Garcia-Galiano D, Borges BC, Burger LL, Boehm U, Elias CF. Leptin receptor null mice with reexpression of LepR in GnRHR expressing cells display elevated FSH levels but remain in a prepubertal state. American journal of physiology Regulatory, integrative and comparative physiology. 2016;**310**(11):R1258-R1266. DOI: 10.1152/ajpregu.00529.2015

[50] Gregory SJ, Kaiser UB. Regulation of gonadotropins by inhibin and activin. Seminars in reproductive medicine. 2004;**22**(3):253-267. DOI: 10.1055/s-2004-831901

[51] Pernasetti F, Vasilyev VV, Rosenberg SB, Bailey JS, Huang HJ, Miller WL, et al. Cell-specific transcriptional regulation of follicle-stimulating hormone-beta by activin and gonadotropin-releasing hormone in the LbetaT2 pituitary gonadotrope cell model. Endocrinology. 2001;**142**(6): 2284-2295. DOI: 10.1210/endo.142.6.8185

[52] Fox RG, Park FD, Koechlein CS, Kritzik M, Reya T. Musashi signaling in stem cells and cancer. Annu Rev Cell Dev Biol. 2015;**31**:249-267. DOI: 10.1146/annurev-cellbio-100814-125446

[53] MacNicol MC, Cragle CE, MacNicol AM. Context-dependent regulation of Musashi-mediated mRNA translation and cell cycle regulation. Cell

Cycle. 2011;**10**(1):39-44. DOI: 10.4161/cc.10.1.14388

[54] Childs GV, Ellison DG, Ramaley JA. Storage of Anterior Lobe Adrenocorticotropin in Corticotropes and a Sub-population of Gonadotropes During the Stress-Nonresponsive Period in the Neonatal Male Rat. Endocrinology. 1982;**110**(5):1676-1692

[55] Moriarty GC, Garner LL. Immunocytochemical studies of cells in the rat adenohypophysis containing both ACTH and FSH. Nature. 1977;**265**(5592): 356-358. DOI: 10.1038/265356a0

[56] Childs GV. Multipotential Pituitary Cells that Contain Adrenocorticotropin (ACTH) and Other Pituitary Hormones. Trends in Endocrinology and Metabolism. 1991;**2**(3):112-117. DOI: 10.1016/s1043-2760(05)80007-4

[57] Childs GV. Growth hormone cells as co-gonadotropes: partners in the regulation of the reproductive system. Trends Endocrinol Metab. 2000;**11**(5):168-175. DOI: 10.1016/s1043-2760(00)00252-6

[58] Childs GV, Unabia G, Rougeau D. Cells that express luteinizing hormone (LH) and follicle-stimulating hormone (FSH) beta-subunit messenger ribonucleic acids during the estrous cycle: the major contributors contain LH beta, FSH beta, and/or growth hormone. Endocrinology. 1994;**134**(2):990-997. DOI: 10.1210/endo.134.2.8299592

[59] Childs GV, Unabia G. Epidermal growth factor and gonadotropin-releasing hormone stimulate proliferation of enriched population of gonadotropes. Endocrinology. 2001;**142**(2):847-853. DOI: 10.1210/endo.142.2.7953

[60] Odle A, Allensworth-James M, Akhter N, Syed M, Haney A, MacNicol M, et al. A Sex-Dependent Tropic Role for Leptin In The Somatotrope As A Regulator of POU1F1 and POU1F1-dependent Hormones. Endocrinology. 2016;**157**(10):3958-3971. DOI: 10.1210/en.2016-1472

[61] Ho Y, Hu P, Peel MT, Chen S, Camara PG, Epstein DJ, et al. Single-cell transcriptomic analysis of adult mouse pituitary reveals sexual dimorphism and physiologic demand-induced cellular plasticity. Protein Cell. 2020. DOI: 10.1007/s13238-020-00705-x

[62] Childs GV, MacNicol AM, MacNicol MC. Molecular Mechanisms of Pituitary Cell Plasticity. Front Endocrinol (Lausanne). 2020;**11**:656. DOI: 10.3389/fendo.2020.00656

[63] Buzi F, Bontempelli AM, Alberti D, Jones J, Pilotta A, Lombardi A, et al. Growth, insulin-like growth factor I (IGF-I), and IGF-binding proteins 1 and 3 in children with severe liver disease before and after liver transplantation: a longitudinal and cross-sectional study. Pediatr Res. 1998;**43**(4 Pt 1):478-483. DOI: 10.1203/00006450-19980 4000-00007

[64] Sone M, Osamura RY. Leptin and the pituitary. Pituitary. 2001;**4**(1-2):15-23. DOI: 10.1023/a:1012978525492

[65] Sone M, Nagata H, Takekoshi S, Osamura RY. Expression and localization of leptin receptor in the normal rat pituitary gland. Cell Tissue Res. 2001;**305**(3):351-356. DOI: 10.1007/s004410100407

[66] Ghilardi N, Ziegler S, Wiestner A, Stoffel R, Heim MH, Skoda RC. Defective STAT signaling by the leptin receptor in diabetic mice. Proc Natl Acad Sci USA. 1996;**93**(13):6231-6235. DOI: 10.1073/pnas.93.13.6231

[67] Carro E, Seoane LM, Senaris R, Casanueva FF, Dieguez C. Leptin

increases in vivo GH responses to GHRH and GH-releasing peptide-6 in food-deprived rats. Eur J Endocrinol. 2000;**142**(1):66-70. DOI: 10.1530/eje.0.1420066

[68] Asada N, Takahashi Y, Honjo M. Effects of 22K or 20K human growth hormone on lipolysis, leptin production in adipocytes in the presence and absence of human growth hormone binding protein. Horm Res. 2000;**54**(4):203-207. DOI: 10.1159/000053260

[69] Allensworth-James M, Odle AK, Haney A, Childs GV. Sex Differences in Somatotrope Dependency on Leptin Receptors in Young Mice: Ablation of LEPR Causes Severe Growth Hormone Deficiency and Abdominal Obesity in Males. Endocrinology. 2015;**156**(9):3253-3264. DOI: 10.1210/EN.2015-1198

[70] Allensworth-James ML, Odle A, Haney A, MacNicol M, MacNicol A, Childs G. Sex-specific changes in postnatal GH and PRL secretion in somatotrope LEPR-null mice. J Endocrinol. 2018;**238**(3):221-230. DOI: 10.1530/JOE-18-0238

Chapter 3

Leptin and Female Reproductive Health

Shyam Pyari Jaiswar and Apala Priyadarshini

Abstract

Leptin is a peptide hormone, secreted primarily by the adipose tissue, placenta being the second leptin-producing tissue in humans. Apart from playing an integral role in food intake regulation and energy balance, leptin is an important signalling molecule affecting human reproduction. Accumulated evidence suggests that leptin has potential roles in the regulation of GnRH and LH secretion, puberty, pregnancy, and lactation. Deregulation of leptin levels has been associated with several reproductive disorders including infertility, recurrent pregnancy loss, and polycystic ovary syndrome. This chapter illustrates the importance of leptin in female reproductive health, its role in the metabolic regulation of reproductive axis and its eventual pathophysiological implications in prevalent reproductive disorders.

Keywords: leptin, pregnancy, reproduction

1. Introduction

Human reproduction is an energy demanding process which requires the complex interaction of biological molecules and neuroendocrine pathways primarily revolving around the hypothalamic–pituitary–ovarian (HPO) axis [1, 2]. The size of body fat and energy stores and the metabolic state of the individual are two of the key elements which determine the appropriate functioning of human reproduction, including the onset of puberty [1, 3].

In a severely undernourished state, the energy stores of the body are deviated to support the indispensable functions for survival, hence compromising the reproductive ability [4, 5].

It has long been observed that the extreme situations of body fat metabolism, that is, obesity and cachexia are both associated with derangement of female reproductive function including infertility, recurrent pregnancy loss (RPL) and polycystic ovary syndrome (PCOS) [1].

The presumptions on the existence of a missing link between the energy homeostasis of the body and female reproductive health culminated in the year 1994, with the discovery of leptin, an adipose tissue derived hormone that maintains the homeostatic control of the body fat stores [1, 6, 7]. Leptin has now been recognised to control and influence the functioning of the HPO axis also exerting a negative feedback effect on the hypothalamus.

2. Leptin: Structure and function

Leptin (derivative of Greek word "leptos" which means thin) is an adipose tissue derived hormone. It a known biomarker of adiposity, its levels rising proportionately with body fat stores [3, 8].

Leptin comprises a 167 amino acid polypeptide chain. This 16 kDa protein is encoded by the obesity gene (Lep^{ob} gene) situated on chromosome 7 [2, 8].

The preliminary function of leptin was recognised to control energy homeostasis via a negative feedback mechanism to the brain, to reduce the intake of food when the body fat stores were sufficient [3, 9].

However, recent literature elucidates that leptin can control and regulate the functioning of HPO axis, has a putative role as a placental hormone and can directly affect the reproductive function of gonads.

In this chapter, the role of leptin in female reproductive health will be illustrated under the following sections:

a. Leptin in normal pregnancy

b. Leptin in pathological pregnancy:

  i. Pre-eclampsia (PE)

  ii. Gestational diabetes mellitus (GDM)

  iii. Fetal growth restriction (FGR)

c. Leptin in puberty and infertility

d. Leptin in menstruation

e. Leptin in PCOS

f. Leptin in recurrent pregnancy loss (RPL).

3. Leptin in normal pregnancy

3.1 Source of leptin in pregnancy

Placenta is the other leptin producing tissue in humans apart from adipose tissue and compelling evidence suggests that both leptin hormone and leptin receptors are expressed in human placenta [1, 8–10]. Leptin is produced by the syncytiotrophoblast cells of the placenta (contribute 95% of total placental leptin) and the vascular endothelial cells on the fetal side (5%) [8, 11, 12]. The amniocytes of the amniotic membrane and the maternal decidua also release leptin into the amniotic fluid [13].

Even though pregnancy is a state of enhanced fat stores, the major proportion of leptin in maternal circulation is contributed by the placenta [1, 11]. Leptin has both endocrine and autocrine actions in the placenta and placental leptin is similar to its adipose tissue derived counterpart in terms of structure and function [10, 11, 14].

Increased blood levels of leptin (by two folds) have been demonstrated in pregnant as compared to non-pregnant women [8]. Presence of leptin has been observed in placenta from 7 weeks of gestation onwards. Leptin levels increase by 30% at as early as 12 weeks of gestation, plateau at mid pregnancy and return to pre-pregnant levels 24 hours after delivery [8, 11]. The clarification for increased leptin concentration during pregnancy is the release of plasma soluble leptin receptors by the placenta which bind the circulating leptin, hence delaying its clearance [1, 11].

3.2 Functions of leptin in pregnancy

3.2.1 In mother

Pregnancy is an anabolic state where adequate energy stores are required to cater to the nutritional demands of the growing fetus. However, pregnancy is a state of leptin resistance and the role of leptin in pregnancy deviates considerably from its classical role of controlling food intake [15, 16].

The functions can be elaborated as follows (**Figure 1**) [8, 17]:

1. Plays an integral role in implantation and formation of blastocyst.

2. Activation of enzymes for lipid oxidation to generate growth substrates in the form of free fatty acids for growing fetus.

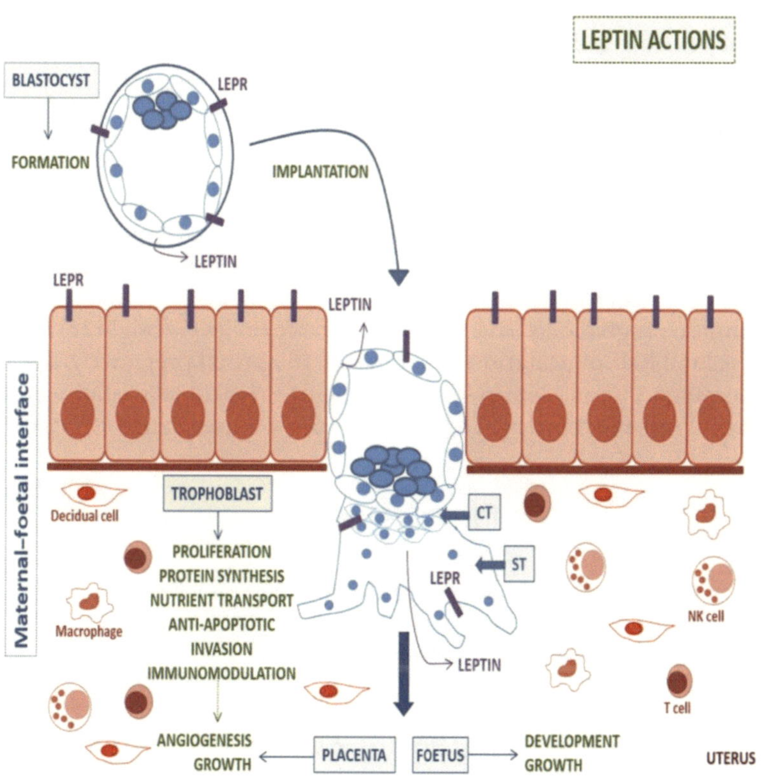

Figure 1.
Actions of leptin seen at maternal-fetal interface. ST, syncytiotrophoblast; CT, cytotrophoblast [17].

3. Placental transfer of these substrates to meet the energy demands of the fetus including amino acid uptake by the fetus.

4. Placental leptin has a paracrine action in the placenta itself. It contributes to placental angiogenesis, induces placental growth and stimulates the trophoblasts to produce hCG.

5. As an immunomodulator, it suppresses maternal immune mediated rejection of the developing fetus [17].

3.2.2 In fetus

Fetal leptin is predominantly fetal in origin and is present in fetal blood from 18 weeks of gestation [8, 18]. Maternal leptin does not cross the placenta to affect fetal functions due to its high molecular weight [19].

However, the umbilical cord blood leptin concentrations correlate strongly with fetal fat mass serving as a good indicator for the same [8, 10, 11, 20]. Fetal leptin levels increase as gestational age increases [21]. Female foetuses have higher serum leptin levels than their male counterparts due to the suppression of leptin by testosterone in males [22].

Leptin receptors have been reported to be expressed in fetal tissues, for example, bone, kidney, and hypothalamus and fetal leptin supports fetal endocrine functions, for example, angiogenesis and erythropoiesis.

4. Leptin in pathological pregnancy

4.1 Leptin and pre-eclampsia (PE)

Pre-eclampsia is a multisystem disorder of unknown aetiology characterised by hypertension ≥140/90 mm Hg after 20 weeks of gestation with proteinuria. Pre-eclampsia complicates around 5% of all pregnancies. The pathophysiology involves defective trophoblastic invasion of maternal spiral arteries leading to reduced placental blood flow and hence hypoxia [23].

Pre-eclamptic pregnancies have higher serum leptin levels (eight folds) specifically in the second half of gestation as compared to normal pregnancy. In PE, plateau of leptin does not occur and leptin levels continue to rise till term, falling only after delivery. The increase in the serum leptin levels are a consequence of placental

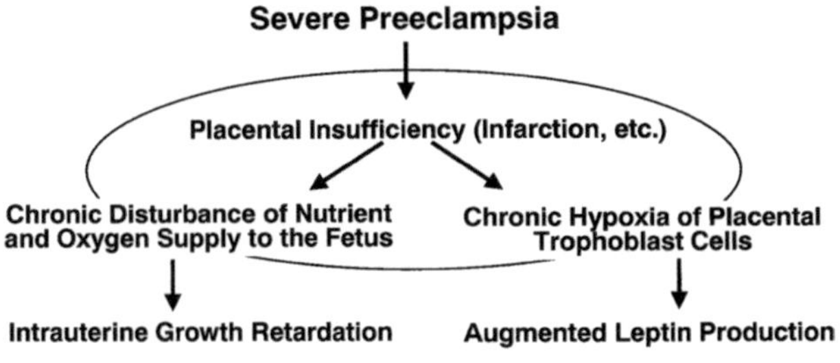

Figure 2.
Schematic diagram representing hyperleptinemia as a consequence of chronic placental hypoxia induced by severe pre-eclampsia [9].

hypoxia induced stress (**Figure 2**). This rise in leptin levels precedes the clinical onset of disease hence can also be considered as a potential predictive marker of PE. Apart from serum, amniotic fluid also shows a higher concentration of leptin than normotensive pregnancies. Leptin being an angiogenic hormone promotes placental vasculogenesis and trans placental nutrient transfer compensating for the placental insufficiency to some extent [8, 11, 17, 24].

The serum leptin levels rise in linear proportion with the severity of the disease [8, 9]. Studies have also suggested that leptin concentrations are higher in term PE as compared to preterm PE [17].

However the cord blood leptin levels are lower which denote a reduced fetal fat mass often associated with PE [11]. Pre eclamptic pregnancies complicated with FGR have higher maternal leptin levels than those without FGR suggesting a greater degree of placental insufficiency [8].

The data available is conflicting and the modulation of leptin in relation to pre-eclampsia is a fertile ground for further studies.

4.2 Leptin and fetal growth restriction (FGR)

Fetal growth restriction may be defined as the failure of the fetus to reach its genetically determined growth potential. FGR complicates 5–10% of all pregnancies and is associated with significant perinatal morbidity and mortality [25].

Studies linking the role of leptin in FGR have yielded conflicting results. A recent meta-analysis involving 1734 women showed no difference in the leptin levels between maternal blood of FGR pregnancies and healthy pregnant women [26].

However evidence suggests that the maternal serum leptin levels are higher in pregnancies complicated with FGR and fetal cord blood levels are lower compared with normal pregnancies. The higher maternal levels are a consequence of increased placental production of leptin triggered by placental insufficiency and hypoxia [27]. The lower cord blood levels reflect a lower fetal fat mass seen in FGR and also suggest a plausible role of leptin as a growth factor [28].

4.3 Leptin and gestational diabetes mellitus

Gestational diabetes mellitus (GDM) is one of the most common metabolic complications occurring during pregnancy with a high risk of maternal and perinatal morbidity, also leading to long term sequelae [29]. It may be defined as glucose intolerance of variable severity with its onset or first recognition during pregnancy [30]. Prevalence of GDM is higher in obese women as compared to women with a normal pre-pregnancy BMI [12].

GDM is associated with increased levels of leptin in the placenta and increased expression of placental leptin receptors. The rise in serum leptin levels has been noted in the first trimester of pregnancy itself, illustrating its possible role as a predictive marker for GDM (4.7 fold greater risk of developing GDM). Not only in serum, higher leptin levels have also been measured in the amniotic fluid of women with GDM, each 1 ng/dl rise in amniotic fluid leptin increasing the risk of developing GDM by 4% [31].

It has been observed the higher umbilical cord leptin levels were present in macrosomic foetuses of diabetic mothers correlating with the increased fetal fat mass. Leptin may also contribute to the increased placental size seen in GDM. Moreover, leptin also stimulates placental protein synthesis and transfer of nutrients to the fetus

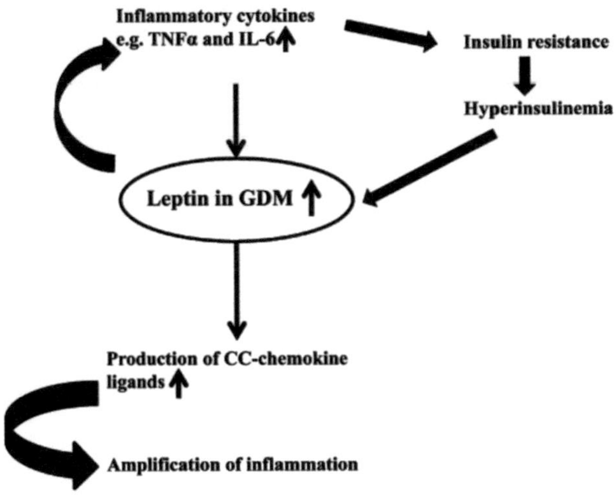

Figure 3.
Association of increased leptin production with chronic inflammatory state, insulin resistance and hyperinsulinemia seen in GDM. TNF-α, tumour necrosis factor alpha; IL-6, interleukin-6 [30].

as can be speculated by increased expression of glycerol transporter aquaporin-9 in the placentae of women with GDM [32].

The enhanced placental production of leptin has also been correlated with a higher production of inflammatory cytokines interleukin-6 and tumour necrosis factor-alpha and therefore linked with the chronic inflammatory state seen in GDM. IL-6 and TNF-α enhance the placental expression of leptin. Leptin in turn stimulates the monocytes for enhanced production of IL-6 and TNF-α resulting in a vicious cycle [11, 17, 30, 33].

The production of leptin is stimulated by hyperinsulinemia seen in GDM. Therefore, increased leptin levels are also associated with the increased insulin resistance seen in GDM during the second half of pregnancy (**Figure 3**) [33].

Studies evaluating novel bioactive therapeutic agents comprising macro and micronutrients which exert anti-inflammatory actions may be a potential cure for inflammation induced leptin resistance at the level of the hypothalamus seen in GDM. This will lead to improved leptin sensitivity at the centre and decreased insulin resistance at the peripheral level [32].

5. Leptin in puberty and infertility

Robust data reveal that obesity is associated with precocious puberty and cachexic women often experience delayed puberty [34]. The association of obesity with puberty as well as infertility led the researchers to investigate the mediator and connecting factor linking obesity with reproduction.

Rat models with deficiency of leptin or leptin receptors failed to attain puberty, elaborating the significance of leptin for reproductive function. The serum levels of leptin rise continuously throughout the entire period of pubertal development. Leptin regulates female pubertal development more closely as compared to males where minimal leptin levels are sufficient to sustain reproductive function [1].

The actions of leptin on various levels of the HPO axis are detailed (**Figure 4**):

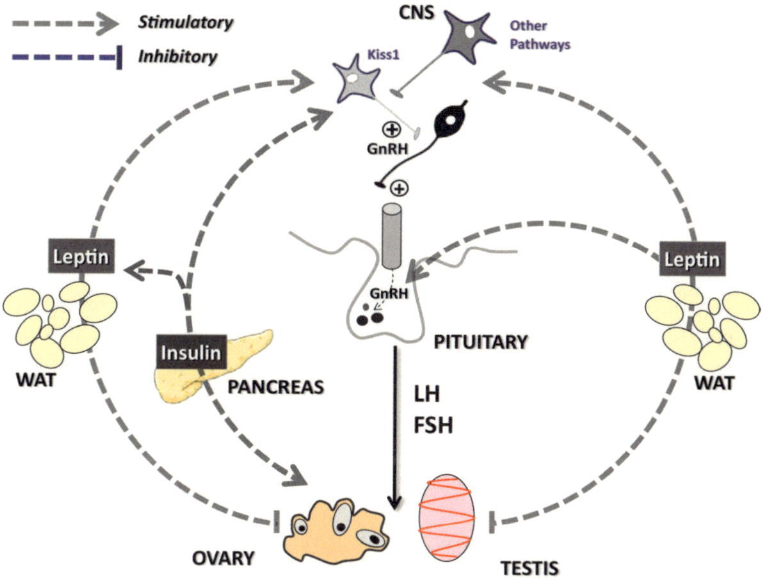

Figure 4.
Figure representing the actions of leptin on the hypothalamic–pituitary–gonadal axis. Both stimulatory and inhibitory effects are depicted. GnRH, gonadotropin releasing hormone; LH, luteinising hormone; FSH, follicle stimulating hormone; WAT, white adipose tissue [1].

5.1 Effects on the central nervous system

The primary site where leptin acts to control the reproductive function is the hypothalamus. Leptin receptors are present on the GnRH producing cells in the hypothalamus [1]. Leptin through its central action on the hypothalamus stimulates the production of GnRH and therefore may be a crucial determinant of the integrity of the HPO axis [35]. In mammals the effect of melatonin is also mediated by leptin, as observed by reduced litter size in leptin deficient mice [36]. The administration of daily dose of leptin to normal female mice resulted in advancement in the timing of opening of the vagina by some days [37].

Kisspeptin, a neuronal substance produced by the kiss1 neurons in the hypothalamus stimulates the release of GnRH. Physical stress conditions result in the inhibition of kiss1 neurons thereby resulting in the suppression of HPO axis. Studies have shown that leptin directly acts on the kiss1 neurons to release kisspeptin hence causing GnRH release [1].

The release of follicle stimulating hormone (FSH) and luteinising hormone (LH) from the pituitary gland is also governed by central pathways involving leptin [38]. Although increased leptin levels are seen in women with excessive body weight, obesity per se is associated with leptin resistance at the level of the hypothalamus. This leptin resistance further aggravates the hyperleptinemia via feedback mechanisms. Although leptin resistance is observed at the centre, the peripheral tissues, for example, the ovaries not only remain sensitive to leptin, but are also subjected to higher levels seen in obesity [35, 39].

5.2 Effects on the ovary

Normal leptin levels (10–20 ng/ml) are required for the synthesis of oestrogen and progesterone from the theca and granulosa cells of the ovary. Leptin is also essential for the normal growth and maturation of the oocyte. The follicular fluid of the maturing Graafian follicle contains leptin, the concentration of which is dependent on the serum leptin concentrations. Higher serum levels of leptin (50–200 ng/ml) were associated with suppression of oocyte maturation and reduced follicular count. Leptin may also play a role in ovulation as can be speculated by a surge in leptin levels occurring at the same time as the LH surge prior to ovulation. Therefore, hyperleptinemia also contributes to infertility by inhibition of ovulation. The role of leptin also extends to the maintenance of corpus luteum after ovulation [3, 38–40].

Hence it can be summarised that decreased leptin levels seen in energy deficient states may be a threat to fertility due to the suppression of HPO axis. However, hyperleptinemia in obese females also causes infertility due to the direct inhibitory action on the gonads.

5.3 Effects on the endometrium

The receptivity of the endometrial epithelium is blunted under the effect of leptin. Studies in mice have revealed that the normal decidualisation of the endometrium is also diminished in obese women. Leptin controls the remodelling of the endometrial epithelium by mediating its proliferation as well as apoptosis [35].

5.4 Effects on the embryo

The effects of leptin on fertility are not confined to the pre-conceptional phase. It also affects the implantation and development of the growing embryo as can be interpreted from lower success rates of IVF in women with hyperleptinemia [39]. Although in vitro studies have demonstrated the positive effects of leptin on growth and proliferation of trophoblastic stem cells, higher levels seen in obese women are a deterrent to the embryonal development [39, 41].

6. Leptin in menstruation

Hyperleptinemia may also be a determinant of menstrual function, again through its effects on the HPO axis [38]. It is well known that heavy exercise and decreased body fat (resulting in lower leptin levels) can lead to cessation of menses. Studies have demonstrated resumption of menses in women with hypothalamic amenorrhoea when treated with recombinant leptin [42, 43].

A cyclical variation has been observed in the serum leptin concentrations correlating with the phases of the menstrual cycle. In the early follicular phase, the concentration of leptin in serum is 14.9 ng/ml, which increases to 20.4 ng/ml in the mid-luteal phase [3]. Data have shown that a mid-cycle surge is seen in leptin levels corresponding to the mid-cycle LH surge. A recent study demonstrated that a 10% rise in leptin level throughout the menstrual cycle resulted in an increase in serum estradiol and luteal progesterone level [44].

The cyclicity of leptin levels in reproductive aged women in contrast to the constant levels in men and post-menopausal females further exemplify the role of leptin in regulation of menstrual cycle [44].

7. Leptin in polycystic ovary syndrome (PCOS)

PCOS is a heterogeneous disease, characterised by chronic oligo/an-ovulation, hyperandrogenism and polycystic ovaries on morphology. It is one of the most common endocrine disorders of women of reproductive age group affecting 5–10% of these women. It is also the most common cause of anovulatory infertility.

Since a vast majority of these patients are obese and have metabolic derangements, several studies have been conducted investigating the role of leptin in PCOS which have yielded conflicting results [1, 17].

It has been observed that the increased LH levels seen in PCOS patients are also associated with increased leptin levels [45]. Since nearly half of these women present with obesity, hyperleptinemia is a common association in PCOS. Several studies have elucidated elevated levels of leptin in PCOS [46, 47]. Others have linked leptin with the insulin resistance seen in PCOS [48]. Leptin has also been associated with the pro-inflammatory and hyperandrogenic state seen in PCOS [49].

Since hyperleptinemia is observed in several clinical manifestations associated with PCOS, it may be speculated that leptin may have a role in the etiopathogenesis of the disease. However, studies directly demonstrating leptin as one of causative factors of PCOS are still sparse.

8. Leptin and recurrent pregnancy loss (RPL)

Recurrent pregnancy loss may be defined as three or more consecutive spontaneous pregnancy losses occurring before the 20th week of gestation irrespective of previous live births [17]. Known causes include anatomical abnormalities, genetic causes, endocrine derangements, environmental factors, and immunological diseases. However, despite a thorough evaluation of the patients, the cause remains unknown in upto 50% of patients. Defects in the leptin signalling pathway have been evaluated as one of the possible causes of idiopathic RPL. Studies have demonstrated raised serum leptin concentrations in women with RPL as compared to controls. In contrast, reduced leptin levels were also observed in women having first trimester abortions. A recent study revealed similar leptin concentration in RPL cases and controls [50–53].

In conclusion, data linking recurrent pregnancy loss with leptin is largely inconclusive, though there is significant evidence suggesting positive association of hyperleptinemia with RPL.

9. Conclusion

It may be concluded that leptin is the cross-talk molecule linking human reproduction and nutrition. More than 25 years after its discovery, leptin is now known to mediate a paraphernalia of functions relating to the reproductive capacity. Leptin exerts its actions in several ways at multiple levels of the pathway of reproduction including the hypothalamus, ovary, and the placenta. It plays a crucial role in essential processes in the establishment of a normal pregnancy such as trophoblastic invasion, placentation, and transfer of nutrients to the developing embryo. The pathological significance of leptin in human reproduction may be elucidated by the fact that deregulation of leptin levels is responsible for the genesis of a wide variety of disorders associated with pregnancy and reproduction including GDM, FGR, PE, PCOS, RPL and infertility. Recombinant leptin therapies and leptin sensitisers should be the ground for further research to address the devastating effects of abnormal leptin levels and leptin resistance on human reproduction.

Author details

Shyam Pyari Jaiswar[1] and Apala Priyadarshini[2]*

1 Department of Obstetrics and Gynecology, King George's Medical University, Lucknow, Uttar Pradesh, India

2 Department of Obstetrics and Gynecology, All India Institute of Medical Sciences, Raebareli, Uttar Pradesh, India

*Address all correspondence to: apalapriyadarshini@gmail.com

References

[1] Vázquez MJ, Romero-Ruiz A, Tena-Sempere M. Roles of leptin in reproduction, pregnancy and polycystic ovary syndrome: Consensus knowledge and recent developments. Metabolism. 2015;**64**(1):79-91. DOI: 10.1016/j.metabol.2014.10.013

[2] Tena-Sempere M, Huhtaniemi I. Gonadotropins and gonadotropin receptors. In: Fauser BCJM, editor. Reproductive Medicine—Molecular, Cellular and Genetic Fundamentals. New York: Partenon Publishing; 2003. pp. 225-244

[3] Childs GV, Odle AK, MacNicol MC, MacNicol AM. The importance of leptin to reproduction. Endocrinology. 1 Feb 2021;**162**(2):bqaa204. DOI: 10.1210/endocr/bqaa204. PMID: 33165520; PMCID: PMC7749705

[4] Kennedy GC, Mitra J. Body weight and food intake as initiating factors for puberty in the rat. The Journal of Physiology. 1963;**166**:408-418

[5] Foster DL, Olster DH. Effect of restricted nutrition on puberty in the lamb: Patterns of tonic luteinizing hormone (LH) secretion and competency of the LH surge system. Endocrinology. 1985;**116**(1):375-381

[6] Friedman J. The long road to leptin. The Journal of Clinical Investigation. 2016;**126**(12):4727-4734. DOI: 10.1172/JCI91578

[7] Zhang Y, Proenca R, Maffei M, Barone M, Leopold L, Friedman JM. Positional cloning of the mouse obese gene and its human homologue. Nature Cell Biology. 1994;**372**:425-432. DOI: 10.1038/372425a0

[8] de Knegt VE, Hedley PL, Kanters JK, Thagaard IN, Krebs L, Christiansen M, et al. The role of leptin in fetal growth during pre-eclampsia. International Journal of Molecular Sciences. 2021;**22**(9):4569

[9] Sagawaa N, Yuraa CS, Itoha H, et al. Role of leptin in pregnancy—A review. Trophoblast Research Supplement. 2002;**16**:S80-S86

[10] Lepercq J, Hauguel De Mouzo S. Leptin during pregnancy. Journal de Gynécologie, Obstétrique et Biologie de la Reproduction. 2002;**31**(2 Pt 1):167-172

[11] Hauguel-de Mouzon S, Lepercq J, Catalano P. The known and unknown of leptin in pregnancy. American Journal of Obstetrics and Gynecology. 2006;**194**(6):1537-1545. DOI: 10.1016/j.ajog.2005.06.064

[12] Powe CE, Allard C, Battista M-C, Doyon M, Bouchard L, Ecker JL, et al. Heterogeneous contribution of insulin sensitivity and secretion defects to gestational diabetes mellitus. Diabetes Care. 2016;**39**:1052-1055

[13] Masuzaki H, Ogawa Y, Sagawa N, Hosoda K, Matsumoto T, Mise H, et al. Nonadipose tissue production of leptin: Leptin as a novel placenta-derived hormone in humans. Nature Medicine. 1997;**3**:1029-1033

[14] Senaris R, Garcia-Caballero T, Casabiell X, Gallego R, Castro R, Considine R, et al. Synthesis of leptin in human placenta. Endocrinology. 1997;**138**:4501-4504

[15] Considine R, Sinha M, Heiman M. Serum immunoreactive leptin concentrations in normal-weight and

obese humans. The New England Journal of Medicine. 1996;**334**:292-295

[16] Khant Aung Z, Grattan DR, Ladyman SR. Pregnancy-induced adaptation of central sensitivity to leptin and insulin. Molecular and Cellular Endocrinology. 2020;**516**:110933. DOI: 10.1016/j.mce.2020.110933

[17] Pérez-Pérez A, Toro A, Vilariño-García T, et al. Leptin action in normal and pathological pregnancies. Journal of Cellular and Molecular Medicine. 2018;**22**(2):716-727

[18] Jaquet D, Leger J, Levy-Marchal C, Oury JF, Czernichow P. Ontogeny of leptin in human fetuses and newborns: Effect of Intrauterine growth retardation on serum leptin concentrations. The Journal of Clinical Endocrinology and Metabolism. 1998;**83**:1243-1246

[19] Smith JT, Waddell BJ. Leptin distribution and metabolism in the pregnant rat: Transplacental leptin passage increases in late gestation Hauguel-de Mouzon, Lepercq, and Catalano 1543 but is reduced by excess glucocorticoids. Endocrinology. 2003;**144**:3024-3030

[20] Lepercq J, Catalano P, Hauguel de Mouzon S. Leptine et grossesse: dogmes, questions et perspectives [Leptin in pregnancy: Facts, questions and future]. Gynécologie, Obstétrique & Fertilité. 2007;**35**(2):89-95. DOI: 10.1016/j.gyobfe.2006.12.015

[21] Karakosta P, Georgiou V, Fthenou E, Papadopoulou E, Roumeliotaki T, Margioris A, et al. Maternal weight status, cord blood leptin and fetal growth: A prospective mother-child cohort study (Rhea study). Paediatric and Perinatal Epidemiology. 2013;**27**:461-471

[22] Helland IB, Reseland JE, Saugstad OD, Drevon CA. Leptin levels in pregnant women and newborn infants: Gender differences and reduction during the neonatal period. Pediatrics. 1998;**101**:e12. DOI: 10.1542/peds.101.3.e12

[23] Spradley FT, Palei AC, Granger JP. Increased risk for the development of preeclampsia in obese pregnancies: Weighing in on the mechanisms. American Journal of Physiology. Regulatory, Integrative and Comparative Physiology. 2015;**309**: R1326-R1343

[24] Anim-Nyame N, Sooranna SR, Steer PJ, Johnson MR. Longitudinal analysis of maternal plasma leptin concentrations during normal pregnancy and pre-eclampsia. Human Reproduction. 2000;**15**:2033-2036

[25] Nardozza LM, Caetano AC, Zamarian AC, Mazzola JB, Silva CP, Marçal VM, et al. Fetal growth restriction: Current knowledge. Archives of Gynecology and Obstetrics. 2017;**295**(5):1061-1077

[26] Goto E. Maternal blood leptin concentration in small for gestational age: A meta-analysis. European Journal of Pediatrics. 2019;**178**(5):763-770

[27] Gurugubelli Krishna R, Vishnu Bhat B. Molecular mechanisms of intrauterine growth restriction. The Journal of Maternal-Fetal & Neonatal Medicine. 2018;**31**(19):2634-2640

[28] Catov JM, Patrick TE, Powers RW, et al. Maternal leptin across pregnancy in women with small- for-gestational-age infants. American Journal of Obstetrics and Gynecology. 2007;**196**: 558.e1-558.e8

[29] Soheilykhah S, Mojibian M, Rahimi-Saghand S, Rashidi M, Hadinedoushan H. Maternal serum leptin

concentration in gestational diabetes. Taiwanese Journal of Obstetrics & Gynecology. 2011;**50**:149-153

[30] Al-Badri MR, Zantout MS, Azar ST. The role of adipokines in gestational diabetes mellitus. Therapeutic Advances in Endocrinology and Metabolism. 2015;**6**(3):103-108

[31] Thagaard IN, Krebs L, Holm JC, et al. Adiponectin and leptin as first trimester markers for gestational diabetes mellitus: A cohort study. Clinical Chemistry and Laboratory Medicine. 2017;**55**:1805-1812

[32] Pérez-Pérez DA, Vilariño-García T, Guadix P, Dueñas JL, Sánchez-Margalet V. Leptin and nutrition in gestational diabetes. Nutrients. 2020;**12**(7):1970

[33] Gennaro G, Palla G, Battini L, Simoncini T, Del Prato S, Bertolotto A, et al. The role of adipokines in the pathogenesis of gestational diabetes mellitus. Gynecological Endocrinology. 2019;**35**(9):737-751

[34] Castellano JM, Bentsen AH, Sánchez-Garrido MA, Ruiz-Pino F, Romero M, Garcia-Galiano D, et al. Early metabolic programming of puberty onset: Impact of changes in postnatal feeding and rearing conditions on the timing of puberty and development of the hypothalamic kisspeptin system. Endocrinology. 2011;**152**:3396-3408

[35] Gambineri A, Laudisio D, Marocco C, Radellini S, Colao A, Savastano S. Female infertility: Which role for obesity? International Journal of Obesity Supplements. 2019;**9**(1):65-72

[36] Lv D, Tan T, Zhu T, Wang J, Zhang S, Zhang L, et al. Leptin mediates the effects of melatonin on female reproduction in mammals. Journal of Pineal Research. 2019;**66**(3):e12559

[37] Chehab FF, Qiu J, Mounzih K, Ewart-Toland A, Ogus S. Leptin and reproduction. Nutrition Reviews. 2002; **60**(10):S39-S46

[38] Baig M, Azhar A, Rehman R, Syed H, Tariq S, Gazzaz ZJ. Relationship of serum leptin and reproductive hormones in unexplained infertile and fertile females. Cureus. 2019;**11**(12):e6524

[39] Broughton DE, Moley KH. Obesity and female infertility: Potential mediators of obesity's impact. Fertility and Sterility. 2017;**107**(4):840-847

[40] Brannian JD, Hansen KA. Leptin and ovarian folliculogenesis: Implications for ovulation induction and ART outcomes. Seminars in Reproductive Medicine. 2002;**20**(2):103-112

[41] Magarinos MP, Sanchez-Margalet V, Kotler M, Calvo JC, Varone CL. Leptin promotes cell proliferation and survival of trophoblastic cells. Biology of Reproduction. 2007;**76**:203-210

[42] Welt CK, Chan JL, Bullen J, et al. Recombinant human leptin in women with hypothalamic amenorrhea. The New England Journal of Medicine. 2004;**351**:987-997

[43] Chou SH, Chamberland JP, Liu X, et al. Leptin is an effective treatment for hypothalamic amenorrhea. Proceedings of the National Academy of Sciences of the United States of America. 2011;**108**: 6585-6590

[44] Ahrens K, Mumford SL, Schliep KC, Kissell KA, Perkins NJ, Wactawski-Wende J, et al. Serum leptin levels and reproductive function during the menstrual cycle. American Journal of Obstetrics and Gynecology. 2014;**210**(3):248.e1-248.e9

[45] Chen X, Jia X, Qiao J, Guan Y, Kang J. Adipokines in reproductive function: A

link between obesity and polycystic ovary syndrome. Journal of Molecular Endocrinology. 18 Mar 2013;**50**(2):R21-37. DOI: 10.1530/JME-12-0247. PMID: 23335807

[46] Rizk NM, Sharif E. Leptin as well as free leptin receptor is associated with polycystic ovary syndrome in young women. International Journal of Endocrinology. 2015;**2015**:927805. DOI: 10.1155/2015/927805. Epub 2015 Jun 9. PMID: 26180527; PMCID: PMC4477211

[47] Brzechffa PR, Jakimiuk AJ, Agarwal SK, et al. Serum immunoreactive leptin concentrations in women with polycystic ovary syndrome. The Journal of Clinical Endocrinology and Metabolism. 1996;**81**:4166-4169

[48] Behboudi-Gandevani S, Ramezani Tehrani F, Bidhendi Yarandi R, et al. The association between polycystic ovary syndrome, obesity, and the serum concentration of adipokines. Journal of Endocrinological Investigation. 2017;**40**:859-866

[49] Escobar-Morreale HF, San Millan JL. Abdominal adiposity and the polycystic ovary syndrome. Trends in Endocrinology and Metabolism. 2007;**18**:266-272

[50] Garrido-Gimenez C, Alijotas-Reig J. Recurrent miscarriage: Causes, evaluation and management. Postgraduate Medical Journal. 2015; **91**(1073):151-162

[51] Zidan HE, Rezk NA, Alnemr AA, et al. Interleukin-17 and leptin genes polymorphisms and their levels in relation to recurrent pregnancy loss in Egyptian females. Immunogenetics. 2015;**67**:665-673

[52] Kratzsch J, Höckel M, Kiess W. Leptin and pregnancy outcome. Current Opinion in Obstetrics & Gynecology. 2000;**12**:501-505

[53] Serazin V, Duval F, Wainer R, Ravel C, Vialard F, Molina-Gomes D, et al. Are leptin and adiponectin involved in recurrent pregnancy loss? The Journal of Obstetrics and Gynaecology Research. 2018;**44**(6):1015-1022

Chapter 4

Role of Leptin in Obesity Management: Current and Herbal Treatment

Sunil T. Galatage, Sakshi N. Gurav, Mahadevi R. Moladi, Tejal R. Podjale, Nikita B. Tejam, Arehalli S. Manjappa, Popat S. Kumbhar, Supriya V. Nikade, Swapnil S. Chopade, Sujit A. Desai, Shweta N. Kalebere and Suresh G. Killedar

Abstract

Obesity is an excessive accumulation of fat in the body associated with numerous complications such as development of hypertension, type 2 diabetes (T2DM), dyslipidemia, sleep apnea, and respiratory disorders; and ultimately life-threatening cardiovascular disease (CVD), stroke, certain types of cancer and osteoarthritis. In 2016, more than 1.9 billion adults aged 18 years and older were overweight. Of these, over 650 million adults were obese, that is over 39% of men and 40% of women were overweight. Rapid rise in obesity cases in both developed and developing countries and people suffering from it needs rapid and complete cure form it without any side effects. Herbal medicine has been used for the treatment of disease for more than 2000 years, and it has proven efficacy. Many studies have confirmed that herbal medicines are effective in the treatment of obesity. Various plants from different families and several phytochemical constituents are responsible for the anti-obesity activity such as fenugreek cinnamon, cardamom, ginger, etc. Present work mainly cover herbal species having leptin-stimulating potential for weight management, importance of leptin, its mechanism of action, current and herbal treatment for effective weight management.

Keywords: obesity, diabetes, leptin, appetite, herbal treatment etc.

1. Introduction

In 2016, more than 1.9 billion adults aged 18 years and older were overweight. Of these over 650 million adults were obese i.e. 39% of adults and over (39% of men and 40% of women) were overweight. Overall, about 13% of the world's adult population (11% of men and 15% of women) were obese in 2016. Obesity is quantities in terms of Body Mass Index (BMI), which is defined as the ratio of the weight and the square of height and is a measure of body adiposity [1]. The incidence and prevalence of obesity, are rising both in developed and developing countries. Although globalization has resulted in substantial improvements in quality of life and food security, as well as reductions in poverty, unintended consequences of globalization are also driving the obesity epidemic. Among the multiple factors contributing to its etiology, the sedentary life styles, white collar jobs, lack of exercise, psychological factors, excess consumption of junk food and the consumption of energy rich diets are the major ones. Obesity is excessive accumulation of fat in the body associated with numerous complications such as development of hypertension, type 2 diabetes (T2DM), dyslipidemia, sleep apnea, and respiratory disorders; and ultimately life-threatening cardiovascular disease (CVD), stroke, certain types of cancer and osteoarthritis. Currently there is rapid rise in obesity and related severe diseases mainly due to drastic changes in lifestyle, living standard and modern diet. However rapid urbanization, economic revolution and free trade liberty are main reasons behind this. Nowadays in low and middle income nations there is drastic change in nutritional values mainly due to getting proteins and fats obtained from animals, added sugars and refined grains. Due to obscure etiology, the pharmacological treatment of obesity has been a particularly challenging task. Reducing body weight by lifestyle alteration is advisable, but sometimes drug intervention is necessary. Combating obesity is going to requires coordinated efforts from the international community, governments, industry, health-care systems, schools, urban planners, agriculture and service sectors, the media, communities and individuals. Further, the cause of concern is the non-availability of drugs for its treatment and the short-term efficacy and limiting side effects of the available drugs. Drugs used for obesity management are mainly classified in to metabolic promoters, digestion and absorption blockers, central appetite suppressants and obesity gene product inhibitors. However drugs used for obesity management specifically affects monoamine neurotransmitters leads to habit forming, dependence or abuse [2]. Anti-obesity drugs have been studied profoundly for decades. The need for adjunctive therapies for weight loss has accelerated the progress in the pharmaceutical industry worldwide. Weight loss drugs may appear to be a solution to obesity. However, possible side effects or adverse drug reactions are always a big public health concern and also a major barrier to the development of new drug products. Obesity, which is broadly refers to excess body fat, and ranked as the fifth foremost reason for death globally. Overweight and obesity are major lifestyle illness that leads to wide variety of chronic diseases, which may include cancers, metabolic syndrome, diabetes, cardiovascular diseases, osteoarthritis, gout, breathing problems etc. The World Health Organization predicted about 30% of death occurring in whole

Weight status	Body mass index in kg/m^2
Under-weight	<18.5
Normal range	18.5–24.9
Over-weight	25.0–29.9
Obese	$\geq$ 30
Obese class-I	30.0–34.9
Obese class-II	35.0–39.9
Obese class-III	$\geq$40

Table 1.
Classification of weight based on body mass index.

world will be initiated with lifestyle disease in 2030 and can be stopped by appropriate identification and conveying associated risk factors. It is therefore essential to detect and diagnose obesity as early as possible [3]. Worldwide more than 1.9 billon adults are overweight and 650 million are obese. Approximately 2.8 million deaths are reported as a result of being overweight and obesity. This is major health related problem in both developed and developing countries. In India more than 135 million individuals were affected by obesity. The study of total body fat accurately requires sophisticated technology. The World Health Organization (WHO) have acquire body mass index, which is calculated by dividing the body weight in kilograms (kg) by the square of the height in meters (m), as a surrogate measure of total body fat (**Table 1**). With this index, obesity is defined when the value is equal to or more than 30 Kg/m^2 [4]. Formula: BMI = $Weight/Height^2$.

2. Leptin

The discovery of leptin 15 years ago generated great excitement that the treatment for obesity had been found, and thus, this prototypical adipocyte-secreted protein/cytokine was named leptin after the Greek word "leptos" for thin. Leptin is a group of 167 amino acids in human leptin gene mainly made up of adipose tissue and enterocytes which mainly regulate energy balance by inhibiting hunger. It is released by white adipose tissue and leptin level is key indicator of body fat. As like other hormones leptin is secreted at regular temporal pattern i.e. highest secretion in early morning and evening. Leptin mainly is an indicator of how much energy stored in fats and caloric intake [5].

2.1 Types of leptin receptors

1. There are mainly three types of leptin receptor i.e. the OBRa, OBRb, and OBRb with formulation (OBRb-*fa*), by measurement of the levels of tyrosine phosphorylation of STAT3 (signal transducers and activators of transcription 3) and MAPK (mitogen-activated protein kinase).

2. This receptors are induced by leptin stimulation of CHO cells stably expressing the OBR (CHO-OBRb, CHO-OBRa, or CHO-OBRb-*fa*cells).

3. As the result of leptin stimulation, enhanced levels of tyrosine phosphorylation of STAT3 [6].

2.2 Mechanism of action of leptin

Leptin (Greek word leptos– thin) also known as "Ob gene" that is located on chromosome number 7. Main role of leptin is to achieve an energy balance in the body. Leptin binds to receptors in brain and performs several actions that may prove that leptin is important in treating obesity.

It works through two distinct types of neurons in arcuate nucleus of hypothalamus.

1. POMC/CART (Pro-opiomelanocortin/cocaine and amphetamine regulated transcripts) neurons

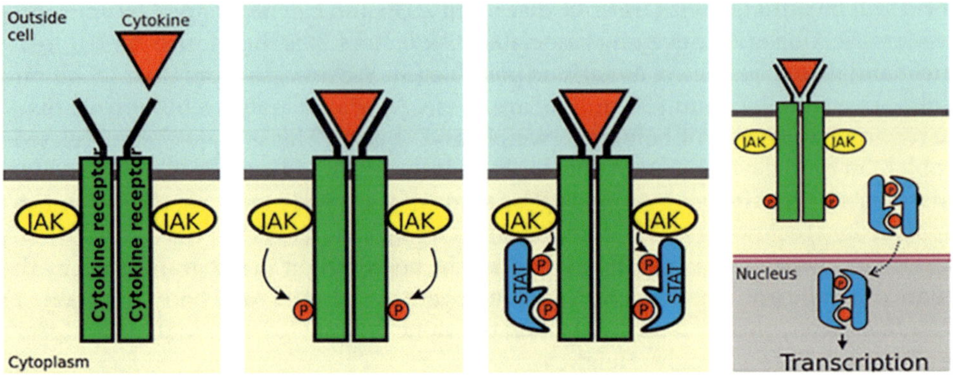

Figure 1.
Mechanism of action of leptin.

2. NPY/AgRP (Neuropeptide Y/Agouti—related peptide) neurons

Leptin stimulates POMC/CART neurons to produce anorexigenic neuropeptide: melanocytes stimulating hormone that results in

1. Endocrine changes

2. Increase sympathetic nerve activity

This stimulates energy expenditure.

Leptin inhibits NPY/AgRP neurons that produce feeding—inducing (orexigenic) neuropeptide: NPY that results in inhibition of food intake.

The binding of leptin to its receptor initiates numerous signal transduction pathways and as result, regulates a range of cellular function in body (**Figure 1**). leptin receptor as a member of type 1 cytokine receptor family, signals via Janus kinase family of tyrosine kinase. Leptin induced dimerization alters the intracellular domain confirmation to increase its affinity for cystolic JAK. After this JAK activate and phosphorylate tyrosine residue, then it bind another free moving protein STAT. This also phosphorylate by JAK. Pairs of phosphorylated STAT dimerize and translocate to the nucleus to regulate gene transcription resulting in a biological response of leptin [7, 8].

3. Pathophysiology

Three parts.

1. Peripheral afferent system (PAS)

2. Control processing.

3. Peripheral efferent system (PES)

Through PAS

3.1 Peripheral appetite suppressing signal

A. It act through secrete leptin and adiponectin.

In obese person the level of adiponectin is low and it involve in thermogenesis.

B. GUT hormone secretes insulin, amylin and glucagon like peptide.

3.2 Peripheral appetite stimulating signal

A. It acts through Gut hormone secrete ghrelin, obestatin. Anorexigenic via ObRb receptor expressed in brain and peripheral tissue which is binding in the hypothalamus, leptin activates a complex neural circuit comprising of anorexigenic (that is appetite suppressing) and orexigenic (that is appetite stimulating) neuropeptide to control food intake. Loss of melanocortin 4 receptor (MC4R) function, a key MCR expressed in the hypothalamus, is the most common genetic cause of obesity in humans [9].

3.3 Through PES

Though PES the regulation is controlled by negative feedback mechanism. Though food intake and energy expenditure. Change in appetite or drastic reduction in hunger mainly due to not only activation neuron via binding to the melanocortin receptor (MCR) by leptin which acts on proopiomelanocortin (POMC) leads to release of melanocyte stimulating hormone (α-MSH) in to synapse but also inhibition of neuropeptide-Y (NPY)/agouti related peptides (AgRP) synthesis in neurons which negatively affects agonistic potential of AgRP on MCR resulting in to suppression of appetite (**Figure 2**) [10].

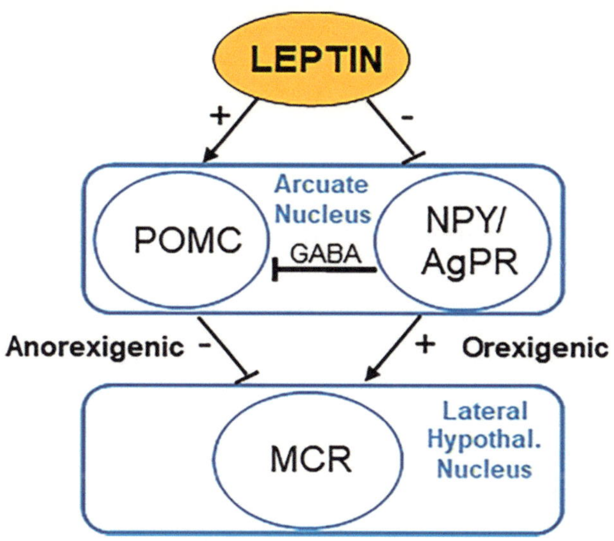

Figure 2.
Regulation of appetite by leptin acting on the nucleus arcuatus of the hypothalamus. Proopiomelanocortin (POMC), neuropeptide Y (NPY), Agouti-related protein (AgRP), melanocortin receptor (MCR), gamma amino butyric acid (GABA).

4. Current treatment for obesity management and its effects

Anti-obesity drugs have been studied profoundly for decades [11–13]. The need for adjunctive therapies for weight loss has accelerated the progress in the pharmaceutical industry worldwide. Weight loss drugs may appear to be a solution to obesity. However, possible side effects or adverse drug reactions are always a big public health concern and also a major barrier to the development of new drug products. Some of the antiobesity drugs commercially available are orlistat, lorcaserin, sibutramine, rimonabant, metformin, exenatide, pramlintide etc. These drugs have a wide variety of severe side-effects including development of cardiovascular problems, restlessness, insomnia, faulty bowel movements, pain in stomach, psychiatric problems etc. Ideally anti-obesity agent would be such as to produce weight loss which can be retained, but with minimal side effects. Medication for short term weight management or selected medications used off label to promote weight loss mentioned in (**Table 2**) and Medication for long term weight management are listed in (**Table 3**).

Drugs	Mechanism	Effect on weight	Adverse effect	Status
Phentermine	Sympathomimetic amine (appetite suppressant)	3.6 kg placebo subtracted weight loss in studies ranging from 2 to 24 weeks	Insomnia, tremor, increase BP and pulse rate, headache, palpitation, constipation.	Diffusion controlled release preparation is available
Diethylpropion	Sympathomimetic amine (appetite suppressant)	3.0 kg placebo subtracted weight loss at 6–52 weeks	Insomnia, tremor, increase BP and pulse rate, headache, palpitation, constipation.	Currently approved drug for short term
Zonisamide	Anti-convulsant drug	5.0% placebo subtracted weight loss at 12 weeks	Increase nervousness, sweating, tremors, gastrointestinal adverse effects, hypersomnia, fatigue and insomnia	Used off—label
Topiramate	Anti- convulsant drug	6.5% placebo subtracted weight loss at 24 weeks	Paresthesia, dizziness, altered taste, fatigue, memory impairment, somnolence, anorexia and abdominal pain	Used off—label

Table 2.
Medication for short term weight management or selected medications used off label to promote weight loss.

Drugs	mechanism	Effect on weight	Adverse effects	status
Orlistat	Pancreatic lipase inhibitor	2.9 kg placebo subtracted weight loss at 1 year	Abdominal pain, bloating, flatulence, oily stools, diarrhea, decrease absorption of fat soluble vitamins	Approved drug for long term weight management
Liraglutide	GLP-1 analogues	7.2 kg Placebo: 2.8 kg	Nausea, and thyroid C-cell focal hyperplasia and medullary thyroid tumor	Approved for treatment of obesity
Tesofensine	Anti-convulsant agent	11.2 kg Placebo: 2 kg	Nausea, dry mouth, headache, insomnia, diarrhea and constipation	Phase 3

Drugs	mechanism	Effect on weight	Adverse effects	status
Cetilistat	Anti-convulsant agent	4.3 kg Placebo: 2.8 kg	Abdominal pain, fecal urgency and diarrhea	Phase 3
Phentermine-topiramate	Unknown	Verage placebo-subtracted weight loss 8.6%	Combination sympathomimetic and carbonic anhydrase inhibitor / Decreases appetite and binge eating behaviors	Approved in 2012
Bupropion/ Naltrexone	Naltrexone is opiate antagonists, and bupropion is an antidepressant	7.2–10.1% (24 weeks)	Nausea, dizziness, insomnia, dry mouth, bowel changes	Approved in 2014
Gelesis100	Superabsorbent hydrogel particles of a cellulose-citric acid matrix / Increases fullness.	6.4% in 6 months	No significant Risk designation	Approved in 2019
Setmelanotide (Imcivree)	Melanocortin 4 receptor agonist	weight loss 12.5–25.6%	Melanocortin-4-receptor agonist / Decreases appetite	Approved in 2020
Semaglutide (Wegovy)	Glucagon Like Peptide-1 receptor agonist	weight loss 8%	Nausea, diarrhea, vomiting, Constipation, abdominal (stomach) pain, headache, fatigue.	Approved in 2021

Table 3.
Drugs/medical devices long term weight management [12–14].

5. Herbal treatment

Herbal medicine has been used for treatment of disease for more than 2000 years, and it has proven efficacy [4, 5, 15–17]. Many studies have confirmed that herbal medicine is effective in the treatment of obesity, but the mechanisms are not clear. In present work an attempt will be done to develop herbal formulation containing different types of spices. It is a doubtless fact that various plants from different families and several phytochemical constituents are responsible for the anti-obesity activity. Current treatment of obesity includes various marketed formulations which have hazardous side effects such as high blood pressure, agitation, diarrhea, sleeplessness, liver damage, rectal bleeding, faster rate palpitations, closed-angle glaucoma, Insomnia etc. which can be overcome by using herbal formulation. Herbal medicine has been used for treatment of disease for more than 2000 years, and it has proven efficacy. Many studies have confirmed that herbal medicine is effective in the treatment of obesity. But the mechanisms are not clear. In present work an attempt will be done to develop herbal formulation containing different types of spices. It is a doubtless fact that various plants from different families and several phytochemical constituents are responsible for the anti-obesity activity[4] Natural herbs gives not only anti-obesity effect but also other health benefits, such as anti-diabetic and anti-hyperlipidemic activities. It is anticipated that the availability of many natural sources will provide a beneficial basis for developing novel anti-obesity products. Nature is loaded with dozens of herbs and spices—from the very common black pepper to the exotic turmeric. Along with amazing health benefits they have to offer, herbs and spices also add flavor and aroma to our food and dishes.

Research has also shown that herbs and spices have the potential to boost metabolism, promote satiety (read: contentment), aid weight management and improve the overall quality of diet. Very few researchers focus on exact molecular level mechanism responsible for anti- obesity activity. Therefore, the growing threat of obesity to global health is encouraging scientists and researchers to put more effort into finding an efficient mechanism of action at molecular level. It is anticipated that there is abundant room for further contributions by researchers to establish the molecular mechanism of new natural anti-obesity agents. Urgency of a novel, nontoxic means needs to be developed to control obesity. Various plant products have been found to be effective in controlling obesity. A good portion of fruits, vegetables, spices and herbs need to be included in the regular diet. Plant derived molecules or phytochemicals are blessed with strong anti-obesogenic, anti-carcinogenic and anti-inflammatory properties. Thus they may serve as a nontoxic and cost-effective method to tackle obesity. These molecules target various pathways that are intricately linked to the process of adipogenesis. This review aims to elucidate the beneficial role of dietary food nutrients in control of obesogenicity. Following are the herbs which stimulate leptin in obesity management.

5.1 Cinnamon

Cinnamomum-verum (cinnamaldehyde)

Cinnamon is most widely used and popular weight loss herbs due to its sugar stabilizing potential which rapidly increase rate of metabolism of fats and rapidly reduces hunger pangs which has excellent for obesity management.

5.2 Ginger

Zingiber officinale (6-gingerol)

Ginger acts as a potential body cleanser which remove the food logged in the digestive system and avoid fat storage resulting in to weight loss and obesity management.

5.3 Cardamom

Elettaria cardamomum (I,8-cineole)

Cardamom boosts metabolism and helps the body burn fat more effectively and Managing conditions like indigestion, constipation, and water retention, elaichi makes for an important weight loss. Cardamom improves rate of metabolism which results in to increasing potential of our body to burn fat which ultimately helpful for weight management.

5.4 Turmeric

Curcuma longa (Curcumin)

Curcumin is safest yellow orange colored material obtained from turmeric having potential role in increase in rate of metabolism, stimulate leptin and adiponectin. Curcumin drastically reduces rate of fat formation and accumulation which ultimately lower total body fat which avoids weight gain.

5.5 Acai berry

Euterpe oleracea containing phenolic acids such as vanillic acid has important role in obesity management. It avoids excessive storage of fat in body and also prevents obesity-induced hepatic steatosis regulating lipid metabolism by increasing cholesterol excretion which is helpful for maintaining weight in control.

5.6 Nettle leaf

Urticadioica (Acetylcholine)

It has tremendous fat burning potential which helpful in maintaining the weight also nettle leaf contains vitamins like C and A which provide nutritional powers along with bold purifying property of nettle leaf.

5.7 Guarana

Paulliniacupana (Caffein)

Guarana improves rate of metabolism which directly results in to obesity control also it suppress genes that aid fat cell production and promote genes that slow it down. Caffein mainly acts on central nervous system prevent overeating due to tension and emotions.

5.8 Cayenne pepper

Capsicum annuum (Capsaicin)

This spice includes a compound called as capsaicin which helps to burn fat and suppresses your hunger cravings. According to a research done by Prudue University—cayenne is effective in weight loss, because it increases body's metabolism activity which causes the body to burn more calories.

5.9 Cumin

Cuminum cyminum (Cumin aldehyde, phellandrene)

Cumin play a vital role in fat burning as it rapidly increases rate of burning calories by increasing rate of metabolism and prominent improvement in rate and extent of digestion. It has also play vital role in boosting immune system.

5.10 Ginseng

Panax ginseng (Ginseng saponin)

Ginseng mainly acts on leptin, insulin and adiponectin which mainly enhance rate metabolism of fats and cholesterol. Ginseng not only play important role in obesity management by acting on angiogenesis but also enhance energy level speed up rate and extent of metabolism.

5.11 Black pepper

Piper nigrum (Piperine)

Piperine is the main bioactive compound that mainly responsible for obesity management. Piperine significantly increases rate of metabolism and burn fat at faster rate mainly due to it improves mRNA expression associated with adipose tissue which is associated with lipogenesis resulting in to improvement in lipid metabolism related to genes specifically in visceral fat.

5.12 Dandelions

Taraxacum (chicoric acid, chlorogenic acid)

Dandelions primarily reduces total cholesterol level and level of fat in liver which is significant in treating obesity related disorders. It also improve rate of digestion and extent of metabolic activities.

5.13 Flax seeds

Linum usitatissimum (Omega 3 fatty acid)

Flaxseeds acts as a bulking agent and gives you a feeling of fullness. Thus, they prevent you from overeating and help you to lose weight.

5.14 Guar gum

Cyamopsis tetragonoloba (Sugars of galactose and maltose)

Guar gum helps in managing diabetes and aids weight loss. It helps to improve the digestion process and gives you a feeling of fullness.

5.15 Garcinia

Garcinia gummi-gutta (Ethyl acetate & hexane moiety)

This fruit promotes appetite suppression and prevents production and deposition of fat. Choose whole food rather than other variants.

5.16 Mustard

Brassica nigra (carotenoids (zeaxanthin, lutein, β-carotene))

Mustard is a very good weight loss herb, as it helps to fasten body's metabolic activity.

5.17 *Cocos nucifera* (caprylic acid)

Coconut oil helps to increase your metabolic speed, which further aids in releasing energy and promoting weight loss.

5.18 Fennel seeds

Foeniculum vulgare (anethole.)

These tiny seeds aid in digestion and help to regulate your hunger. Besides, it also helps in cleansing your liver.

5.19 Psyllium

Plantago ovate (hemicellulose, arabinoxylans)

This is a very safe weight loss agent. These seeds make you feel fuller for a longer time and slow down the absorption of simple carbs.

5.20 Hibiscus

Hibiscus rosa-sinensis (anthraquinones)

Hibiscus is loaded with various obesity fighting agents like chromium, ascorbic acid and hydroxycitric acid (HCA).

6. Conclusion

Nowadays there is drastic rise in Incidences and prevalence of obesity in both developed and developing countries and people suffering from it need rapid and complete cure form it without any side effects. Herbal treatment stimulating leptin acts as competent alternative to current treatment without any side effects using resources form natural origin.

Acknowledgements

The authors are thankful to Department of Pharmaceutics Gajanan Maharaj College of Pharmacy Mahagaon, and Trustees of Sant Gajanan Maharaj College of Pharmacy Mahagaon for providing required guidance and support.

Conflict of interest

The authors declare no conflict of interest.

Notes/thanks/other declarations

Special thanks to Shvtej S. Galatage for continuous support throughout the work.

Abbreviations

AgRP	agouti-related protein
BMI	body Mass Index
CART	cocaine and amphetamine regulated transcripts neurons
T2DM	type 2 diabetes mellitus
CVD	cardiovascular disease
GABA	gamma aminobutyric acid
MAPK	mitogen-activated protein kinase
MCR	melanocortin receptor
NPY	Neuropeptide Y Agouti-related
OBRa, OBRb, OBRbfa	Obesity Receptor a, b and fa respectively
PAS	Peripheral Afferent Nervous System
PES	Peripheral Efferent Nervous System

POMC	Proopiomelanocortin
WHO	World Health Organization
STAT3	signal transducers and activators of transcription 3

Author details

Sunil T. Galatage[1*], Sakshi N. Gurav[1], Mahadevi R. Moladi[1], Tejal R. Podjale[1], Nikita B. Tejam[1], Arehalli S. Manjappa[2], Popat S. Kumbhar[2], Supriya V. Nikade[1], Swapnil S. Chopade[2], Sujit A. Desai[3], Shweta N. Kalebere[4] and Suresh G. Killedar[1]

1 Sant Gajanan Maharaj College of Pharmacy, Mahagoan, Maharashtra, India

2 Tatyasaheb Kore College of Pharmacy, Maharashtra, India

3 Annasaheb Dange College of D Pharmacy, Ashta, Maharashtra, India

4 Genesis Institute of Pharmacy, Kolhapur, Maharashtra, India

*Address all correspondence to: gsunil201288@gmail.com

References

[1] Parikh N, Brahmbhatt R. Herbal approach for treatment of obesity Indo American. Journal of Pharmaceutical Sciences. 2018;**05**(03):1694-1703

[2] Yanfei S, Mingyue S. Herbal medicine for the treatment of obesity: An overview of scientific evidence from 2007 to 2017. Evidence-Based Complementary and Alternative Medicine. 2017;**2017**:1-18

[3] Singh C, Geetha A. Review on herbal approach towards the treatment of obesity. Journal of Pharma Research. 2015;**4**(6):248-251

[4] Karri S, Sharma S. Natural anti-obesity agents and their therapeutic role in management of obesity: A future trend perspective. Biomedicine & Pharmacotherapy. 2019;**110**:224-338

[5] Kelesidis T, Kelesidis L, Chou S, Mantzoros CS. Narrative review: The role of leptin in human physiology: Emerging clinical applications. Annals of Internal Medicine. 2010;**152**(2):93-100

[6] Srivastava N, Lakhan R. Patho-physiology and genetics of obesity. Indian Journal of Experimental Biology. 2007;**45**:929-936

[7] Mamata D. Formulation and evaluation of poly herbal anti-diabetic tablet dosage form. International Journal of Ayurvedic & Herbal Medicine. 2017;7(6):2956-2962

[8] Rai P, Dambal A. Development of an anti-obesity polyherbal formulation containing *Terminalia arjuna*, Lagen-ariasiceraria and *Piper nigrum*. The Pharma Innovation Journal. 2015;**3**(11):33-37

[9] Chien M-Y, Ku Y-H, Chang J-M, Yang C-M, Chen C-H. Effects of herbal mixture extracts on obesity in rats fed a high-fat diet. Journal of Food and Drug Analysis. 2016;**24**(3):594-601

[10] Nam M-H, Lee S-W, Na H-Y, Yoo J-H, Paik S-H, Ahn KS, et al. Herbal acupuncture for the treatment of obesity. Journal of Acupuncture and Meridian Studies. 2016;**9**(2):49-57

[11] Jain D, Bavage P. Evaluation of anti-obesity effect of fattolin, a polyherbal formulation in progesterone induced obesity in mice. Indian Journal of Pharmaceutical Education and Research. 2016;**50**(3):391-396

[12] Patil M, Kagathara V. Effect of polyherbal formulation in obesity associated diabetes. International journal of pharmacy and pharmaceutical science. 2010;**2**(3):180-186

[13] Safaei M, Sundararajan EA, Driss M, Boulila W, Shapi A. A Systematic Literature Review on Obesity: Understanding the causes and consequences of obesity and reviewing various machine learning approaches used to predict obesity. Computers in Biology and Medicine. 2021;**136**:1-17

[14] Tchang BG, Kumar R, Aronne LJ. Pharmacologic Treatment of Overweight and Obesity in Adults. Semantic Scholar; 2000. Corpus ID: 232839857

[15] Flak JN, Myers MG. Minireview: CNS mechanisms of leptin action. Molecular Endocrinology. 2016;**30**(1):3-12

[16] Obradovic M, Sudar-Milovanovic E, Soskic S, Essack M, Arya S, Stewart AJ, et al. Leptin and obesity: Role and clinical implication. Frontiers in Endocrinology. 2021;**12**:1-14

[17] Kang JG, Park C-Y. Anti-obesity drugs: A review about their effects and safety. Diabetes Metabolism Journal. 2012;**36**(1):13-25

Section 2

Obesity Consequences and Management

Chapter 5

The Multiple Consequences of Obesity

Indu Saxena, Amar Preet Kaur, Suwarna Suman, Abhilasha, Prasenjit Mitra, Praveen Sharma and Manoj Kumar

Abstract

Increase in body weight due to excess accumulation of fat can lead to obesity, a chronic, progressive, relapsing, multifactorial, neurobehavioral disease caused by adipose tissue dysfunction. Obesity often results in adverse biomechanical, metabolic, psychosocial, and economic consequences. In humans, effects of obesity are diverse and interrelated and can be classified on the basis of organ/organ system affected. Physical problems associated with weight gain are musculoskeletal problems, respiratory problems, lower limb venous diseases, skin-related problems, and stress incontinence in females. Metabolic conditions caused by obesity include gout, insulin resistance and metabolic syndrome, type 2 diabetes mellitus, certain cancers, CVD, fatty liver, gall bladder disease, etc. Obesity is known to affect the reproductive health. Hypogonadism and pseudo-gynecomastia are more common in males with obesity. Decreased fertility is reported in both the sexes. Polycystic ovarian syndrome (PCOS), anovulation, endometrial hyperplasia, and increased risk of complications in pregnancy have been reported in females. Persons with obesity have increased healthcare expense, pay more insurance premium, take more illness-related leaves, thus suffering economic loss due to their condition. Persons with obesity are often considered legitimate targets for teasing and bullying, which may cause social isolation, depression, eating disorders, etc. Obesity affects the morbidity and mortality. This chapter deals with the different consequences of obesity.

Keywords: obesity, metabolic syndrome, insulin resistance, type 2 diabetes mellitus, obesity-related health

1. Introduction

Living organisms are constitutionally wired to store energy for survival in periods of scarcity. Eel and salmon are reported to survive long periods without food [1–3]. The excess intake of calories leads to energy accumulation in the form of fat, glycogen, or starch. Plants store energy reserves as starch and oil. We were unable to find reports of adverse consequences of excess energy storage in plants and lower organisms. The stored energy helps the organism to tide over periods of calorie scarcity and during hibernation, aestivation, or migration in animals. In higher organisms, deposition of excess calories results in impairment of body functions with adverse

IntechOpen

Type of problems	Examples of associated conditions
Physical problems	1. Musculoskeletal disorders a. Decreased mobility b. Loss of balance c. Osteoarthritis d. Gout
	2. Respiratory problems a. Decreased lung compliance b. Increased risk of asthma c. Sleep apnea
	3. Lower limb venous disease a. Thrombosis b. Varicose veins c. Venous insufficiency
	4. Skin-related problems
	5. Stress incontinence in females
Metabolic disorders	1. Hyperglycemia
	2. Dyslipidemia
	3. Gout Hyperglycemia increases risk of skin infections, eye diseases, and kidney diseases. Both hyperglycemia and dyslipidemia cause insulin resistances, leading to increased risk of type 2 diabetes, cardiovascular disease, stroke, and cancers.
Gut-associated diseases	1. Cholelithiasis
	2. Pancreatitis
	3. Fatty liver
	4. Gastroesophageal reflux disease
Reproductive Health Issues	A. Males 1. Hypogonadism
	2. Gynecomastia
	3. Decreased fertility
	B. Females
	1. Polycystic Ovarian Syndrome (PCOS)
	2. Anovulation
	3. Endometrial hyperplasia
	C. Increased risk of complications in pregnancy
	1. Gestational diabetes
	2. Preeclampsia
	3. Cesarian section
Economic issues	1. Increased expense on obesity-related diseases
	2. Decreased pay
	3. Decreased job opportunity

Mental and social issues	1. Social stigma
	2. Bullying
	3. Binge eating
	4. Depression
Quality of life and mortality	1. Increased risk of morbidity, mortality decreased quality of life

Table 1.
Multiple consequences of obesity.

effects on health and longevity. Obesity with adverse health effects has been reported in zebrafish [4], reptiles [5, 6], and birds [7].

Energy in humans is stored as glycogen or triacylglycerols (TAGs). Relative to the amount of calories that can be stored as triacylglycerols (TAGs), only a small amount of calories can be stored as glycogen. An adult liver can store up to 120 g glycogen, while the skeletal muscles can store up to 400 g glycogen. Triacylglycerols are hydrophobic energy-dense molecules that can be stored in large amounts in the adipocytes. Adipose tissue is the loose collection of adipocytes in a mesh of collagen fibers, deposited at various sites in the body. Preadipocytes, fibroblasts, vascular endothelial cells, adipose tissue macrophages, and small blood vessels are also present in the adipose tissue.

Increased mass of adipose tissue, abnormal site of deposition, or abnormal size of adipocytes can result in adverse consequences on health and quality of life (**Table 1**).

2. Physical problems associated with obesity

These result from the abnormally high weight of the affected person and are closely related to each other and to the other consequences of obesity including metabolic dysfunction and insulin resistance. For convenience, we have classified them into musculoskeletal disorders, skin-related problems, respiratory problems, lower-limb venous diseases, and urinary incontinence.

2.1 Musculoskeletal disorders

These include decreased mobility, loss of balance, and osteoarthritis, which are associated with abnormal increase in body weight (**Figure 1**).

2.1.1 Decreased functional mobility

Obesity is one of the major causes for the loss of functional mobility. Altered posture and gait resulting from abnormal fat deposition, compromised bone strength, pain, and breathlessness compromise the mobility [8], which must be taken into account by treating physicians advising increased physical activity for weight loss. Decreased mobility results in further increase in weight.

2.1.2 Loss of balance

Increased weight, decreased mobility, and altered posture result in loss of balance, increasing the risk of falls and injury [9]. In spite of the cushioning effect of the fat

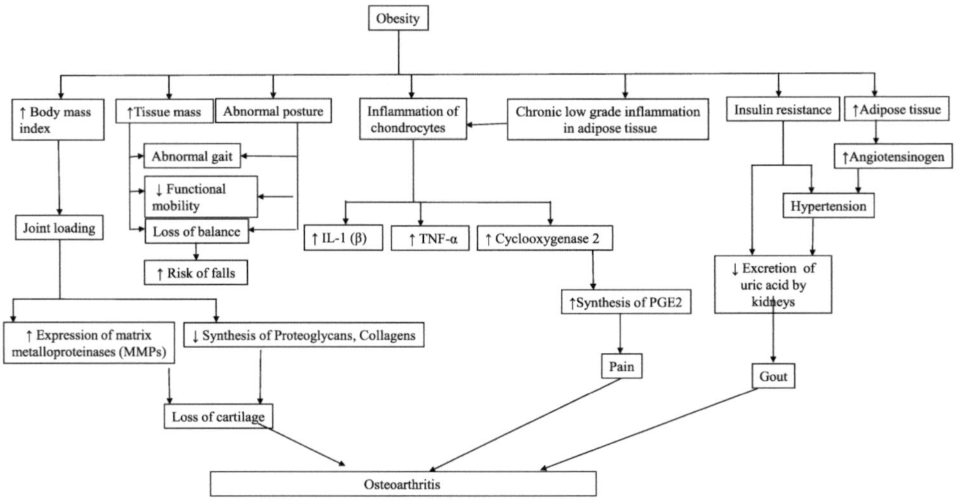

Figure 1.
Association of obesity with musculoskeletal disorders.

mass, falls in patients with obesity are more serious and require higher treatment costs and specialized care [10].

2.1.3 Osteoarthritis (OA)

Progressive loss of articular cartilage and formation of osteophytes (bony spurs usually caused by local inflammation) result in osteoarthritis [11]. Obesity is a risk factor for OA of knee, hands, and wrist (but not of hip) [12]; thus excessive body weight alone cannot fully explain the increased incidence of OA in people with obesity. Increased body mass index (BMI) in obesity results in altered gait and increased strain on the knee, causing biomechanical joint loading [13]. This is associated with increased expression of matrix metalloproteinases in chondrocytes and increased degradation of proteoglycans [14]. Synthesis of DNA, proteoglycans, and collagen is decreased, contributing to the loss of cartilage in joints [14]. Chondrocytes subjected to high loading show increased expression of pro-inflammatory cytokines including TNF-α and IL-1(β), along with an increased expression of cyclooxygenase-2 leading to increased PGE2 (responsible for inflammatory pain) synthesis [15].

Increase in the amount of adipose tissue leads to metabolic dysfunction: obesity-related sarcopenia, deposition of intramuscular lipid, and chronic low-grade systemic inflammation, all of which contribute to osteoarthritis [16].

2.1.4 Gout

Insulin resistance, often seen in patients with obesity, causes decreased excretion of uric acid, leading to hyperuricemia [17, 18]. Adipose tissue is known to express all the components of renin-angiotensin system (RAS), including angiotensinogen [19]. The resulting hypertension may cause glomerular arteriolar damage and reduce uric acid excretion. Hyperuricemia and gout have been associated with osteoarthritis [20, 21].

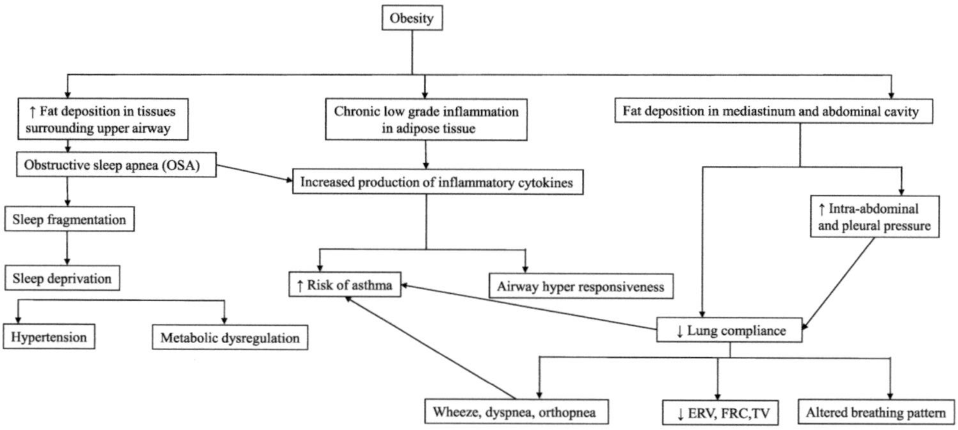

Figure 2.
Association of obesity with respiratory disorders.

2.2 Respiratory problems

Obesity is associated with various respiratory problems that are correlated with each other (**Figure 2**).

2.2.1 Reduced compliance of lungs

Increased fat deposition in the mediastinum and abdominal cavity increases intra-abdominal and pleural pressure, thus reducing compliance of the lungs. Altered breathing pattern, with decrease in expiratory reserve volume (ERV), functional reserve capacity (FRC), and tidal volume (TV), with slight increase in mean respiratory rate have been reported in subjects with obesity [22, 23], Obesity has little effect on the residual volume (RV) and total lung capacity (TLC) [24].

2.2.2 Obesity and asthma

The relationship between obesity and asthma has been established by a meta-analysis involving more than 300,000 adults [25]. The expression of adipokines secreted by adipose tissue is different in persons with obesity. Decreased expression of adiponectin (anti-inflammatory adipokine) and increased expression of leptin (pro-inflammatory adipokine) have been reported in asthmatic patients with obesity [26]. Leptin, an anorexigenic hormone, increases metabolic rate and is involved in surfactant production and neonatal lung development [27]. Sood et al. [28] have reported a strong association between high BMI and high levels of serum leptin with asthma in adults.

Inflammatory cytokines such as TNF-α, IL-8, and monocyte chemoattractant protein-1 (MCP-1) have also been reported to be raised in persons with obesity. However, their role in asthma associated with obesity is not clear [29]. In older patients, abdominal obesity and metabolic syndrome have been reported to be associated with restrictive lung disease [30].

2.2.3 Obstructive sleep apnea (OSA)

The prevalence of obstructive sleep apnea in adult persons with obesity is about 45%, compared with 25% in persons with normal weight [31]. Increased fat deposit in tissues surrounding the upper airway decreases the size of lumen and increases collapsibility of the upper airway. OSA may cause sleep fragmentation, which may lead to sleep deprivation [32]. Since experimental sleep deprivation and self-reported short sleep have been linked with metabolic dysregulation, it is possible that OSA may also be a contributing factor in metabolic dysregulation associated with obesity.

2.3 Lower limb venous diseases

Venous diseases (blood clots, deep vein thrombosis, superficial venous thrombosis or phlebitis, chronic venous insufficiency or CVI, varicose and spider veins, and venous stasis ulcers) may be caused by one or more of the following factors: immobility (as in bed-ridden patients) leading to stagnation of blood), blood vessel injury caused by trauma/needles/intravenous catheters/infections, central venous hypertension, conditions that increase the blood coagulation, and pregnancy. Different cancers are associated with deep vein thrombosis.

Varicose veins and chronic venous insufficiency are more common in aged women compared with men. Obesity has been found to be associated with all types of lower limb venous diseases (**Figure 3**). Willenberg et al. [33] showed that lower limb venous flow parameters are different in healthy persons with and without obesity. Various

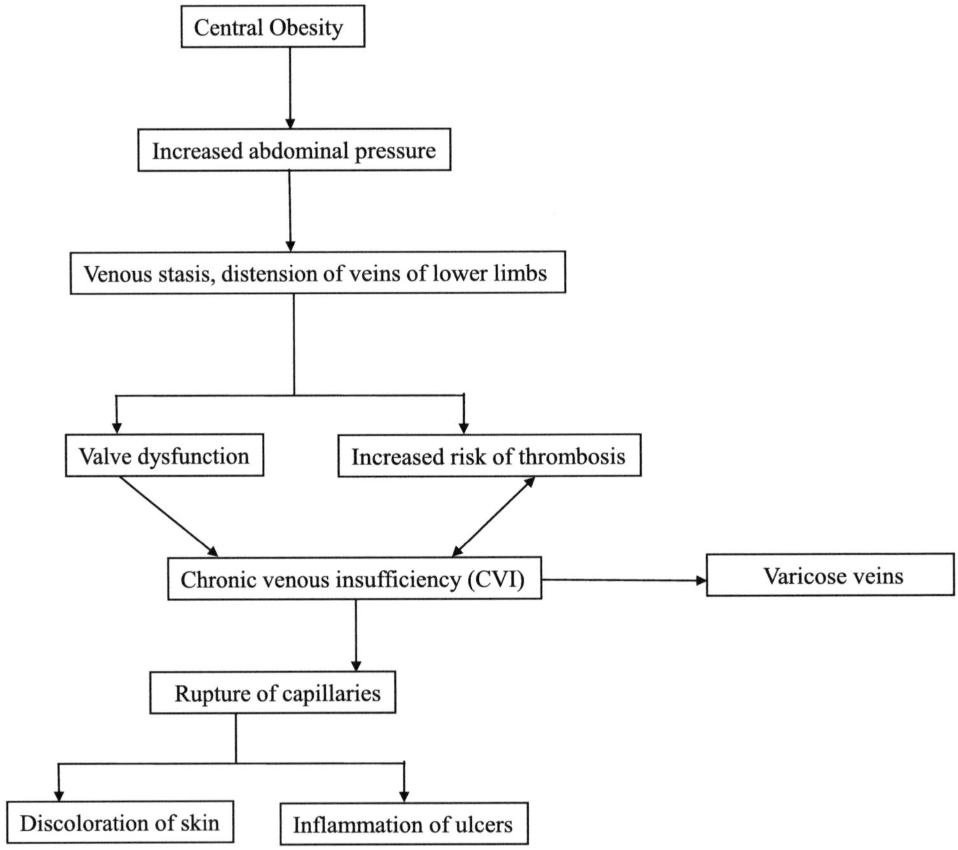

Figure 3.
Obesity as a cause of lower limb venous diseases.

epidemiological studies show that obesity is associated with chronic venous disease, phlebitis, and thromboembolism [34–37]. Untreated CVI results in increased pressure and swelling leading to rupture of capillaries. The skin may appear reddish-brown and becomes sensitive to bumps and scratches. Burst capillaries may lead to inflammation and even ulcers.

Increased intra-abdominal pressure caused by central obesity is transmitted to the extremities via femoral veins leading to resistance to venous return, producing venous valvular insufficiency. The self-perpetuating cycle of worsening venous insufficiency causes venous stasis and distension of veins in the lower limb. Obesity produces a chronic low-grade inflammation, which damages the affected veins and increases the risk of thromboembolism [33].

2.4 Skin problems

Different problems of the integumentary system associated with obesity can be classified on the basis of their pathophysiologic origin (**Figure 4**). Skin lesions associated with mechanical causes include striae, lipodystrophy, plantar hyperkeratosis, and venous insufficiency. Acanthosis nigricans and skin tags or acrochordons are due to insulin resistance. Obesity-related hyperandrogenism may cause acne, hirsutism, and androgenic alopecia. Skin folds created by obesity increase the risk of intertrigo and infections.

2.4.1 Mechanical causes of dermatologic manifestations associated with obesity

Striae or stretch marks are a type of scarring of the dermis associated with stretching of the dermis. Striae distensae may appear as a consequence of pregnancy, puberty, or obesity and appear on abdomen, breasts (in females), and shoulders (in body builders). They are more common in females [38]. Striae atrophicans due to thinning of the skin may appear in adrenal gland disorders [39].

Other dermatological conditions with mechanical causes include intertrigo, conditions associated with chronic venous insufficiency, and lymphedema [40]. Intertrigo

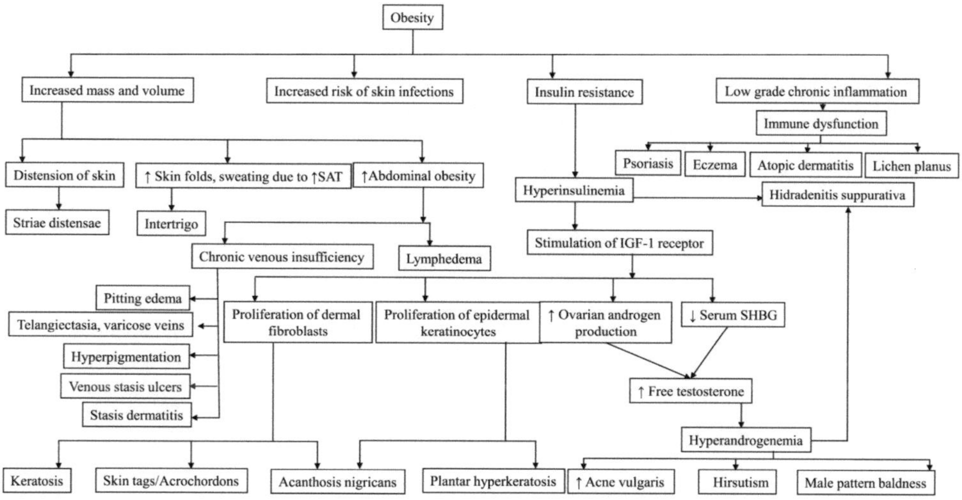

Figure 4.
Dermatological manifestations associated with obesity.

is an inflammation of skin resulting from friction between opposing skin surfaces of skin folds. It may have an infectious component. Axilla, groin, intergluteal, and inframammary areas may be involved [41]. Hot, humid climates and obesity (BMI > 30 kg/m^2) are known to promote intertrigo. Persons with obesity tend to sweat more.

Dermatologic sequelae of chronic venous insufficiency (discussed above) are often seen in patients with obesity and include pitting edema, varicose veins, telangiectasia, hyperpigmentation, venous stasis ulcers, and scaling of the skin (stasis dermatitis) [42].

Blocking or damage of the lymphatic system resulting in accumulation of lymph in soft tissues, especially legs or arms, is called lymphedema. Obesity is a risk factor for secondary lymphedema [40].

2.4.2 Obesity-related endocrine disorders of skin

These include skin tags, acanthosis nigricans, keratosis pilaris, hidradenitis suppurativa and hirsutism, and plantar hyperkeratosis.

a. Skin tags or acrochordons. Skin tags are soft cutaneous growths, usually benign, more commonly seen in persons with obesity, metabolic syndrome, type 2 diabetes, or in persons with family history of skin tags [43]. They occur in both males and females, usually later on in life, but are less common after the seventh decade. The polypoid lesions are skin-colored, brown, or red, 1–5 mm in size (rarely larger) with a loose edematous fibrovascular core, and may be attached to a fleshy stalk. They are more common in skin folds: axilla, groin, eyelids, and neck [44]. Although not painful, they can cause trouble by getting caught in clothing or jewelry, resulting in itching or bleeding. However, skin tags in large numbers may be seen in patients with Birt-Hogg-Dube (BHD) syndrome and tuberous sclerosis, where they appear around the neck: the molluscum pendulum necklace sign [45, 46].

b. Acanthosis nigricans (AN). Hyperpigmented velvety plaques usually in body folds, neck, knuckles, and scalp may be seen in patients with obesity. The condition was first reported more than an hundred years ago in the Atlas for Rare Skin Diseases. The term acanthosis nigricans was proposed by Paul Gerson Unna and published in 1891 in a case report by Sigmund Pollitzer [47]. Obesity-associated AN was previously called pseudo acanthosis nigricans; however, this term is incorrect. This is because the initial cases identified in Europe were associated with abdominal or pelvic malignancies. Association of AN with obesity was first reported by Robertson and Tasker in 1947 [48]. Like acrochordons, AN is also associated with insulin resistance often seen in obesity. Probably, the hyperinsulinemia seen in insulin resistance leads to direct and indirect activation of the insulin-like growth factor receptor, triggering proliferation of the dermal fibroblast and epidermal keratinocyte [49]. Friction and perspiration may also be involved in the development of AN [50].

c. Keratosis pilaris (chicken skin) is a benign condition of the skin in which sterile papules occur on the skin (collections of dead skin cells). Though these papules may occur anywhere on the body (except palms and soles), they are more common on the posterior aspect of upper arms, anterior aspects of thighs, face, and buttocks [51].

d. Hidradenitis suppurativa or acne inversa is a chronic painful condition of the terminal follicular epithelium in the apocrine gland–bearing skin (groin, bottom, axilla, breasts) [51]. It affects about 1% of the population and is strongly associated with smoking and obesity. It is also linked with hyperandrogenemia, as many patients have acne and hirsutism [52].

e. Hirsutism, acne vulgaris, and androgenic alopecia seen in some female patients with obesity (with or without polycystic ovarian syndrome, PCOS) are due to hyperandrogenemia, often associated with peripubertal obesity [51–54]. Increased insulin production (hyperinsulinemia) due to insulin resistance in obesity increases IGF-1 levels and augments ovarian androgen production [55]. Hyperinsulinemia produces a decrease in serum level of steroid hormone binding globulin (SHBG), resulting in a further increase in the level of free testosterone. Treatments that reduce insulin levels usually correct hyperandrogenemia and ovulatory dysfunction [56].

f. Plantar hyperkeratosis (thickening of skin over metatarsophalangeal joints, caused due to increased pressure and mechanical stress placed on the feet) is seen in almost 50% patients with obesity [40]. Increased circulating levels of IGF-1 seen in hyperinsulinemia lead to overactivation of IGF-1 receptors on fibroblasts and keratinocytes. The abnormal IGF-1 signaling causes cellular hyperproliferation (**Figure 4**).

2.4.3 Increased risk of skin infections

Obesity has been associated with an increased risk of skin, respiratory tract, and urinary tract infections [57]. An increased risk of community-acquired infections has been reported by Harpsoe et al. [58] in both overweight and underweight women. Obesity alters the function of skin, sebum, and sweat glands, affects the structure of collagen and subcutaneous fat, and slows wound healing. A number of skin infections that are more common in persons with obesity include candidiasis, candida folliculitis, furunculosis, tinea cruris, and folliculitis. Cellulitis is less common [42].

2.4.4 Obesity-associated immune disorders affecting skin

Normal adipose tissue in a nonobese person has a population of anti-inflammatory/regulatory immune cells: M2-macrophages and regulatory T cells. These are replaced by pro-inflammatory cells: M1 macrophages, Th1, Th17, and cytotoxic T cells in adipose tissue in persons with obesity [59]. Systemic immune adaptations in obesity include increased number of circulating monocytes, neutrophils, Th1, Th17, and Th22 cells. The pro-inflammatory cytokines produced by pathogenic adipose tissue (IL-1β, IL-6, IL-17, and IFN-γ) result in a chronic low-grade inflammation. Skin conditions such as psoriasis, atopic dermatitis, and eczema are strongly associated with obesity [60]. Hashba et al. [61] have suggested the association of lichen planus with obesity.

2.5 Urinary incontinence (UI)

Urinary incontinence may be of different types: stress incontinence when pregnancy, childbirth, etc., weaken the muscles supporting and controlling bladder; urge incontinence caused by involuntary action of bladder muscles; and mixed incontinence that shares the causes of both stress and urge incontinence. Thyroid problems, uncontrolled diabetes, and medicines such as diuretics can worsen the problem of UI. High BMI, especially BMI higher than 40 kg/m^2, has been strongly associated with stress predominant incontinence including mixed incontinence [62]. Central obesity increases the abdominal pressure, which increases the bladder pressure and urethral mobility, leading to UI. Chronic strain and stretching seen in pregnancy and abdominal obesity weaken the muscles and other structures of the pelvic floor. Surgical and non-surgical weight loss has been reported to decrease incontinence and improved quality of life.

3. Metabolic disorders associated with obesity

3.1 Organization of the adipose tissue

Adipose tissue is a loose connective tissue in which about half the cells are adipocytes, the remaining is stromal vascular fraction containing preadipocytes, fibroblasts, endothelial cells, and macrophages [63]. The adipose tissue may be considered the largest endocrine gland in the body.

Based on the metabolic features of the adipocytes, adipose tissue (AT) can be white adipose tissue (WAT), which stores excess energy as fat, and brown adipose tissue (BAT), which dissipates stored energy as heat (**Figure 5**). Both WAT and BAT are present in mammals and are formed throughout life. In humans, WAT development begins during early to mid-gestation period. WAT adipocytes contain a large single (unilocular) droplet of triacylglycerols occupying 90% of the cell volume, with the cytoplasm and the nucleus squeezed to the periphery. Adipocytes of BAT are smaller, multilocular, and contain mitochondria and uncoupling protein-1 (UCP-1), which is involved in non-shivering thermogenesis. The brown appearance of BAT is due to high vasculature and high mitochondrial content. It has a high density of noradrenergic parenchymal fibers. BAT is 5–10 times more vascularized than WAT. A third type of adipose tissue, the beige or brite (brown in white) adipose tissue with paucilocular adipocytes is dispersed in the WAT [64–66]. Browning of WAT has been suggested under the influence

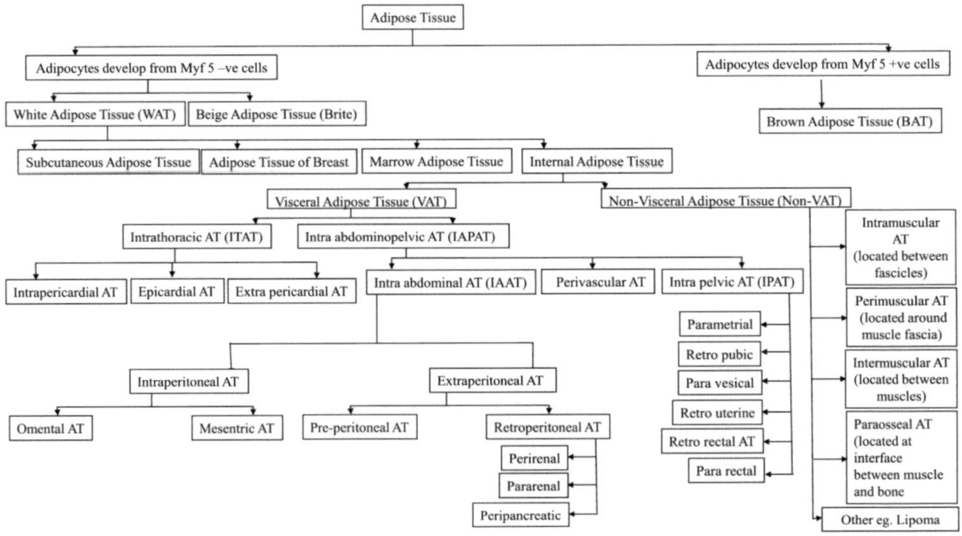

Figure 5.
Types of adipose tissue.

of the hormone irisin, which is produced by the skeletal muscle during exercise [67]. Adipocytes of WAT and beige adipose tissue are predominantly derived from the Myf 5 negative progenitor cells, while adipocytes of BAT are predominantly from Myf 5 positive progenitor cells. Myf 5 or myogenic factor 5 is a gene for transcriptional factor expressed during embryonic myogenesis [68]. Brown and beige AT show anatomical decline with aging and protect from obesity and type 2 diabetes mellitus (T2DM).

Based on the location of the white adipose tissue, it is broadly classified as subcutaneous and visceral (**Figure 5**). The subcutaneous adipose tissue (SAT) stores excess energy, provides insulation from heat and cold, and functions as an endocrine organ. Visceral adipose tissue (VAT) provides a protective padding around organs. Specialized adipose tissue is associated with the bone marrow, breast, retroorbital adipose tissue, and epicardium [69]. In persons having the same BMI, females tend to have more adipose tissue than males. Females also have more subcutaneous adipose tissue (SAT) compared with males. Localized fat pads, e.g., the synovia are considered as SAT. The SAT of lower trunk and gluteal-thigh region is further organized in two separate layers: the superficial SAT, SSAT (evenly distributed around the circumference of the abdomen), and the deep SAT, DSAT (most of which is located in the posterior half of the abdomen). The SSAT and DSAT are separated by the fascia of Scarpa. SSAT has a higher expression of metabolic regulatory genes, while DSAT has a higher level of expression of inflammatory genes and higher lipolytic activity. Thus, higher volume of DSAT is associated with higher levels of free fatty acids [70].

3.2 Specialized adipose tissue

Bone marrow contains adipose tissue called the marrow adipose tissue (MAT), which increases in amount in periods of calorie restriction, in contrast to adipose tissue present at other sites in the body. Exercise results in decrease in the size of MAT, as well as of the adipocytes present in MAT. Adipocytes of MAT develop from the mesenchymal stem cells.

3.3 Diseases associated with adipose tissue

In some persons there is a variable lack of adipose tissue, which may be generalized or specific (abnormal distribution of adipose tissue). This condition is called lipodystrophy. Lack of sufficient adipose tissue results in increased levels of fatty acids in blood, as they cannot be stored as TGs in the adipocytes. Raised levels of fatty acids cause lipotoxicity, characterized by ectopic fat deposition in the muscle, liver, and pancreas, thus contributing to T2DM [71].

3.3.1 Development of insulin resistance

The mechanism of development of insulin resistance is complicated and is influenced by diverse factors, including the location and type of adipose tissue that increases in mass.

Depending on the location, WAT is further classified into different types (**Figure 5**) [72, 73]. Excess calorie intake leads to enlargement of adipocytes (hypertrophy) as well as increase in the number of adipocytes (hyperplasia) [74]. The new adipocytes may develop from preadipocytes or from adipocytes of BAT. Adipogenesis through differentiation of progenitor cells to adipocytes occurs through transcription factors such as peroxisome proliferator-activated receptor-γ

(PPAR-γ), and CCAAT/enhancer binding protein-α [75]. Increase in the size of the adipocytes is associated with insulin resistance and inflammation. Adipose hypertrophy seen in morbid adiposity results in heterogeneity of cell size within the same depot of adipose tissue, with cell size ranging from 20 microns to 300 microns [76]. Usually, SAT contains more preadipocytes compared with VAT, so adipose hypertrophy is less in SAT [77]. Normal adipose tissue produces adipokines (leptin, adiponectin) that regulate appetite and energy metabolism and cytokines. Pro-inflammatory cytokines include TNF-α, visfatin, resistin, angiotensin II, serum amyloid alpha, plasminogen activator inhibitor, and IL-6, while anti-inflammatory cytokines include apelin, transforming growth factor beta (TGFβ), IL-10, IL-4, IL-13, and IL-1 receptor antagonist (IL-1Ra) [78]. Male hormones promote hypertrophy, while female hormones promote hyperplasia [79]. In lean adipose tissue, the adipose cells are 5–10% of all cells in the tissue; in obese adipose tissue, this number is as high as 60% [80]. Although the life span of adipocytes is about 8 years, increase in size beyond a critical cell size and nutrient excess produce endoplasmic reticulum stress, hypoxia, and death of adipocyte, attracting infiltration of macrophages. This is more in VAT. Adipocyte remnants are absorbed by macrophages, which become activated. In lean adipose tissue, the adipose tissue macrophages (ATMs) are predominantly M2 (anti-inflammatory) type. Pathologic adipose has greater number of M1 ATMs, which are pro-inflammatory and produce cytokines in large amounts after absorbing dead adipocytes. This results in chronic low-grade inflammation and insulin resistance.

In some persons with obesity, excess calories are preferentially stored in SAT, which does not produce inflammation. This type of obesity is also called metabolically healthy obesity (MHO) [81]. In contrast, increase in VAT is associated with abnormal blood lipid profile, i.e., dyslipidemia, insulin resistance, metabolic syndrome, type 2 diabetes, and hypertension. This type of obesity is called metabolically unhealthy obesity (MUHO) and is due to deposition of intraabdominal fat.

Hypertrophic stressed adipocytes are unable to take up free fatty acids, which are therefore diverted to other non-fat-storing organs such as muscle, liver, pancreas, and heart, where they are stored as ectopic fat. This results in impaired glucose uptake by muscle cells, decreased glucose utilization by liver and adipose causing hypertriglyceridemia, hyperglycemia, reduced amounts of HDL cholesterol, increased amounts of LDL and VLDL cholesterol, increased proportion of small, dense LDL particles, and insulin resistance. Products of fatty acid metabolism such as long-chain fatty acyl-Co A, diacyl glycerol (DAG), and ceramide are harmful to cells and aggravate insulin resistance by causing phosphorylation of the serine residues on the insulin receptor substrate (IRS) [82]. In skeletal muscle, lipid can be stored in adipocytes between muscle fibers, or as cytosolic triacylglycerols within the muscle cells (intramyocellular lipids, IMCLs). IMCLs are an adaptive response in endurance athletes and are present in close proximity to mitochondria. Increased IMCL stores in insulin resistance or T2DM is a consequence of raised free fatty acid levels in blood and impaired fatty acid oxidation in the muscle [83]. This may also be due to mitochondrial dysfunction.

Recent evidence suggests the role of leptin resistance and hyperleptinemia of obesity causes production of reactive oxygen species (ROS) and increases oxidative stress, promoting the risk of hypertension, heart disease, and cancer [84–86]. Endoplasmic reticulum stress, protein tyrosine phosphatase 1B, and suppressor of cytokine 3 (SOC3) signaling mediate leptin resistance and are also involved in insulin resistance [87].

3.3.2 Type 2 diabetes

Insulin resistance in the liver, adipose, and muscles coupled with ectopic fat in the pancreas contributes to hyperglycemia and T2DM. Deposition of ectopic fat in the pancreas is seen in almost two-thirds of patients with obesity. Most of this is due to adipocyte infiltration into pancreatic tissue rather than accumulation of intracellular lipid. Ectopic pancreatic fat is associated with an increased risk of T2DM and cardiovascular disease (CVD). Increased lipolysis and inflammation caused by ectopic pancreatic fat are also reported to promote acute pancreatitis [88].

3.3.3 Fatty liver

Hepatic insulin resistance caused by DAG and ceramide promotes lipotoxicity, ectopic fat deposition, insulin resistance, and steatosis, leading to nonalcoholic fatty liver disease (NAFLD) [89].

3.3.4 Obesity and cardiovascular disease

Excess free fatty acids reaching the heart can be stored as epicardial adipose tissue (EAT), also called pericardial fat (present between the visceral and parietal pericardia), or surrounding the blood vessels (perivascular adipose tissue or PVAT). Although the cardiac muscle uses free fatty acids for obtaining energy, when delivered in excess these fatty acids are stored as ectopic fat in the cardiac myocyte, disrupting its function. Higher levels of LDL and VLDL receptors are expressed in the epicardial tissue from patients with T2DM. The PVAT produces adipokines and many molecules that affect vascular reactivity: monocyte chemotactic protein-1 (MCP-1)], nitric oxide, prostacyclin, and angiotensin II. PVAT present around the thoracic aorta resembles BAT, while the PVAT around the abdominal aorta resembles WAT [90, 91]. Healthy PVAT is largely anti-inflammatory, while dysfunctional PVAT promotes atherosclerosis.

3.3.5 Obesity and cancer

Different types of cancers associated with obesity include breast, endometrial, prostrate, pancreatic, adenocarcinoma of esophagus, colon cancer, meningioma, and cancers of ovary, kidney, thyroid, liver, etc. [92–94]. Though different mechanisms have been proposed, chronic inflammation is a major factor for cancer initiation and progression. Excess nutrients activate metabolic signaling pathways such as c-Jun N-terminal kinase (JNK), nuclear factor κ B (NFκB), and protein kinase R that may promote development of neoplasm [95, 96]. Synthesis of IGF-1 is stimulated by insulin. IGF-1 promotes tumor growth via the PI3K/Akt/mTOR and the Ras/Raf/MAPK pathways [96]. IL-6, a pro-inflammatory cytokine produced during adipose tissue inflammation, activates the androgen receptor and promotes cell survival and proliferation in prostate cancer [97]. Aromatase, the rate-limiting enzyme of estrogen synthesis, is also stimulated by inflammatory cytokines and PGE2 [98–101].

Risk of gallstones is increased in obesity. Chronic gall bladder inflammation from gallstones may predispose to cancer of the gall bladder [102]. Similarly, chronic inflammation of hepatitis may increase the risk of liver cancer [103].

Cancer survivorship, including cancer progression, prognosis, recurrence, and quality of life are reported to be worsened by obesity [104, 105]. Obesity is associated with an increased risk of treatment-related lymphedema in breast cancer survivors and incontinence in prostate cancer survivors (treated with radial prostatectomy) [106, 107]. Risk of local recurrence was higher in obese/overweight male patients with stage II or stage III renal cancer [108]. Similarly, obesity increases the risk of mortality in patients with multiple myeloma [109].

3.3.6 Eye diseases associated with obesity

Ocular manifestations of obesity are less known and not well documented. Its association with age-related cataract, glaucoma, age-related maculopathy, and diabetic retinopathy has been reported [110, 111]. Cortical and posterior subcapsular or PSC cataracts have been most consistently associated with obesity. Obesity-induced leptin resistance and hyperlipidemia promote formation of reactive oxygen species, which are involved in cataract formation. Other complications of obesity: insulin resistance, hyperglycemia, diabetes, diabetes, and hypertension (see above) are known to be risk factors for cataract.

Increased retroorbital adipose tissue seen in obesity has been reported to be associated with increased intraocular pressure (IOP) [112, 113]. Raised IOP may be a risk factor for glaucoma. The AREDS (Age-Related Eye Disease Study) Report [114] has reported an association between obesity and age-related macular degeneration. (AMD) Oxidative stress secondary to hyperleptinemia may cause damage to lipids in Bruch membrane and secretion of excessive vascular endothelial growth factor (VEGF), which elicit invasion of neovascularization in Bruch membrane in neovascular AMD [115]. Inflammation may also play a role in AMD development. Diabetic retinopathy, a common complication of T2DM (which is associated with diabetes), can result in loss of vision [116]. Other diseases of the eye that may be associated with obesity include retinal vein occlusion, oculomotor nerve palsy, recurrent lower eyelid entropion, keratoconus, papilledema, floppy eyelid syndrome and benign intracranial hypertension (pseudotumor cerebri) [117–121].

4. Gut-associated diseases

Besides fatty liver and pancreatitis (discussed above), obesity is associated with increased risk of cholelithiasis (gall bladder stones) and gastroesophageal reflux disease (GERD).

4.1 Cholelithiasis

About 90% gallstones are cholesterol stones while the rest are made of calcium bilirubinate, calcium complexes, mucin glycoproteins, or unconjugated bilirubin. Obesity and metabolic syndrome are two risk factors for the development of cholelithiasis, other factors being genetics, age, gender, parity, and presence of hepatitis C virus infection and chronic kidney disease [122]. Recent study by Su et al. [123] shows that obesity reduces the age of onset of gallstone formation. Energy-dense food such as increased consumption of refined carbohydrates and saturated fats with decreased intake of fiber, and medicines such as estrogen and progesterone can promote cholelithiasis [124]. Rapid weight loss of more than 1.5 kg/week can also promote gallstone formation [125].

4.2 Gastroesophageal reflux disease (GERD)

Heartburn and regurgitation are typical manifestations of GERD. Epidemiologic data show an association of obesity with GERD and Barrett's esophagus, a condition in which the lower part of the esophagus is damaged by repeated exposure to stomach acid [126, 127].

5. Effect of obesity on reproductive health

Obesity has been shown to cause sub-fecundity and infertility in both sexes [128–130]. Overweight and obesity result in changes in the hypothalamus-pituitary-gonadal (HPG) axis in both men and women, affecting hormone levels and gametogenesis.

5.1 Reproductive problems in males

Chronic inflammation along with insulin and leptin resistance is associated with increase in adipose tissue (see above), affecting reproductive issues.

5.1.1 Hypogonadism and pseudo-gynecomastia

Insulin resistance may be responsible for obesity-induced hypogonadism in males. Male obesity secondary hypogonadism or MOSH is caused by hyperestrogenism, metabolic endotoxemia, and hyperleptinemia. Hyperestrogenism decreases pituitary secretion of luteinizing hormone through a negative feedback action that impairs the synthesis and production of testosterone from Leydig cells. Hypercaloric diet with excess lipids causes breakdown of the normal leaky gut, facilitating passage of bacterial endotoxin from gut lumen into the blood stream (metabolic endotoxemia). Some animal studies suggest that bacterial endotoxin (Lipopolysaccharides-LPS) reduces testicular function by binding toll-like receptor 4 (TLR4) on Leydig cells, stimulating production of inflammatory cytokines [131–134].

Obesity is associated with elevated levels of leptin and leptin resistance. Leptin prevents the neuropeptide Y (NPY) neurons from inhibiting the release of GnRH. Leptin resistance results in reduced release of GnRH, FSH, and LH and impairs spermatogenesis [135].

Kisspeptin, a hypothalamic peptide encoded by the KiSS1 gene, is an important neuromodulator involved in HPG axis and fertility control. Most kisspeptin cells are localized at the hypothalamic level in humans. Kisspeptin and its G-protein-coupled receptor (KISS 1R or GPR-54) increase the delivery of GnRH into portal circulation, resulting in enhanced secretion of LH and FSH from the anterior pituitary. Decreased endogenous kisspeptin secretion is seen in obesity-related hypogonadotropic hypogonadism (HH) [136–139]. Increased leptin levels are associated with decreased total and free testosterone levels in males.

Hyperinsulinemia results in decreased production of sex hormone binding globulin (SHBG) by the hepatocytes, causing increased availability of free testosterone for reaction by aromatase in the adipose tissue. Aromatase converts testosterone to estradiol [140], further decreasing testosterone level with increase in estrogen level. This may result in pseudo-gynecomastia, with excess adipose deposition in breast area [134]. Sleep apnea associated with obesity disrupts the nocturnal rise in testosterone [134].

High waist circumference is associated with erectile dysfunction due to atherogenic effect on peripheral vasculature [141]. Low ejaculatory volume and oligo-zoospermia have been noted in males with increased BMI and waist circumference [142]. Increased testicular heat, elevated inflammatory mediators, and increased presence of reactive oxygen species in men with obesity affect the quality of sperms [143].

5.2 Reproductive problems in females

Earlier onset of menarche has been reported in adolescent females with overweight or obesity, compared with their normal-weight counterparts. The association of obesity with menstrual disorders, infertility, and recurrent miscarriages was recognized early [144, 145].

Insulin resistance promotes hyperandrogenemia and decreases the level of steroid hormone binding globulin (SHBG) resulting in elevated levels of free testosterone (discussed above). Aromatization of testosterone to estrogens by aromatase in the adipose tissue suppresses the release of gonadotrophin from the pituitary [140]. Elevated levels of leptin impair follicle development, ovulation, and oocyte maturation in women with obesity [146, 147].

5.2.1 Polycystic ovarian syndrome (PCOS)

This hormonal disorder is one of the most common endocrine disorder in premenopausal women, is also associated with obesity, metabolic syndrome, and T2DM. Irregular periods, anovulatory cycles, oligo-amenorrhea, excess androgen, hirsutism, and polycystic ovaries are the main characteristics of PCOS [148, 149]. Most women with PCOS have elevated levels of plasma free fatty acids, are insulin resistant, and have compensatory hyperinsulinemia. High levels of free fatty acids induce mitochondrial dysfunction, inflammation, oxidative stress, and immune disorders [150]. High levels of plasma free fatty acids cause increased synthesis of androgens in the ovary as well as in the zona reticularis of the adrenal gland. Insulin stimulates androgenesis by stimulating P450c17 activity in zona reticularis of the adrenal gland to produce DHEA and androstenedione [151]. Hyperinsulinemia causes decreased expression of SHBG by hepatocytes (see above), thus further increasing free testosterone levels. Aromatase (CYP19A1) in adipocytes as well as in the tissue of endometriosis converts androgens to estradiol, which inhibits the secretion of gonadotropin releasing hormone, resulting in decreased release FSH and LH from the pituitary. This affects maturation of follicles, production of estrogen, ovulation, maintenance of function of corpus luteum.

Women with PCOS may have problems in conceiving and increased risk of gestational diabetes and miscarriage or premature birth. Impairment of the hypothalamus-pituitary-gonadal (HPG) axis and follicular environment caused by obesity results in fertility problems, miscarriages, and complications in pregnancy.

5.2.2 Anovulation and quality of oocyte

Ovulation disorders account for at least 30% cases of infertility. Menstrual cycle without the release of ovum is called anovulatory cycle. Women with obesity have higher rates of anovulatory menstrual cycles [152, 153], the exact mechanism of which is not known. Common causes of anovulation include hyperandrogenism (as in PCOS, congenital adrenal hyperplasia, androgen-producing tumors), hyperprolactinemia, anorexia, excessive strenuous exercise, stress, thyroid dysfunction, primary pituitary dysfunction, premature ovarian failure, and certain medications. Obesity and strenuous exercise are known to alter profiles of insulin and adiponectin, thus impairing fertility in women. Obese women remain sub-fertile even in the absence of ovulatory dysfunction [154, 155].

Obesity affects the quality of sperm, ovum, embryo, placenta, and the uterine environment. The competence of the oocyte is defined in terms of its ability to become fertilized and support embryo development. Oocyte competence may be influenced by obesity. Machtinger et al. [156] have shown that oocytes from women with obesity are smaller in size, have more abnormal spindles and chromosome misalignment than those from women with normal BMI. Negative outcomes for women undergoing in vitro fertilization (IVF) are more common in women with higher BMI, due to the poor oocyte quality, lower preimplantation rate, and uterine receptivity [157]. Decreased rate of conception, infertility, early pregnancy loss, and reduced success of assisted reproductive technology (ART) have been reported in females with obesity [158].

High serum levels of insulin, insulin resistance, high levels of glucose, lactate, triglycerides, and C-reactive protein in the follicular fluid have a negative impact on oocyte maturation.

Mitochondria of the oocyte must be fully functional, as ATP generated by them are required for oocyte maturation and blastocyst formation. High levels of fuel molecules (glucose, free fatty acids, triglycerides, and cholesterol) in environment increase intracellular lipid accumulation and cause damage to the endoplasmic reticulum and mitochondria. Mice fed on high-fat diet have oocytes with accumulated lipid, increased reactive oxygen species (ROS), and have altered structure of mitochondria [159].

5.2.3 Endometrial hyperplasia

Abnormally thickened lining of the uterus due to disordered proliferation of endometrial glands or endometrial hyperplasia is caused by excess androgen with a relative deficiency of progesterone [160]. Untreated endometrial hyperplasia may develop into endometrial cancer [161]. Endogenous estrogen excess may occur in anovulatory cycles (during perimenopause or PCOS), obesity, and estrogen secreting tumors of the ovary. The most common symptom of endometrial hyperplasia is abnormal uterine bleeding.

5.3 Obesity-related complications in pregnancy

Women with obesity have a higher risk of miscarriage, gestational diabetes, preeclampsia, premature delivery, cesarean section, and post-partum hemorrhage. Maternal obesity with poor glycemic control may result in fetal macrosomia and associated complications. Twenty percent less detection of fetal anomalies has been reported in women with obesity [162].

5.3.1 Risk of miscarriage

A Danish cohort study [163] involving more than 5000 women reported a hazard ratio for miscarriage of 1.23 for women with obesity conceiving spontaneously. Risk of miscarriage is higher in women with obesity who conceive with IVF, even when using donor eggs from women with normal BMI.

5.3.2 Gestational diabetes

Schummers et al. [164] studied 226,000 singleton pregnancies in British Columbia. They have reported an incidence of gestational diabetes of 7.9%. The risk of gestational diabetes was doubled with a BMI > 30, and more than tripled at BMI > 40 kg/m^2.

5.3.3 Risk of preeclampsia

Women with overweight have double the risk of preeclampsia, while women with obesity have triple the risk, compared with women with normal BMI [164, 165]. Increased physical activity during pregnancy may reduce the risk of both gestational diabetes and preeclampsia.

5.3.4 Preterm labor

Obesity has been shown to increase the risk of preterm delivery [165, 166]. This may be due to increased levels of circulating cytokines and inflammatory proteins in women with obesity.

5.3.5 Cesarean section

The rate of Cesarean section increases with increase in maternal BMI [165, 167]. There is also an increased risk of wound infection, dehiscence, post-partum hemorrhage, and deep vein thrombosis. Duration of labor is longer in women with obesity. There is an increased risk of fetal distress, instrumental delivery, and shoulder dystocia in women with obesity.

6. Economic consequences of obesity

Obesity is a risk factor for various diseases (see above). Expenses on medicine, loss of pay due to absence from work caused by illness, reduced job opportunities, etc., lead to constraint on family budget [168].

6.1 Direct expenses

These include the medical expenses on obesity-related diseases. Expense on medicines for hypertension, type 2 diabetes, dyslipidemia, kidney diseases, stroke; and medical expenses incurred on hospitalization for various conditions affect the family budget as well as the budget of the country [169].

6.2 Indirect expenses

Absence from work due to disease results in decreased pay and early mortality affects the family income. Kjellberg et al. [170] report a 2% decrease in income, 3% increase in social transfer payments, and a 4% increase in healthcare costs per BMI point above 30. Thus, the indirect costs constitute the greatest proportion of total costs associated with obesity. Lee et al. [171] have reported that women with higher BMI are 0.33 times less likely to have service jobs, earn 9% lower monthly wages, and are half as likely to have jobs with bonuses compared with those with normal BMI.

7. Mental and social issues

Obesity is considered a social stigma in most societies. People with obesity are considered responsible for their condition and are often the victims of teasing and bullying, at all ages, from preschool through adolescence to adulthood [172–176].

7.1 Bullying

Bullying is intentional unprovoked aggression that may be physical (hitting, shoving), mental (name calling, spreading rumors, social exclusion, fat shaming on social media) or both, which causes harm to the victim. It involves an imbalance of physical or psychological power. Weight-based victimization is more common at younger age, but may be observed in adults also [177]. It has been noted that pre-adolescent or adolescent boys with overweight or obesity who are stronger than their peer may show bullying behavior, victimizing those who are physically weaker than them [178].

7.2 Binge eating

Binge eating disorder (BED) is a type of disordered eating in which the individual consumes a relatively large amount of food in a short span of time, compared with other people of the same age, gender, and weight. BED affects 1–3% of the general population. People with BED are 3–6 times more likely to be overweight or obese than persons without eating disorders [179]. Around 30% persons with BED report a history of childhood obesity [180].

7.3 Depression

Meta-analysis conducted by Luppino et al. [181] shows a reciprocal link between depression and obesity. Obesity increases the risk of depression, and depression is predictive of developing obesity. Both obesity and depression are common and both are risk factors for cardiovascular diseases [182]. Depression is also an important cause of premature mortality, primarily due to suicide.

8. Quality of life and mortality

Obesity and the associated diseases affect the quality of life and influence the length of life span [183].

8.1 Decreased quality of life

Health-related quality of life encompasses physical, mental, and social health and is influenced by factors such as socioeconomic status, culture, and environment of the person concerned. The degree of obesity is inversely proportional with the quality of life, as persons with higher BMI values are more likely to have obesity-associated diseases [184].

8.2 Risk of mortality

At least 2.8 million people die annually as a consequence of being overweight or obese. Many complications of obesity are mentioned above that deteriorate the quality of life and may promote early death. Most of the deaths are a direct consequence of cardiovascular problems or cancer [185].

9. Conclusion

Obesity is a condition that can compromise health and is closely associated with various medical conditions caused by increased body mass, metabolic derangement, psychological effects, or economic or social aspects. Awareness about the causes and consequences of obesity should be created among the general public so that persons with obesity may receive timely care with empathy.

Conflict of interest

None.

Author details

Indu Saxena[1*], Amar Preet Kaur[1], Suwarna Suman[2], Abhilasha[3], Prasenjit Mitra[4], Praveen Sharma[5] and Manoj Kumar[6]

1 Department of Biochemistry, All India Institute of Medical Sciences Gorakhpur, Gorakhpur, Uttar Pradesh, India

2 Department of Ophthalmology, All India Institute of Medical Sciences Johdpur, Johdpur, Rajasthan, India

3 Department of Biochemistry, All India Institute of Medical Sciences Patna, Patna, Bihar, India

4 Sanjay Gandhi Post Graduate Institute of Medical Sciences, Chandigarh, India

5 Department of Biochemistry, All India Institute of Medical Sciences Jodhpur, Jodhpur, Rajasthan, India

6 Maharshi Vashishtha Autonomous State Medical College, Basti, India

*Address all correspondence to: indu.saxena@rediffmail.com

References

[1] Wang T, Hung CCY, Randall DJ. The comparative physiology of food deprivation: From feast to famine. Annual Review of Physiology. 2006;**68**:223-225

[2] Van Ginneken VJT, Antonissen E, Muller UK, Booms R, Eding E, Verreth J, et al. Eel migration to the sargasso: Remarkably high swimming efficiency and low energy costs. The Journal of Experimental Biology. 2005;**208**:1329-1335

[3] Boetius I, Boetius J. Lipid and protein content in Anguilla anguilla during growth and starvation. Dana. 1985;**4**:1-17

[4] Oka T, Nishimura Y, Zang L, Hirano M, Shimada Y, Wang Z, et al. Diet-induced obesity in zebrafish shares common pathophysiological pathways with mammalian obesity. BMC Physiology. 2010;**10**:21. DOI: 10.1186/1472-6793-10-21

[5] Hackbarth R. Reptile Diseases. Neptune City (NJ): TFH Publications; 1990

[6] Warwick C. Reptilian disease in relation to artificial environments, with special reference to ethology. International Colloquium on Pathology and Medicine of Reptiles and Amphibians. 1991;**4**:107-119

[7] Beaufrère H, Nevarez JG, Holder K, Pariaut R, Tully TN, Wakamatsu N. Characterization and classification of psittacine atherosclerotic lesions by histopathology, digital image analysis, transmission and scanning electron microscopy. Avian Pathology. 2011;**40**(5):531-544

[8] Forhan M, Gill SV. Obesity, functional mobility and quality of life. Best Practice & Research Clinical Endocrinology & Metabolism. 2013;**27**:129-137. DOI: 10.1016/j.beem.2013.01.003

[9] Finkelstein EA, Chen H, Prabhu M, Trogdon JG, Corso PS. The relationship between obesity and injuries among U.S. adults. American Journal of Health Promotion. 2007;**21**:460-468

[10] Capodaglio P, Cimolin V, Tacchini E, et al. Balance control and balance recovery in obesity. Current Obesity Reports. 2012;**1**:166-173. DOI: 10.1007/s13679-012-0018-7

[11] Abramson SB, Attur M. Developments in the scientific understanding of osteoarthritis. Arthritis Research. 2009;**11**:227-236

[12] Grotle M, Hagen KB, Natvig B, Dahl FA, Kvien TK. Obesity and osteoarthritis in knee, hip and/or hand: An epidemiological study in the general population with 10 years follow-up. BMC Musculoskeletal Disorders. 2008;**9**(1):1-5

[13] Widmyer MR, Utturkar GM, Leddy HA, Coleman JL, Spritzer CE, Moorman CT III, et al. High body mass index is associated with increased diurnal strains in the articular cartilage of the knee. Arthritis and Rheumatism. 2013;**65**(10):2615-2622

[14] Fujisawa T, Hattori T, Takahashi K, Kuboki T, Yamashita A, Takigawa M. Cyclic mechanical stress induces extracellular matrix degradation in cultured chondrocytes via gene expression of matrix metalloproteinases and interleukin-1. The Journal of Biochemistry. 1999;**125**(5):966-975

[15] Fermor B, Weinberg JB, Pisetsky DS, Misukonis MA, Fink C,

Guilak F. Induction of cyclooxygenase-2 by mechanical stress through a nitric oxide-regulated pathway. Osteoarthritis and Cartilage. 2002;**10**(10):792-798

[16] Collins KH, Herzog W, MacDonald GZ, Reimer RA, Rios JL, Smith IC, et al. Obesity, metabolic syndrome, and musculoskeletal disease: Common inflammatory pathways suggest a central role for loss of muscle integrity. Frontiers in Physiology. 2018;**9**:112. DOI: 10.3389/fphys.2018.00112

[17] Roddy E, Choi HK. Epidemiology of gout. Rheumatic Diseases Clinics of North America. 2014;**40**(2):155-175

[18] Ter Maaten JC, Voorburg A, Heine RJ, Ter Wee PM, Donker AJ, Gans RO. Renal handling of urate and sodium during acute physiological hyperinsulinaemia in healthy subjects. Clinical Science (London, England). 1997;**92**(1):51-58

[19] Karlsson C, Lindell K, Ottosson M, Sjöström L, Carlsson B, Carlsson LM. Human adipose tissue expresses angiotensinogen and enzymes required for its conversion to angiotensin II. The Journal of Clinical Endocrinology and Metabolism. 1998;**83**(11):3925-3929. DOI: 10.1210/jcem.83.11.5276

[20] Roddy E, Doherty M. Gout and osteoarthritis: A pathogenetic link? Joint, Bone, Spine. 2012;**79**(5):425-427

[21] Ma CA, Leung YY. Exploring the link between uric acid and osteoarthritis. Frontiers in Medicine (Lausanne). 2017;**4**:225. DOI: 10.3389/fmed.2017.00225

[22] Leone N, Courbon D, Thomas F, Bean K, Jégo B, Leynaert B, et al. Lung function impairment and metabolic syndrome: The critical role of abdominal obesity. American Journal of Respiratory and Critical Care Medicine. 2009;**179**(6):509-516

[23] Ochs-Balcom HM, Grant BJ, Muti P, Sempos CT, Freudenheim JL, Trevisan M, et al. Pulmonary function and abdominal adiposity in the general population. Chest. 2006;**129**(4):853-862

[24] Jones RL, Nzekwu MM. The effects of body mass index on lung volumes. Chest. 2006;**130**(3):827-833

[25] Beuther DA, Sutherland ER. Overweight, obesity, and incident asthma: A meta-analysis of prospective epidemiologic studies. American Journal of Respiratory and Critical Care Medicine. 2007;**175**(7):661-666

[26] Sideleva O, Suratt BT, Black KE, Tharp WG, Pratley RE, Forgione P, et al. Obesity and asthma: An inflammatory disease of adipose tissue not the airway. American Journal of Respiratory and Critical Care Medicine. 2012;**186**(7):598-605

[27] De Blasio MJ, Boije M, Kempster SL, Smith GC, Charnock-Jones DS, Denyer A, et al. Leptin matures aspects of lung structure and function in the ovine fetus. Endocrinology. 2016;**157**(1):395-404

[28] Sood A, Ford ES, Camargo CA Jr. Association between leptin and asthma in adults. Thorax. 2006;**61**(4):300-305

[29] Dixon AE, Peters U. The effect of obesity on lung function. Expert Review of Respiratory Medicine. 2018;**12**(9):755-767. DOI: 10.1080/17476348.2018.1506331

[30] Fimognari FL, Pasqualetti P, Moro L, Franco A, Piccirillo G, Pastorelli R, et al. The association between metabolic syndrome and restrictive ventilatory dysfunction in older persons. The Journals of Gerontology. Series A, Biological Sciences and Medical Sciences. 2007;**62**(7):760-765

[31] Benotti P, Wood GC, Argyropoulos G, Pack A, Keenan BT, Gao X, et al. The

impact of obstructive sleep apnea on nonalcoholic fatty liver disease in patients with severe obesity. Obesity (Silver Spring). 2016;**24**(4):871-877. DOI: 10.1002/oby.21409

[32] Romero-Corral A, Caples SM, Lopez-Jimenez F, Somers VK. Interactions between obesity and obstructive sleep apnea: Implications for treatment. Chest. 2010;**137**(3):711-719. DOI: 10.1378/chest.09-0360

[33] Willenberg T, Schumacher A, Amann-Vesti B, Jacomella V, Thalhammer C, Diehm N, et al. Impact of obesity on venous hemodynamics of the lower limbs. Journal of Vascular Surgery. 2010;**52**(3):664-668. DOI: 10.1016/j.jvs.2010.04.023

[34] Danielsson G, Eklof B, Grandinetti A. L. Kistner R. The influence of obesity on chronic venous disease. Vascular and Endovascular Surgery. 2002;**36**(4):271-276

[35] Davies HO, Popplewell M, Singhal R, Smith N, Bradbury AW. Obesity and lower limb venous disease - The epidemic of phlebesity. Phlebology. 2017;**32**(4):227-233. DOI: 10.1177/0268355516649333

[36] Ageno W, Piantanida E, Dentali F, Steidl L, Mera V, Squizzato A, et al. Body mass index is associated with the development of the post-thrombotic syndrome. Thrombosis and Haemostasis. 2003;**89**:305-309

[37] Hansson PO, Eriksson H, Welin L, Svärdsudd K, Wilhelmsen L. Smoking and abdominal obesity: Risk factors for venous thromboembolism among middle-aged men: The study of men born in 1913. Archives of Internal Medicine. 1999;**159**(16):1886-1890

[38] Kasielska-Trojan A, Sobczak M, Antoszewski B. Risk factors of striae gravidarum. International Journal of Cosmetic Science. 2015;**37**(2):236-240

[39] Oakley AM, Patel BC. Stretch Marks. Treasure Island (FL): StatPearls Publishing; 2021. p. 2021. Available from: https://www.ncbi.nlm.nih.gov/books/NBK436005/

[40] Waldman RA, Kettler AH. Dermatologic manifestations of obesity: Part I mechanical causes. Journal of Obesity and Weight-loss Medication. 2016;**1**:010

[41] Kalra MG, Higgins KE, Kinney BS. Intertrigo and secondary skin infections. American Family Physician. 2014;**89**(7): 569-573

[42] Scheinfeld NS. Obesity and dermatology. Clinics in Dermatology. 2004;**22**(4):303-309. DOI: 10.1016/j.clindermatol.2004.01.001

[43] El Safoury OS, Ibrahim M. A clinical evaluation of skin tags in relation to obesity, type 2 diabetes mellitus, age, and sex. Indian Journal of Dermatology. 2011;**56**(4):393-397. DOI: 10.4103/0019-5154.84765

[44] Pandey A, Sonthalia S. Skin Tags. Treasure Island (FL): StatPearls Publishing; 2021. p. 2021

[45] Zabawski E, Styles A, Goetz D, Cockerell C. Asymptomatic facial papules and acrochordons of the thighs Birt-Hogg-Dube syndrome. Dermatology Online Journal. 1997;**3**(2):6

[46] Sachs C, Lipsker D. The molluscum pendulum necklace sign in tuberous sclerosis complex: A case series a pathognomonic finding? Journal of the European Academy of Dermatology and Venereology. 2017;**31**(11):e507-e508

[47] Pollitzer S. Acanthosis nigricans: A symptom of a disorder of the

abdominal sympathetic. Journal of the American Medical Association. 1909;**53**(17):1369-1373

[48] Robinson SS, Tasker S. Acanthosis nigricans juvenilis associated with obesity; report of a case, with observations on endocrine dysfunction in benign acanthosis nigricans. Archives of Dermatology and Syphilology. 1947;**55**(6):749-760

[49] Kutlubay Z, Engin B, Bairamov O, Tüzün Y. Acanthosis nigricans: A fold (intertriginous) dermatosis. Clinics in Dermatology. 2015;**33**(4):466-470

[50] Schilling WH, Crook MA. Cutaneous stigmata associated with insulin resistance and increased cardiovascular risk. International Journal of Dermatology. 2014;**53**(9):1062-1069

[51] Waldman RA, Kettler AH. Dermatologic manifestations of obesity: Part 2 endocrine abnormalities. Australian Journal of Dermatology. 2016;**3**(3):1053-1059

[52] Sayed CJ, Hsiao JL, Okun MM. Hidradenitis suppurativa foundation Women's health subcommittee. Clinical epidemiology and Management of Hidradenitis Suppurativa. Obstetrics and Gynecology. 2021;**137**(4):731-746. DOI: 10.1097/AOG.0000000000004321

[53] Burt Solorzano CM, Knudsen KL, Anderson AD, Hutchens EG, Collins JS, Patrie JT, et al. Insulin resistance, hyperinsulinemia, and LH: Relative roles in peripubertal obesity-associated hyperandrogenemia. The Journal of Clinical Endocrinology and Metabolism. 2018;**103**(7):2571-2582. DOI: 10.1210/jc.2018-00131

[54] McCartney CR, Prendergast KA, Chhabra S, Eagleson CA, Yoo R, Chang RJ, et al. The association of obesity and hyperandrogenemia during the pubertal transition in girls: Obesity as a potential factor in the genesis of postpubertal hyperandrogenism. The Journal of Clinical Endocrinology and Metabolism. 2006;**91**(5):1714-1722. DOI: 10.1210/jc.2005-1852

[55] Napolitano M, Megna M, Monfrecola G. Insulin resistance and skin diseases. The Scientific World Journal. 2015;**1**:247-250. DOI: 10.1155/2015/479354

[56] Poretsky L, Cataldo NA, Rosenwaks Z, Giudice LC. The insulin-related ovarian regulatory system in health and disease. Endocrine Reviews. 1999;**20**:535-582

[57] Kaspersen KA, Pedersen OB, Petersen MS, Hjalgrim H, Rostgaard K, Møller BK, et al. Obesity and risk of infection: Results from the Danish blood donor study. Epidemiology. 2015;**26**(4):580-589. DOI: 10.1097/EDE.0000000000000301

[58] Harpsøe MC, Nielsen NM, Friis-Møller N, Andersson M, Wohlfahrt J, Linneberg A, et al. Body mass index and risk of infections among women in the Danish National Birth Cohort. American Journal of Epidemiology. 2016;**183**(11):1008-1017. DOI: 10.1093/aje/kwv300

[59] Kane H, Lynch L. Innate immune control of adipose tissue homeostasis. Trends in Immunology. 2019;**40**:857-872. DOI: 10.1016/j.it.2019.07.006

[60] Nakamizo S, Honda T, Kabashima K. Obesity and inflammatory skin diseases. Trends in Immunotherapy. 2017;**3**(1):98. DOI: 10.24294/ti.v3.i1.98

[61] Hashba H, Bifi J, Thyvalappil A, Sridharan R, Sreenivasan A, Mathew P. Prevalence of metabolic syndrome in

patients with lichen planus: A cross-sectional study from a tertiary care center. Indian Dermatology Online Journal. 2018;**9**(5):304-308. DOI: 10.4103/idoj.IDOJ_27_18

[62] Subak LL, Richter HE, Hunskaar S. Obesity and urinary incontinence: Epidemiology and clinical research update. The Journal of Urology. 2009;**182**(Suppl. 6):S2-S7. DOI: 10.1016/j.juro.2009.08.071

[63] Bays HE, Gonzalez-Campoy JM, Bray GA, Kitabchi AE, Bergman DA, Schorr AB, et al. Pathogenic potential of adipose tissue and metabolic consequences of adipocyte hypertrophy and increased visceral adiposity. Expert Review of Cardiovascular Therapy. 2008;**6**(3):343-368

[64] Cinti S. The adipose organ at a glance. Disease Models & Mechanisms. 2012;**5**(5):588-594. DOI: 10.1242/dmm.009662

[65] Ishibashi J, Seale P. Medicine Beige can be slimming. Science. 2010;**328**:1113-1114

[66] Petrovic N, Walden TB, Shabalina IG, Timmons JA, Cannon B, Nedergaard J. Chronic peroxisome proliferator-activated receptor gamma (PPARgamma) activation of epididymally derived white adipocyte cultures reveals a population of thermogenically competent, UCP1-containing adipocytes molecularly distinct from classic brown adipocytes. Journal of Biological Chemistry. 2015;**285**(10):7153-7164. DOI: 10.1074/jbc.M109.053942

[67] Boström P, Wu J, Jedrychowski MP, Korde A, Ye L, Lo JC, et al. A PGC1-α-dependent myokine that drives brown-fat-like development of white fat and thermogenesis. Nature. 2012;**481**(7382):463-468

[68] Shan T, Liang X, Bi P, Zhang P, Liu W, Kuang S. Distinct populations of adipogenic and myogenic Myf5-lineage progenitors in white adipose tissues. Journal of Lipid Research. 2013;**54**(8):2214-2224. DOI: 10.1194/jlr.M038711

[69] Zwick RK, Guerrero-Juarez CF, Horsley V, Plikus MV. Anatomical, physiological, and functional diversity of adipose tissue. Cell Metabolism. 2018;**27**(1):68-83. DOI: 10.1016/j.cmet.2017.12.002

[70] Monzon JR, Basile R, Heneghan S, Udupi V, Green A. Lipolysis in adipocytes isolated from deep and superficial subcutaneous adipose tissue. Obesity Research. 2002;**10**(4):266-269

[71] Bays H, Mandarino L, DeFronzo RA. Role of the adipocyte, free fatty acids, and ectopic fat in pathogenesis of type 2 diabetes mellitus: Peroxisomal proliferator-activated receptor agonists provide a rational therapeutic approach. The Journal of Clinical Endocrinology and Metabolism. 2004;**89**(2):463-478. DOI: 10.1210/jc.2003-030723

[72] Available from: https://analyzedirect.com/documents/guides/adipose_tissue_classification_and_quantification.pdf

[73] Shen W, Wang Z, Punyanita M, Lei J, Sinav A, Kral JG, et al. Adipose tissue quantification by imaging methods: A proposed classification. Obesity Research. 2003;**11**(1):5-16. DOI: 10.1038/oby.2003.3

[74] Hausman DB, DiGirolamo M, Bartness TJ, Hausman GJ, Martin RJ. The biology of white adipocyte proliferation. Obesity Reviews. 2001;**2**:239-254

[75] Wang Q, Imam MU, Yida Z, Wang F. Peroxisome proliferator-activated receptor gamma (PPARγ) as a target for concurrent management of diabetes and obesity-related cancer. Current Pharmaceutical Design.

2017;**23**:3677-3688. DOI: 10.2174/1381612 82366617070412510

[76] Rey-López JP, de Rezende LF, Pastor-Valero M, Tess BH. The prevalence of metabolically healthy obesity: A systematic review and critical evaluation of the definitions used. Obesity Reviews. 2014;**15**:781-790. DOI: 10.1111/obr.12198

[77] Stenkula KG, Erlanson-Albertsson C. Adipose cell size: Importance in health and disease. American Journal of Physiology—Regulatory, Integrative and Comparative Physiology. 2018;**315**:R284-R295

[78] Misra A, Vikram NK. Clinical and pathophysiological consequences of abdominal adiposity and abdominal adipose tissue depots. Nutrition. 2003;**19**:457-466

[79] Ouchi N, Parker JL, Lugus JJ, Walsh K. Adipokines in inflammation and metabolic disease. Nature Reviews. Immunology. 2011;**11**(2):85-97

[80] Weisberg SP, McCann D, Desai M, Rosenbaum M, Leibel RL, Ferrante AW. Obesity is associated with macrophage accumulation in adipose tissue. The Journal of Clinical Investigation. 2003;**112**:1796-1808. DOI: 10.1172/ JCI200319246

[81] Blouin K, Nadeau M, Perreault M, Veilleux A, Drolet R, Marceau P, et al. Effects of androgens on adipocyte differentiation and adipose tissue explant metabolism in men and women. Clinical Endocrinology. 2010;**72**(2):176-188

[82] Morino K, Petersen KF, Shulman GI. Molecular mechanisms of insulin resistance in humans and their potential links with mitochondrial dysfunction. Diabetes. 2006;**55**(Supplement 2):S9-S15

[83] Snel M, Jonker JT, Schoones J, Lamb H, de Roos A, Pijl H, et al. Ectopic fat and insulin resistance: Pathophysiology and effect of diet and lifestyle interventions. International Journal of Endocrinology. 2012;**2012**(7):983814. DOI: 10.1155/ 2012/983814

[84] Morawietz H, Bornstein SR. Leptin, endothelin, NADPH oxidase, and heart failure. Hypertension. 2006;**47**(5):e20-e21

[85] Barone I, Giordano C, Bonofiglio D, Andò S, Catalano S. Leptin, obesity and breast cancer: Progress to understanding the molecular connections. Current Opinion in Pharmacology. 2016;**31**:83-89. DOI: 10.1016/j.coph.2016.10.003

[86] Saxena NK, Taliaferro-Smith L, Knight BB, et al. Bidirectional crosstalk between leptin and insulin-like growth factor-I signaling promotes invasion and migration of breast cancer cells via transactivation of epidermal growth factor receptor. Cancer Research. 2008;**68**:9712-9722. DOI: 10.1158/0008-5472.CAN-08-1952

[87] Mori H, Hanada R, Hanada T, Aki D, Mashima R, Nishinakamura H, et al. Socs3 deficiency in the brain elevates leptin sensitivity and confers resistance to diet-induced obesity. Nature Medicine. Jul 2004;**10**(7):739-743

[88] Noel P, Patel K, Durgampudi C, Trivedi RN, de Oliveira C, Crowell MD, et al. Peripancreatic fat necrosis worsens acute pancreatitis independent of pancreatic necrosis via unsaturated fatty acids increased in human pancreatic necrosis collections. Gut. 2016;**65**:100-111

[89] Sarwar R, Pierce N, Koppe S. Obesity and nonalcoholic fatty liver disease: Current perspectives. Diabetes, Metabolic Syndrome and Obesity: Targets and Therapy. 2018;**11**:533-542. DOI: 10.2147/DMSO.S146339

[90] Chait A, den Hartigh LJ. Adipose tissue distribution, inflammation and its metabolic consequences, including diabetes and cardiovascular disease. Frontiers in Cardiovascular Medicine. 2020;**7**:22. DOI: 10.3389/fcvm.2020.00022

[91] Qi XY, Qu SL, Xiong WH, Rom O, Chang L, Jiang Z-S. Perivascular adipose tissue (PVAT) in atherosclerosis: A double-edged sword. Cardiovascular Diabetology. 2018;**17**(134):1-20. DOI: 10.1186/s12933-018-0777-x

[92] Hursting SD, Digiovanni J, Dannenberg AJ, et al. Obesity, energy balance, and cancer: New opportunities for prevention. Cancer Prevention Research (Philadelphia, Pa.). 2012;**5**:1260-1272

[93] Bhaskaran K, Douglas I, Forbes H, et al. Body- mass index and risk of 22 specific cancers: A population-based cohort study of 5.24 million UK adults. Lancet. 2014;**384**:755-765

[94] Niedermaier T, Behrens G, Schmid D, Schlecht I, Fischer B, Leitzmann MF. Body mass index, physical activity, and risk of adult meningioma and glioma: A meta-analysis. Neurology. 2015;**85**(15):1342-1350. DOI: 10.1212/WNL.0000000000002020

[95] Solinas G, Karin M. JNK1 and IKKbeta: Molecular links between obesity and metabolic dysfunction. The FASEB Journal. 2010;**24**:2596-2611

[96] Nakamura T, Furuhashi M, Li P, Cao H, Tuncman G, Sonenberg N, et al. Double-stranded RNA-dependent protein kinase links pathogen sensing with stress and metabolic homeostasis. Cell. 2010;**140**:338-348

[97] Iyengar NM, Hudis CA, Dannenberg AJ. Obesity and cancer: Local and systemic mechanisms. Annual Review of Medicine. 2015;**66**:297-309

[98] Lonergan PE, Tindall DJ. Androgen receptor signaling in prostate cancer development and progression. Journal of Carcinogenesis. 2011;**10**:20

[99] Subbaramaiah K, Morris PG, Zhou XK, et al. Increased levels of COX-2 and prostaglandin E2 contribute to elevated aromatase expression in inflamed breast tissue of obese women. Cancer Discovery. 2012;**2**:356-365

[100] Irahara N, Miyoshi Y, Taguchi T, et al. Quantitative analysis of aromatase mRNA expression derived from various promoters (I.4, I.3, PII and I.7) and its association with expression of TNF-alpha, IL-6 and COX-2 mRNAs in human breast cancer. International Journal of Cancer. 2006;**118**:1915-1921

[101] Brown KA, McInnes KJ, Hunger NI, et al. Subcellular localization of cyclic AMP-responsive element binding protein-regulated transcription coactivator 2 provides a link between obesity and breast cancer in postmenopausal women. Cancer Research. 2009;**69**:5392-5399

[102] Randi G, Franceschi S, La Vecchia C. Gallbladder cancer worldwide: Geographical distribution and riskfactors. International Journal of Cancer. 2006;**118**(7):1591-1602

[103] Bishayee A. The role of inflammation and liver cancer. Advances in Experimental Medicine and Biology. 2014;**816**:401-435

[104] Calle EE, Rodriguez C, Walker-Thurmond K, Thun MJ. Overweight, obesity, and mortality from cancer ina prospectively studied cohort of U.S. adults. New England Journal of Medicine. 2003;**348**(17):1625-1638

[105] Schmitz KH, Neuhouser ML, Agurs-Collins T, Zanetti KA, Cadmus-Bertram L, Dean LT, et al. Impact of obesity on cancer survivorship and the potential relevance of race and ethnicity. Journal of the National Cancer Institute. 2013;**105**(18):1344-1354. DOI: 10.1093/jnci/djt223

[106] Paskett ED, Dean JA, Oliveri JM, Harrop JP. Cancer-related lymphedema risk factors, diagnosis, treatment, and impact: A review. Journal of Clinical Oncology. 2012;**30**(30):3726-3733

[107] Gacci M, Sebastianelli A, Salvi M, et al. Role of abdominal obesity for functional outcomes andcomplications in men treated with radical prostatectomy for prostate cancer: Results of the MulticenterItalian report on radical prostatectomy (MIRROR) study. Scandinavian Journal of Urology. 2014;**48**(2):138-145

[108] Meyerhardt JA, Tepper JE, Niedzwiecki D, et al. Impact of body mass index on outcomes and treatment-related toxicity in patients with stage II and III rectal cancer: Findings from intergroup trial 0114. Journal of Clinical Oncology. 2004;**22**(4):648-657

[109] Teras LR, Kitahara CM, Birmann BM, et al. Body size and multiple myeloma mortality: A pooled analysisof 20 prospective studies. British Journal of Haematology. 2014;**166**(5):667-676

[110] Zang EA, Wynder EL. The association between body mass index and the relative frequencies of diseases in a sample of hospitalized patients. Nutrition and Cancer. 1994;**21**:247-261

[111] Cheung N, Wong TY. Obesity and eye diseases. Survey of Ophthalmology. 2007;**52**(2):180-195

[112] Klein BE, Klein R, Linton KL. Intraocular pressure in an American community. The beaver dam eye study. Investigative Ophthalmology & Visual Science. 1992;**33**:2224-2228

[113] Mori K, Ando F, Nomura H, et al. Relationship between intraocular pressure and obesity in Japan. International Journal of Epidemiology. 2000;**29**:661-666

[114] Age-Related Eye Disease Study Research Group. Risk factors associated with age-related macular degeneration. A case-control study in the age-related eye disease study: Age-related eye disease study report number 3. Ophthalmology. 2000;**107**:2224-2232

[115] Spaide RF, Armstrong D, Browne R. Continuing medical education review: Choroidal neovascularization in age-related macular degeneration--what is the cause? Retina. 2003;**23**:595-614

[116] van Leiden HA, Dekker JM, Moll AC, et al. Blood pressure, lipids, and obesity are associated with retinopathy: The Hoorn study. Diabetes Care. 2002;**25**:1320-1325

[117] Wong TY, Larsen EK, Klein R, et al. Cardiovascular risk factors for retinal vein occlusion and arteriolar emboli: The atherosclerosis risk in Communities & Cardiovascular Health studies. Ophthalmology. 2005;**112**:540-547

[118] Teuscher AU, Meienberg O. Ischaemic oculomotor nerve palsy. Clinical features and vascular risk factors in 23 patients. Journal of Neurology. 1985;**232**:144-149

[119] Raina J, Foster JA. Obesity as a cause of mechanical entropion. American Journal of Ophthalmology. 1996;**122**:123-125

[120] Krispel CM, Keltner JL, Smith W, Chu DG, Ali MR. Undiagnosed papilledema in a morbidly obese patient

population: A prospective study. Journal of Neuro-Ophthalmology. 2011;**31**:310-315

[121] Kristinsson JK, Carlson AN, Kim T. Keratoconus and obesity-a connection? Investigative Ophthalmology & Visual Science. 2003;**44**:812

[122] Venneman NG, van Erpecum KJ. Pathogenesis of gallstones. Gastroenterology Clinics of North America. 2010;**39**:171-183

[123] Py S, Hsu YC, Cheng YF, Kor CT, Su WW. Strong association between metabolically-abnormal obesity and gallstone disease in adults under 50 years. BMC Gastroenterol. 2019;**19**:117. DOI: 10.1186/s12876-019-1032-y

[124] Lammert F, Gurusamy K, Ko CW, Miquel JF, Mendez-Sanchez N, Portincasa P, et al. Gallstones. Nature Reviews Disease Primers. 2016;**2**:16024. DOI: 10.1038/nrdp.2016.24

[125] Pariente A, Erlinger S. Cholelithiasis and obesity: Epidemiology, pathophysiology, clinical manifestations and prevention. Hepato-Gastro Oncologie Digestive. 2017;**24**(1):18-25. DOI: 10.1684/hpg.2016.1395

[126] El-Serag HB, Hashmi A, Garcia J, Richardson P, Alsarraj A, Fitzgerald S, et al. Visceral abdominal obesity measured by CT scan is associated with an increased risk of Barrett's oesophagus: A case-control study. Gut. 2014;**63**(2):220-229

[127] Emerenziani S, Rescio MP, Guarino MP, Cicala M. Gastro-esophageal reflux disease and obesity, where is the link? World Journal of Gastroenterology. 2013;**19**(39):6536-6539. DOI: 10.3748/wjg.v19.i39.6536

[128] Eisenberg ML, Kim S, Chen Z, Sundaram R, Schisterman EF, Buck Louis GM. The relationship between male BMI and waist circumference on semen quality: Data from the LIFE study. Human Reproduction. 2014;**29**(2):193-200. DOI: 10.1093/humrep/det428

[129] Amiri M, Ramezani TF. Potential adverse effects of female and male obesity on fertility: A narrative review. International Journal of Endocrinology and Metabolism. 2020;**18**(3):e101776. DOI: 10.5812/ijem.101776

[130] Glenn T, Harris AL, Lindheim SR. Impact of obesity on male and female reproductive outcomes. Current Opinion in Obstetrics and Gynecology. 2019;**31**(4):201-206. DOI: 10.1097/GCO.0000000000000549

[131] De Lorenzo A, Noce A, Moriconi E, Rampello T, Marrone G, Di Daniele N, et al. MOSH syndrome (male obesity secondary hypogonadism): Clinical assessment and possible therapeutic approaches. Nutrients. 12 Apr 2018; **10**(4):474. DOI: 10.3390/nu10040474

[132] Tremellen K. Gut endotoxin leading to a decline IN Gonadal function (GELDING) - a novel theory for the development of late onset hypogonadism in obese men. Basic and Clinical Andrology. 2016;**26**(1):1-13

[133] Dohle GR, Arver S, Bettocchi C, Jones TH, Kliesch S. EAU guidelines in male hypogonadism. European Association of Urology. 2015;**3**:242-252

[134] Costanzo PR, Pacenza NA, Aszpis SM, Suárez SM, Pragier UM, Usher JGS, et al. Clinical and etiological aspects of gynecomastia in adult males: A multicenter study. BioMed Research International. 2018;**1**:1-7. DOI: 10.1155/2018/8364824

[135] Isidori AM, Caprio M, Strollo F, et al. Leptin and androgens in male

obesity: Evidence for leptin contribution to reduced androgen levels. The Journal of Clinical Endocrinology and Metabolism. 1999;**84**:3673-3680

[136] Hrabovszky E, Ciofi P, Vida B, et al. The kisspeptin system of the human hypothalamus: Sexual dimorphism and relationship with gonadotropin-releasing hormone and neurokinin B neurons. European Journal of Neuroscience. 2010;**31**:1984-1998

[137] Ohtaki T, Shintani Y, Honda S, et al. Metastasis suppressor gene KiSS-1 encodes peptide ligand of a G-protein-coupled receptor. Nature. 2001;**411**:613-724

[138] Dhillo WS, Chaudhri OB, PattersonM,etal.Kisspeptin-54stimulates the hypothalamic-pituitary gonadal axis in human males. The Journal of Clinical Endocrinology and Metabolism. 2005;**90**:6609-6615

[139] George JT, Veldhuis JD, Tena-SempereM, MillarRP, AndersonRA. Exploring the pathophysiology of hypogonadism in men with type 2 diabetes: Kisspeptin-10 stimulates serum testosterone and LH secretion in men with type 2 diabetes and mild biochemical hypogonadism. Clinical Endocrinology. 2013;**79**:100-104

[140] Cohen PG. The hypogonadal-obesity cycle: Role of aromatase in modulating the testosterone-estradiol shunt—A major factor in the genesis of morbid obesity. Medical Hypotheses. 1999;**52**:49-51

[141] Janiszewski PM, Janssen I, Ross R. Abdominal obesity and physical inactivity are associated with erectile dysfunction independent of body mass index. The Journal of Sexual Medicine. 2009;**6**:1990-1998

[142] Sermondade N, Faure C, Fezeu L, Shayeb AG, Bonde JP, Jensen TK, et al. BMI in relation to sperm count: An updated systematic review and collaborative meta-analysis. Human Reproduction Update. 2013;**19**(3):221-231

[143] Tunc O, Bakos HW, Tremellen K. Impact of body mass index on seminal oxidative stress. Andrologia. 2011;**43**:121-128

[144] Silvestris E, de Pergola G, Rosania R, Loverro G. Obesity as disruptor of the female fertility. Reproductive Biology and Endocrinology. 2018;**16**(1):22. DOI: 10.1186/s12958-018-0336-z

[145] Broughton DE, Moley KH. Obesity and female infertility: Potential mediators of obesity's impact. Fertility and Sterility. 2017;**107**(4):840-847. DOI: 10.1016/j.fertnstert.2017.01.017

[146] Practice Committee of the American Society for Reproductive Medicine. Obesity and reproduction: A committee opinion. Fertility and Sterility. 2015;**104**(5):1116-1126

[147] Duggal PS, Van Der Hoek KH, Milner CR, Ryan NK, Armstrong DT, Magoffin DA, et al. The in vivo and in vitro effects of exogenous leptin on ovulation in the rat. Endocrinology. 2000;**141**(6):1971-1976. DOI: 10.1210/endo.141.6.7509

[148] Dunaif A. Insulin resistance and the polycystic ovary syndrome: Mechanism and implications for pathogenesis. Endocrine Reviews. 1997;**18**(6):774-800. DOI: 10.1210/edrv.18.6.0318

[149] Cano F, Garcia-Velasco JA, Millet A, Remohi J, Simon C, Pellicer A. Oocyte quality in polycystic ovaries revisited: Identification of a particular subgroup of women. Journal of Assisted Reproduction and Genetics. 1997;**14**(5):254-261. DOI: 10.1007/BF02765826

[150] Carpentier AC. Postprandial fatty acid metabolism in the development of lipotoxicity and type 2 diabetes. Diabetes & Metabolism. 2008;**34**(2):97-107

[151] Tee MK, Dong Q, Miller WL. Pathways leading to phosphorylation of p450c17 and to the posttranslational regulation of androgen biosynthesis. Endocrinology. 2008;**149**(5):2667-2677

[152] Parihar M. Obesity and infertility. Reviews in Gynaecological Practice. 2003;**3**:120-126

[153] Giviziez CR, Sanchez EG, Approbato MS, Maia MC, Fleury EA, Sasaki RS. Obesity and anovulatory infertility: A review. JBRA Assisted Reproduction. 2016;**20**(4):240-245. DOI: 10.5935/1518-0557.20160046

[154] Wise LA, Rothman KJ, Mikkelsen EM, Sorensen HT, Riis A, Hatch EE. An internet-based prospective study of body size and time-to-pregnancy. Human Reproduction. 2010;**25**:253-264

[155] Gesink Law DC, Maclehose RF, Longnecker MP. Obesity and time to pregnancy. Human Reproduction. 2007;**22**:414-420

[156] Machtinger R, Combelles CM, Missmer SA, Correia KF, Fox JH, Racowsky C. The association between severe obesity and characteristics of failed fertilized oocytes. Human Reproduction. 2012;**27**(11):3198-3207

[157] Bellver J, Ayllon Y, Ferrando M, Melo M, Goyri E, Pellicer A, et al. Female obesity impairs in vitro fertilization outcome without affecting embryo quality. Fertility and Sterility. 2010;**93**:447-454

[158] Luke B, Brown MB, Stern JE, Missmer SA, Fujimoto VY, Leach R. SART writing group. Female obesity adversely affects assisted reproductive technology (ART) pregnancy and live birth rates. Human Reproduction. 2011;**26**(1):245-252

[159] Igosheva N, Abramov AY, Poston L, Eckert JJ, Fleming TP, Duchen MR, et al. Maternal diet-induced obesity alters mitochondrial activity and redox status in mouse oocytes and zygotes. PLoS One. 2010;**5**(4):e10074

[160] Parkash V, Fadare O, Tornos C, WG MC. Committee Opinion No. 631: Endometrial Intraepithelial Neoplasia. Obstetrics & Gynecology. 2015; **126**(4):897. DOI: 10.1097/AOG.0000000000001071

[161] Siegel RL, Miller KD, Jemal A. Cancer statistics. A Cancer Journal for Clinicians. 2018;**68**(1):7-30. DOI: 10.3322/caac.21442

[162] American College of Obstetricians and Gynecologists. ACOG practice bulletin no 156: Obesity in pregnancy. Obstetrics & Gynecology. 2015;**126**:e112-e126

[163] Hahn KA, Hatch EE, Rothman KJ, Mikkelsen EM, Brogly SB, Sørensen HT, et al. Body size and risk of spontaneous abortion among Danish pregnancy planners. Paediatric and Perinatal Epidemiology. 2014;**28**(5):412-423

[164] Schummers L, Hutcheon JA, Bodnar LM, Lieberman E, Himes KP. Risk of adverse pregnancy outcomes by prepregnancy body mass index: A population-based study to inform prepregnancy weight loss counseling. Obstetrics and Gynecology. 2015; **125**(1):133

[165] Marchi J, Berg M, Dencker A, Olander EK, Begley C. Risks associated with obesity in pregnancy, for the

mother and baby: A systematic review of reviews. Obesity Reviews. 2015;**16**(8):621-638

[166] Lutsiv O, Mah J, Beyene J, McDonald SD. The effects of morbid obesity on maternal and neonatal health outcomes: A systematic review and meta-analyses. Obesity Reviews. 2015;**16**(7):531-546

[167] Weiss JL, Malone FD, Emig D, Ball RH, Nyberg DA, Comstock CH, et al. Obesity, obstetric complications and cesarean delivery rate–a population-based screening study. American Journal of Obstetrics and Gynecology. 2004;**190**(4):1091-1097

[168] Spieker EA, Pyzocha N. Economic impact of obesity. Primary Care. 2016;**43**(1):83-95. DOI: 10.1016/j.pop.2015.08.013

[169] Thompson D, Edelsberg J, Colditz GA, Bird AP, Oster G. Lifetime health and economic consequences of obesity. Archives of Internal Medicine. 1999;**159**(18):2177-2183. DOI: 10.1001/archinte.159.18.2177

[170] Kjellberg J, Tange LA, Ibsen R, Højgaard B. The socioeconomic burden of obesity. Obesity Facts. 2017;**10**: 493-502. DOI: 10.1159/000480404

[171] Lee H, Ahn R, Kim TH, Han E. Impact of obesity on employment and wages among young adults: Observational study with panel data. International Journal of Environmental Research and Public Health. 2019;**16**(1):139. DOI: 10.3390/ijerph16010139

[172] Leeper L. Body size stigmatization in preschool children: The role of control attributions. Journal of Pediatric Psychology. 2004;**29**:613-620

[173] Klesges RC, Haddock CK, Stein RJ, Klesges LM, Eck LH, et al. Relationship between psychosocial functioning and body fat in preschool children: A longitudinal investigation. Journal of Consulting and Clinical Psychology. 1992;**60**:793-796

[174] Pierce JW, Wardle J. Cause and effect beliefs and self-esteem of overweight children. Journal of Child Psychology and Psychiatry. 1997;**38**:645-650

[175] Van Geel M, Vedder P, Tanilon J. Are overweight and obese youths more often bullied by their peers? A meta-analysis on the relation between weight status and bullying. International Journal of Obesity. 2014;**38**:1263-1267

[176] Puhl RM, Brownell KD. Bias, discrimination, and obesity. Obesity Research. 2001;**9**:788-805

[177] Bacchini D, Licenziati MR, Garrasi A, Corciulo N, Driul D, Tanas R, et al. Bullying and victimization in overweight and obese outpatient children and adolescents: An Italian multicentric study. PLoS One. 2015;**10**(11):e0142715. DOI: 10.1371/journal.pone.0142715

[178] Griffiths LJ, Wolke D, Page AS, Horwood P. Obesity and bullying: Different effects for boys and girls. Archives of Disease in Childhood. 2006;**91**:121-125

[179] Kessler RC, Berglund PA, Chiu WT, Deitz AC, Hudson JI, Shahly V, et al. The prevalence and correlates of binge eating disorder in the World Health Organization world mental health surveys. Biological Psychiatry. 2013;**73**(9):904-914

[180] Jacobi C, Hayward C, de Zwaan M, Kraemer HC, Agras WS. Coming to terms with risk factors for eating disorders: Application of risk terminology and suggestions for a general

taxonomy. Psychological Bulletin. 2004;**130**(1):19-65

[181] Luppino FS, de Wit LM, Bouvy PF, et al. Overweight, obesity, and depression: A systematic review and meta-analysis of longitudinal studies. Archives of General Psychiatry. 2010;**67**(3):220-229. DOI: 10.1001/archgenpsychiatry.2010.2

[182] Penninx BW, Beekman AT, Honig A, Deeg DJ, Schoevers RA, van Eijk JT, et al. Depression and cardiac mortality: Results from a community-based longitudinal study. Archives of General Psychiatry. 2001;**58**(3):221-227

[183] Taylor VH, Forhan M, Vigod SN, McIntyre RS, Morrison KM. The impact of obesity on quality of life. Best Practice & Research. Clinical Endocrinology & Metabolism. 2013;**27**(2):139-146

[184] Stephenson J, Smith CM, Kearns B, et al. The association between obesity and quality of life: A retrospective analysis of a large-scale population-based cohort study. BMC Public Health. 2021;**21**(1):1-9. DOI: 10.1186/s12889-021-12009-8

[185] De Gonzalez AB, Hartge P, Cerhan JR, Flint AJ, Hannan L, MacInnis RJ, et al. Body-mass index and mortality among 1.46 million white adults. NEJM. 2010;**363**(23):2211-2219

Chapter 6

Personalized Strategy of Obesity Prevention and Management Based on the Analysis of Pathogenetic, Genetic, and Microbiotic Factors

Svitlana Drozdovska, Olena Andrieieva, Valeriya Orlenko, Igor Andrieiev, Victoriya Pastukhova, Iuliia Mazur, Olha Hurenko and Anastasiia Nahorna

Abstract

This chapter reviews the issue of overweight management, which is one of the major challenges faced by most countries today. The causes of obesity include genetic and epigenetic factors, a lack of physical activity, eating disorders, and gut microbiota status. Physical exercise is the main means of prevention and management of overweight and obesity. The effectiveness of exercise programs for obese people typically varies around 80%, but it can be increased by taking into account biochemical, genetic, epigenetic, and microbiome markers, which allows choosing the most appropriate type of exercise according to individual characteristics. The pathogenetic preconditions for reducing exercise tolerance were examined based on the existing imbalance of adipokines, cytokines, and incretins. The association between genotype and weight loss induced by different diets and types of exercise was discussed along with obesity epigenetic markers. The effects of dietary choice on the microbiome composition and its contribution to the development of systemic inflammation in obese people were assessed. The weight management exercise program for middle-aged women was presented. The structure and value of the factors that determine the physical condition of overweight middle-aged women were described. These data provide the basis for designing a sound exercise program for weight management.

Keywords: gene polymorphisms, obesity, exercise training, personalized approach, health-enhancing physical exercise

1. Introduction

Obesity is one of the modern world challenges, which has become epidemic and has negatively affected population health. Obesity and overweight, which in most cases accompany metabolic syndrome and type 2 diabetes, are among the independent risk factors for overall mortality, including death from cardiovascular disease and cancer [1]. In recent years, special attention has been given to the sedentary lifestyle of people of almost all ages, as it is proven that lack of physical activity is an independent significant factor in deteriorating health. A meta-analysis of studies examining the relationship between physical activity and overall mortality showed that a higher level of total physical activity of any intensity and less time spent in sedentary behaviors are associated with a significant reduction in the risk of overall mortality [2].

In addition to physical inactivity, eating disorders, and intestinal microbiota status, the causes of obesity include genetic factors, such as gene polymorphisms and epigenetic modifications. Weight loss training programs are the major means of obesity prevention, cardiovascular fitness improvement, and body mass reduction. However, the effectiveness of these programs ranges from 79–83%. The outcomes of exercise training aimed at weight loss in overweight and obese adults depend on individual characteristics of the body, such as morphological and metabolic features, developed under the influence of hereditary and environmental factors throughout life. A number of informative biochemical, genetic, epigenetic, and microbiotic markers can be used to determine the most effective mode of exercise training according to individual metabolic characteristics.

The current situation in the world only exacerbates it drawing attention to the increased risk of COVID-19-related death in overweight and obese people. The problem of being overweight in light of the current epidemic situation is further exacerbated as the quarantine restrictions, which are periodically imposed by state and municipal authorities, contribute to the spread of hypodynamia among the population. The stress provoked by the epidemic situation triggers destructive eating behaviors with excessive calorie density. Hypodynamia and excessive calorie density make them gain weight even more and lead to greater health risks. The urgency of this problem stipulates the need to develop a personalized approach to designing physical exercise programs for obese people and assess the impact of individual markers of obesity on the effectiveness of such programs.

2. Imbalance of adipokines, cytokines, and incretins as a pathogenetic risk factor for reduced exercise tolerance

The progressive increase in obesity prevalence during the second half of the last century has put adipose tissue at the center of scientific interest. It is now seen not only as a passive reservoir for the accumulation of energy reserves but as a metabolically active endocrine organ that secretes hormones and cytokines. Adipose tissue cytokines and adipokines are involved in the regulation of many vital processes, the imbalance of which results in the development of insulin resistance, metabolic syndrome, diabetes, and cardiovascular complications. Many studies confirm that the presence of metabolic syndrome or any of its components correlates with the level of pro-inflammatory cytokines [3].

Our studies showed a significant increase in IL-6 (interleukin 6), TNF-α (tumor necrosis factor alpha), and OPG (osteoprotegerin) in subjects with overweight and obesity irrespective of the presence of carbohydrate metabolism disorders confirming the significant role of overweight and obesity in the development of nonspecific inflammation, one of the main pathogenetic risk factors for metabolic disorders development (**Table 1**). We wanted to pay special attention to a new cytokine identified in obese people.

Cytokine	No diabetes mellitus (n = 50)				Type 2 diabetes mellitus (n = 58)			
	No obesity (n = 19)	Obesity (n = 31)	t	p	No obesity (n = 20)	Obesity (n = 38)	t	p
TNF-alpha	12.1 ± 1.2	22.0 ± 1.4	5.2	0.001	13.6 ± 0.5	24.8 ± 1.5	7.3	0.001
IL-1	13.6 ± 2.3	11.5 ± 0.6	0.9	0.433	10.5 ± 0.4	12.1 ± 1.0	1.6	0.127
IL-6	17.4 ± 3.3	36.4 ± 0.7	5.6	0.001	13.5 ± 2.7	38.1 ± 2.0	7.3	0.001
S IL-6R	294.6 ± 31.3	333.4 ± 17.6	1.1	0.317	365.0 ± 54.2	354.1 ± 25.2	1.3	0.252
Osteoprotegerin	8.7 ± 0.8	23.9 ± 2.2	6.6	0.001	7.4 ± 1.3	23.4 ± 2.6	5.5	0.001

Note: p—statistical significance of the difference between the groups with and without obesity.

Table 1.
Mean cytokine levels (pg/mL) in obese patients.

The glycoprotein OPG, which belongs to the tumor necrosis factor receptor superfamily, was initially identified as an inhibitor of bone resorption, however other important regulatory functions of OPG have been later identified. The OPG/RANKL (NF-κB ligand receptor) axis has been shown to play a significant regulatory role in the skeletal, immune, and vascular systems, including vascular calcification that accompanies atherosclerosis. Elevated OPG levels are associated with the incidence and prevalence of coronary heart disease. Moreover, increased OPG is considered as an independent risk factor for overall vascular mortality in obese adults and IR (insulin resistant) [4]. Our data showed that the OPG level was the most sensitive proinflammatory cytokine. This is confirmed by other authors. Kotanidou et al. (2018) reported that obese individuals show an increase in serum OPG already during puberty, and a key factor in the regulation of OPG is IR, which accompanies even the initial metabolic disorders on the background of excessive body weight [5].

We also investigated the levels of some hormones, which we believe play a key role in the regulation of appetite, neurophysiological relationships between the gut-brain axis and muscles, and physical activity (**Table 2**).

The most significant changes were observed in insulin and leptin. Hyperinsulinemia as a consequence of insulin resistance and hyperleptinemia are the most common hormonal disorders in the background of being overweight. These data are confirmed by numerous studies. Leptin is one of the most well-known adipose tissue hormones; it is very sensitive to energy consumption, especially in energy-deficient conditions. It has been shown that a reduction in the serum leptin was observed before fat loss even after 2–3 days of a low-calorie diet. Decreased leptin levels can cause a number of biological and hormonal responses, including the decreased activity of the sympathetic nervous system, hypothalamic gonadotropin-releasing hormones, IGF-I (insulin growth factor I), GH (increased production of growth hormone), and ACTH (adrenocorticotropic hormone). Conversely, hyperleptinemia, which is common in overweight people, is associated with leptin resistance. At night, the leptin level is 30% higher [4]. In the presence of obesity, the level of leptin is increased many times, and a 10% decrease in body weight decreases its blood content by 50%. According to modern ideas, leptin sends a signal to the hypothalamus by activating specific leptin receptors, which are located in different parts of the brain – hypothalamus, cerebellum, cortex, hippocampus, thalamus, and vascular plexus of the cerebral capillary endothelium [6].

An important regulator of leptin secretion is hyperinsulinemia. Adipocytes produce leptin in response to increased postprandial insulin levels in healthy people and patients with metabolic syndrome. Based on numerous studies, we can conclude that the feedback mechanism between the level of insulin secretion by β-cells and fat and muscle cells utilizing glucose depends only on leptin action because leptin receptors are present in the islets of Langerhans of the pancreas, so there is a direct relationship between the concentration of insulin and its effect on the secretion of hormones by adipocytes. Normally, due to the increase in insulin secretion, production of leptin increases that inhibits the secretion and release of insulin by the feedback mechanism [7].

It should be noted that in our study we did not find a significant difference in cortisol levels between patients with normal body weight and obesity. However, it is well known that over time, elevated glucocorticoid levels can lead to increased skeletal muscle protein breakdown, adipose tissue lipolysis, and hepatic gluconeogenesis accompanied by decreased glucose utilization. These effects increase circulating blood glucose levels, thus contributing to insulin resistance and hyperinsulinemia.

Hormone	No diabetes mellitus (n = 50)				Type 2 diabetes mellitus (n = 58)			
	No obesity (n = 19)	Obesity (n = 31)	t	p	No obesity (n = 20)	Obesity (n = 38)	t	p
Insulin (μUnits/mL)	5.5 ± 0.7	8.9 ± 0.3	5.1	0.001	6.4 ± 0.3	14.3 ± 1.4	5.4	0.001
Leptin (ng/mL)	18.2 ± 4.4	32.3 ± 3.8	2.4	0.020	18.4 ± 6.2	39.8 ± 3.9	2.6	0.014
Cortisol (nmol/L)	427.6 ± 45.7	461.5 ± 41.5	0.5	0.632	425.7 ± 43.9	440.9 ± 26.5	0.3	0.759

Note: p—statistical significance of the difference between the groups with and without obesity.

Table 2.
Mean hormone levels in obese patients.

In recent years, there has been increasing information about the effects of incretins, which are a group of gut-derived hormones, on the regulation of body weight. Modern pharmacological therapy of obesity is associated with the introduction of GLP-1 (glucagon-like peptide-1) agonists, the level of which is significantly reduced in overweight and obese people irrespective of disorders of carbohydrate metabolism. Incretin hormones, such as GLP-1 and GIP (glucose-dependent insulinotropic peptide), are secreted from the gastrointestinal tract into the portal circulatory system in response to nutrients. In a nutrient-dependent manner, incretins have been shown to contribute to lowering blood glucose levels by increasing insulin secretion, decreasing glucagon secretion, and decreasing the rate of gastric emptying. The main effect of GLP-1 is glucose-dependent stimulation of insulin secretion by pancreatic beta cells. GLP-1 slows down the rate of gastric emptying, which helps to reduce fluctuations in postprandial glycemia [8, 9]. GLP-1 also enhances the feeling of satiety and reduces food intake, by providing prolonged stimulation of mechanoreceptors and satiation receptors. Decreased food intake may be mediated by a direct effect of GLP-1 on sensory neurons located in the upper gastrointestinal tract or by a direct effect on the central nervous system because GLP-1 receptors are present in the hypothalamic centers that regulate food intake.

Physical activity combined with a balanced diet is the basis for the prevention and normalization of weight gain and obesity. No modern guidelines for weight correction, impaired carbohydrate metabolism, prevention, and treatment of cardiovascular complications can be provided without a primary emphasis on the need for physical activity. At least 150 min per week of moderate-intensity physical activity is the minimum required to ensure active metabolism of basic, carbohydrate and fat metabolism. For example, the American Diabetes Association currently provides the following recommendations for physical activity/exercise for people with carbohydrate metabolism disorders. Daily exercise, or at least not allowing more than 2 days to elapse between exercise sessions, is recommended to enhance insulin action. Adults with type 2 diabetes should ideally perform both aerobic and resistance exercise training for optimal glycemic and health outcomes. Structured lifestyle interventions that include at least 150 min/week of physical activity and dietary changes resulting in weight loss of 5–7% are recommended to prevent or delay the onset of type 2 diabetes in populations at high risk and with prediabetes [10]. To date, the influence of physical activity on the pathogenetic risk factors of overweight and obesity has been proven, including optimization of the secretion of adipose tissue hormones, incretins and reduction of low-gradient nonspecific inflammation [11, 12].

The most convincing data on the effects of physical activity on adipose tissue hormones concern leptin. It has been shown that short-term exercise does not affect leptin levels in healthy people. However, longer and more intense exercises (≥60 min), which are associated with increased energy expenditure (≥800 kcal), lead to a decrease in leptin levels [13, 14]. In general, lifestyle changes that result in weight loss contribute to the normalization of serum insulin and leptin levels [15].

An inverse relationship was also found between physical activity and proinflammatory cytokine levels in obesity, diabetes, and metabolic syndrome. It is believed that the positive effect of exercise, which is partly mediated by changes in the profile of adipokines, is an increase in anti-inflammatory cytokines with a decrease in proinflammatory ones. This effect was described at the level of gene expression, protein ligands, and receptor binding [16]. For example, exercises increase insulin sensitivity by lowering TNF-α, C-reactive protein, and increasing adiponectin. Interleukin-6 is the first cytokine that appears in the bloodstream during exercise, and its levels increase exponentially in response to exercise [17]. The increase in IL-6 levels in plasma caused by exercise correlates with the muscle mass, as well as with the mode, duration and, especially, the intensity of exercise. Infusion of recombinant human IL-6 (rhIL-6) in humans simulates the IL-6 response to exercise and prevents an increase in plasma TNF-α [18]. Inhibition of IL-6-induced TNF-α production has also been shown in cultured human monocytes. Furthermore, IL-6 stimulates the release of other anti-inflammatory cytokines, including IL-10 and IL-1Ra. These and other experiments suggest that the anti-inflammatory effects of exercise are partly mediated by IL-6 levels [19].

It has also been shown that normal physical activity can affect glucose-induced GLP-1 secretion [20]. The more time spent in physical activity, the more pronounced is the glucose-induced GLP-1 response irrespective of insulin sensitivity. This indicates a positive effect of normal moderate-intensity physical activity on GLP-1 secretion that may help improve glucose regulation and reduce the risk of type 2 diabetes [21, 22]. Therefore, physical activity contributes not only to weight normalization but also improves metabolic disorders characteristic of obese and overweight people.

3. Role of genetic factors in weight loss efficiency

The common reasons are believed to be unhealthy eating habits and low physical activity, but undoubtedly body weight is also influenced by genetic factors that account for 40–70% variance in BMI [23]. Besides, there are marked inter-individual differences in terms of weight loss even if energy consumption and expenditure are supervised [24].

A plethora of studies has shown that SNPs (single nucleotide polymorphisms) of certain genes are associated with weight, waist circumference, distribution, and types of fat tissue. Moreover, an accumulating number of epidemiological evidence indicate that genetic pressure could be one of the leading factors in the obesity epidemic spread due to the assortative mating and increased number of offspring in individuals with higher BMI [25]. Thus, obesity-associated genetic variants could become more common in the population, thus demanding new weight-loss strategies that take into consideration the interaction between genetic factors, diet, and physical activity. Only a rare number of genetic mutations can lead to unavoidable obesity, hence, the impact of genetics on BMI could be diminished by environmental and behavioral factors [25]. Identification of genetic factors determining individual susceptibility to weight loss can be used to choose the appropriate intensity and mode of weight loss program intervention and diet macronutrient composition or to suggest alternative treatment methods, such as surgery or pharmacological intervention.

Obesity is an extreme form of fat tissue accumulation. According to thermodynamics laws, even low continuous excess of calories income over calories expenditure causes obesity development [26], although the reasons for increased or decreased dietary intake could be different.

The long-term efficiency of weight loss is considerably determined by dietary habits that include nutritional composition, timing, quantity, and quality of food intake. The genetic predictors influencing the nervous system function define nutritional behavior and can lead to monogenic obesity forms. For example, SNPs of the *MC4R* (melanocortin 4 receptor), *BDNF* (brain-derived neurotrophic factor), and *FTO* (fat mass and obesity-associated) genes are associated with hyperphagia and increased fat macronutrient intake [25]. From this perspective, designing an individual nutrition plan taking into consideration genetically predetermined dietary habits is important to improve long-term adherence to the prescribed diet.

All successful weight loss programs are focused on reducing caloric intake through the alteration of macronutrient composition (i.e., low-carb vs. low-fat diet, high-protein diet) [27], although different methods of creating a calorie deficit may be chosen depending on an individual's genetic profile (**Figure 1**).

FTO is one of the most studied obesity-related genes and its genetic variants are associated with higher total energy and fat intake, reduced satiety, and craving for calories dense food [26, 28], which partially can be explained by a higher level of appetite-related hormones (ghrelin and leptin) [29]. High-protein diets could be a useful tool in managing satiety [27] and reduction of appetite-related hormones in case of *FTO*-associated obesity. For example, carriers of risk allele *FTO* rs1558902 experience a greater weight loss in response to a 2-year high-protein diet intervention program; and, generally, higher content of protein in a diet is preventive against weight gain for this risk allele carrier [30]. Furthermore, the carriers of rs1558902 SNP experience more metabolic benefits from high-fat diets compared to low-fat diets [31]. Putting together this data allows for designing a diet plan for the rs1558902 risk allele carriers with the highest adherence (high protein), weight loss, and health improvement (high fat) properties.

Several other SNPs are also associated with a greater weight loss in response to a high-fat diet plan, including *HNF1A* (hepatocyte nuclear factor-1 alpha) gene rs7957197 minor T allele, *TNF-α* gene rs1800629 minor A allele, and *CYP2R1 (*cytochrome P450 2R1*)* gene rs10741657 minor A allele [32]. The last association may suggest that a high amount of dietary high-quality fat also contains other essential nutrients, such as vitamin D, that could be beneficial for people prone to its deficiency. Similarly, monounsaturated fats are well known for their anti-inflammatory properties in obesity [33] and a diet plan full of these fats is beneficial for IL-6 polymorphism rs1800795 associated with the higher inflammatory process [32].

However, despite the increased satiety properties, a high-fat, high-protein plan is not a universal approach. Often the carriers of genes variants that impair insulin

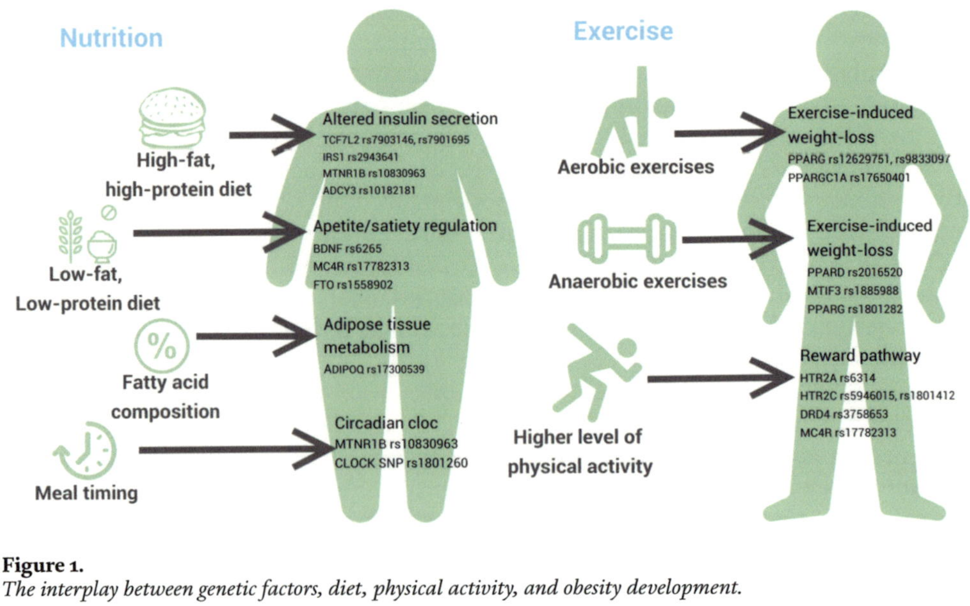

Figure 1.
The interplay between genetic factors, diet, physical activity, and obesity development.

secretion benefit more from low-fat diets. For instance, the *ADCY3* (adenylate cyclase 3) gene codes for an adenylate cyclase protein, which is responsible for the formation of cyclic AMP, a secondary messenger involved in insulin secretion, decreased mTOR signaling and lipogenesis, and promoted thermogenesis and fatty acid oxidation. The minor allele of *ADCY3* rs10182181 SNP has been shown to correlate with increased BMI. The carriers of this allele lost more weight with low-fat diets in comparison to high-protein diets [34]. Such improvement can be explained by a higher percentage of carbohydrates in a diet and its positive influence on insulin signal function. The same is known for the two *TCF7L2* (transcription factor 7-like 2) SNPs rs7903146 and rs7901695—the individuals with these risk alleles for type 2 diabetes undergo lower weight loss with a high-fat diet [32, 35, 36] and experience more metabolic benefits from lower protein intake. Likewise, the carriers of the *MTNR1B* (melatonin receptor 1B) risk allele rs10830963, which is associated with increased fasting glucose and type 2 diabetes, experience greater weight loss with a low-fat diet [37]. Similar results are obtained with the *IRS1* (insulin receptor substrate 1) genetic variant related to insulin resistance and increased BMI. Those with the SNP risk allele rs2943641 lose more weight with the high-carbohydrate low-fat diet, while the low-carbohydrate high-fat diet is more suitable for the noncarriers [38].

Additionally, different macronutrient compositions should be considered for the carriers of different *PPARG2* (peroxisome proliferator-activated receptor gamma) rs1801282 and *PPM1K* (protein phosphatase 1 K) rs1440581 polymorphisms. The GG and GC genotypes (obesity-related G allele carriers) of the *PPARG2* gene lose more fat following a low-fat diet, whereas individuals with the CC genotype experience greater weight loss with a high-fat nutrition plan [39]. Although *PPM1K* is the gene coding for a protein participating in the branched-chain amino acid metabolism, its SNP rs1440581 T allele correlates with higher fasting glucose and higher BMI and is associated with greater fat loss following a high-fat diet [32], while a low-fat diet has more benefits for individuals with the CC genotype [40].

Moreover, the composition of dietary fats, that is, the proportion of saturated, poly-, and monounsaturated fats, can be critical for a successful weight loss for the specific genotypes. *ADIPOQ* is a gene that encodes for adiponectin, the most ubiquitous protein hormone that is secreted by the adipose tissue. The level of serum adiponectin is correlated with BMI and has 80% heritability [41]. Its expression can be affected by the rs17300539 SNP located in the proximal promoter region. A risk variant of this gene is associated with higher BMI, although the genetic impact on body weight becomes negligible when the level of dietary intake of MUFA (monounsaturated fatty acids) is reduced to less than 13% of energy intake [28]. However, for another *ADIPOQ* SNP rs266729 located in the promoter region, two studies revealed no benefits for weight loss in the minor risk allele carriers with different body compositions [41, 42]. Although individuals with all genotypes showed an improvement in body weight and parameters of glucose homeostasis, non-risk allele carriers showed better response.

The timing of meals can also be an important part of weight-loss strategies since some of the circadian rhythm signaling proteins are associated with increased BMI and diabetes. For example, G allele of *MTNR1B* (melatonin receptor 1B) rs10830963 was found to be associated with higher BMI and higher resting glucose levels, however, the association was more significant in early sleep timing compared to late sleep timing [43]. This allele was associated with elevated melatonin levels early in the morning, thus simultaneous food intake additionally elevates blood glucose levels and may disturb circadian rhythm regulation. Similarly, weight loss resistance is the case for carriers of the C allele of *CLOCK* (basic helix–loop–helix-PAS transcription factor) SNP rs1801260 is also associated with higher activity in the second half of the day [44]. This data suggests the disturbance of the natural circadian rhythm due to modern lifestyle. This knowledge could help align meal timing with the natural cycle so that carriers of the risk allele could experience more weight loss by scheduling their breakfast later in the day.

While dietary lifestyle changes are a key weight loss factor, individuals experience more metabolic and health benefits when those are combined with physical activity intervention [24]. Although WHO recommends a minimal 150 min per week of moderate exercise for health improvement, a number of studies have shown that such amount of physical activity is not sufficient for clinically significant weight loss, thus indicating the need for increased physical activity to 225–420 min per week. It is decidedly more likely to lose more weight with increased physical activity, however, the optimal level of physical exercise still should be determined (**Figure 1**). Furthermore, various types of exercises are available, for example, anaerobic, aerobic, and interval training, all of which affect body composition and metabolism in different ways and could be beneficial to different genotypes [45].

The PPAR (peroxisome proliferator-activated receptors) family genes are involved in lipolysis and lipogenesis, the efficiency of energy utilization, and mitochondrial biogenesis [45]. Some SNPs located in these genes are often associated with different weight loss outcomes in response to physical activity intervention. According to our data, SNPs (rs12629751, rs9833097) of the *PPARG* gene are associated with greater fat mass loss and improvement in cardiometabolic health. Another member of the peroxisome receptors family *PPARGC1A* is induced by physical activity and associated with an increased lipid oxidation rate. Our results showed that the polymorphism of this gene rs17650401 is correlated with the efficiency of fat mass loss following a moderate exercise intervention program [45].

As was mentioned, different types of physical activity would be beneficial for individuals with different genotypes (**Figure 1**). Well-known *PPARG* polymorphism Pro12Ala has no or even negative effects on weight loss in response to the aerobic training program [46]. Moreover, individuals with the high-risk SNP of *PPARD* gene rs2016520 also showed less weight loss after a moderate aerobic exercise program [47]. The 12Ala allele is associated with strong abilities and is responsible for the transition to an anaerobic energy supply during exercise [48], so carriers of this obesity-related allele can benefit more from the anaerobic intervention programs or high-intensity interval training. This is the case for the obesity-related SNP rs1885988 of the MTIF3 (mitochondrial translational initiation factor 3) gene, where intensive lifestyle interventions lead to more weight loss in risk-allele carriers [49].

Interestingly, the predisposition to physical activity seems to be heritable. The majority of genes responsible for this trait are involved in behavior control, mood, and reward pathway function. For instance, *MC4R* genes are associated with a low level of physical activity [50], therefore, the risk-allele carriers could be discouraged with high-intensity or high-impact exercise. In contrast, some polymorphisms are related to exercise adherence and even correlated with exercise dose (rs6314 *HTR2A,* 5-hydroxytryptamine receptor 2A), duration (rs5946015 *HTR2C* and rs3758653 *DRD4,* dopamine receptor D4), and intensity (rs1801412 *HTR2C*) [51], consequently, they can determine a better outcome from the higher level of physical activity.

Plenty of studies has indicated that there is a wide inter-individual variation in response to diet and physical activity weight-loss programs. Personalization of dietary and physical activity recommendations could be a powerful tool for planning the most appropriate weight loss plan taking into account subjective feeling of satiety (*FTO* variants), metabolic characteristics (polymorphisms associated with disrupted insulin signaling), meal schedule (*MTNR1B* and *CLOCK*), required level and type of physical activity (*PPAR* family genes), and long-term adherence to designed physical activity plan (MC4R, HTR genes, DRD4). Altogether genotyping data could be used for managing and preventing obesity with a higher level of success.

3.1 Personalization of health-promoting fitness programs for young women based on PPARG gene polymorphism

To personalize health-promoting fitness programs for young women, a study was conducted that included an assessment of women's physical fitness before and after the implementation of two 4-month health-promoting fitness programs (aerobic and resistance workouts). The personalized approach presupposed genotyping women according to Pro/Ala polymorphism of the PPARG gene. At the beginning of the pedagogical experiment, we formed two groups of women, the experimental group 1 (EG1) (resistance training, n = 24) and the experimental group 2 (EG2) (aerobic training, n = 20).

The results of the study showed the dependence of young women's physical fitness on their genotype for the above-mentioned polymorphism as a result of undergoing fitness programs by them. Resistance workouts caused significant changes in body composition, with a slight decrease in body weight and girth for women with Pro/Ala and Ala/Ala genotypes, while among women with Pro/Pro genotype, there was a significant decrease in body weight and girth. The level of physical fitness in women with Pro/Pro genotype increased by 11.1%, and in women with Pro/Ala and Ala/Ala genotype by 10.5% ($p < 0.05$) under the influence of the strength fitness program.

The patterns of the changes in the parameters of physical condition differed between the women with Pro/Pro genotype and Pro/Ala and Ala/Ala genotypes, who participated in aerobic training. Aerobic training resulted in significant changes in the bodyweight of young women in both subgroups.

Identification of genetic markers allows applying a differentiated approach in the development of fitness programs, which stipulates choosing the structure of the program, the ratio of aerobic and resistance activities, exercise intensity, and pulse regimes depending on the polymorphism of the *PPARG* gene [52].

3.2 Microbiome and obesity

The global obesity epidemic has stimulated a great interest in studying the effects of microbial metabolome on the metabolic profile and maintenance of the energy homeostasis of an individual. The study by Turnbaugh et al. was one of the first that showed the relationship between the gut microbiota and increased body weight [53]. These and other similar findings formed a basis for the development of ideas about the mechanisms of microbiome influence on metabolic pathways.

The introduction of new technologies based on the achievements of genomics, transcriptomics, proteomics, metabolomics, and bioinformatics, in the last decade, has revolutionized and expanded the understanding of the structure and function of the human microbiome, as well as of its key role in regulating metabolic processes in the macroorganism, absorption of nutrients, endogenous synthesis of essential enzymes, vitamins, and biologically active compounds [54].

3.3 Functional significance of microbial enterotypes

The microbiome consists of about 100 trillion microorganisms that exist in a symbiotic relationship with human hosts [55] and can be classified into four enterotypes: Bacteroides, Prevotella, Ruminococcus, and Firmicutes, which have different dominant classifications, pathways, functions, and correlations between coexisting genera. The Bacteroides enterotype metabolizes carbohydrates and proteins with enzymes involved in glycolysis and pentose phosphate pathways. Prevotella and Ruminococcus contribute to the transport and absorption of monosaccharides by enriching the membrane and binding gut mucin to hydrolyze it. Enterotypes use different strategies to obtain energy from substrates present in the gut ecosystem. The specific composition of enterotypes responds to special mechanisms of metabolism of carbohydrates, amino acids, and fatty acids, which determine the frequency of obesity and obesity-related metabolic diseases [56].

16S rRNA microbiome sequencing identified the relationship between microbial diversity and different physiopathological conditions and allowed to observe the behavior of different types and genera of bacteria in combination with different phenotypes, different types of diets, and, in particular, obesity [57]. It is assumed that the microbiome can regulate the extraction of energy substrates from food and energy balance of the body, thus promoting the development of obesity or protecting against it. This hypothesis was confirmed in a study by Gordon, which reported an increase in fat content in the body of gnotobiotic (germfree) rats after fecal transplantation from obese rats [58]. Some studies have shown an increase in the percentage of Firmicutes and a decrease in the percentage of Bacteroidetes in obese humans compared to humans and underweight rats [59], while the others did not find significant changes in microbial composition between the two groups, and some even reported the opposite results. The relationship between the gut microbiome and metabolic disorders was first proven in the laboratory of Jeffrey I. Gordon at the Washington University School of Medicine in St. Louis. The authors demonstrated that leptin-resistant mice, characterized by increased appetite and obesity, have a deficiency of Bacteroidetes and an increased relative proportion of Firmicutes compared with control animals [60].

3.4 Relationship between obesity and the ratio of Bacteroides and Firmicutes in fecal samples

Dysbiosis in obesity is often characterized by a decrease in microbial diversity, changes in the relative numbers of major enterotypes, such as Firmicutes and Bacteroidetes, and/or an increase in pathogenic microorganisms. In a study of 18 obese male volunteers, the percentage of total fecal bacteria identified as Bacteroides did not differ between obese subjects and a normal weight control group [57]. These results contrast with similar studies but are quite consistent taking into account significant inter-individual differences.

Despite the disagreement, the ratio of Firmicutes to Bacteroidetes was studied and associated with susceptibility to disease [60], particularly an increase in the number of Firmicutes and a decrease in Bacteroidetes were observed in obese patients and type 2 diabetics [61]. The ratio of Firmicutes and Bacteroidetes in the fecal samples of healthy adults was 10/1 and in obese patients was 100/1. Thus, obesity was shown to be associated with an increase in the number of Firmicutes and a decrease in fecal Bacteroidetes [62]. Also, the predominance of Firmicutes in the gut microbiota was constantly observed in obese subjects in the study of Lei et al. [60], and the number of Proteobacteria was related to a large number of genera Bacteroides, Prevotella, and Ruminococcus that is positively correlated with a healthy intestinal microbiota. Some authors believe that an important factor associated with obesity is not the ratio of Bacteroidetes to Firmicutes in the gut microbiota, but the amount of short-chain fatty acids produced by it [63].

3.5 Microbiota-derived metabolites

Microbial metabolites are able to affect the metabolic functions of the host and play a key role in the pathophysiology of metabolic diseases. Bacteria of the gut microbiome produce a large number of enzymes that catalyze the depolymerization of complex carbohydrates as well as the degradation of indigestible components of chyme to SCFA (short-chain fatty acids), which are not only energy substrates but can also serve as messengers participating in the immune and systemic inflammatory response [64] and affecting intestinal motility and vascular tone. Many human and animal studies have shown a clear relationship between gut microflora, SCFAs, and obesity.

Bile acids are also one of the most important microbial products with bioactivity in stimulating the secretion of gut hormones, as intestinal bacteria are involved in the deconjugation of bile acids, which are endogenous ligands of the FXR (nuclear Farnezoid receptor), found in various tissues, such as liver, intestines, kidneys, adipose tissue, and immune cells. Bile acid signaling through FXR plays a role in maintaining lipid and glucose homeostasis. Studies have shown that FXR-deficient mice have impaired insulin signaling with impaired regulation of glucose homeostasis and elevated blood cholesterol and triglyceride levels [65]. Among the microbiota-derived metabolites, TMAO (trimethyl N-oxide) should also be mentioned, which is an important modulating factor in various diseases and significantly affects platelet hyperactivity, abnormal plasma lipid levels, obesity, and insulin resistance [66].

However, the main end product of the hydrolysis of indigestible carbohydrates is SCFA, that is, acetic (acetate), propionic (propionate), and butyric (butyric) acids, which are the most common and make up >95% of the total content of SCFAs and are produced in an approximate molar ratio of 60:20:20, reaching a combined concentration of more than 100 mM in the intestinal lumen [67], and act as the main energy supply for intestinal epithelial cells and, therefore, can increase the protection of the mucous barrier [68]. As the primary metabolic end product, gram-negative Bacteroidetes produce acetate and propionate, while the type Firmicutes produce mostly butyrate [69]. Several animal and human studies have found elevated concentrations of SCFAs in feces (particularly propionate) in obese individuals compared to normal-weight subjects [70] and, at the same time, recent data suggest that butyrate and propionate may promote healthy metabolism by activating IGN (intestinal gluconeogenesis) [71], which plays a dual role in maintaining energy homeostasis—regulating food intake and increasing insulin sensitivity. Propionate can directly initiate gut-brain communication by acting as an agonist of FFAR3 (free fatty acid receptor 3) to induce IGN with a positive effect on host physiology [65]. SCFAs are not only involved in energy metabolism but also perform a signaling function by activating GPRs (G-protein bound receptors) or FFAR2 (free fatty receptor 2). As reported, propionic acid is the most powerful activator of this receptor [53]. GPRs are expressed in most cells of the gastrointestinal tract, as well as in adipose tissue and immune cells. High-level expression of this receptor was found in the endocrine L-cells of the ileum and colon, which produce GLP-1 and PYY (peptide YY), and, in this way, SCFAs can modulate the secretion of incretins and regulate the onset of satiety and appetite, thus affecting the metabolic mechanisms of obesity [72].

3.6 The role of dietary intervention

Accumulated data from numerous meta-analyzes shows that macronutrients, especially proteins, fats, and insoluble fiber, have a profound effect on the structure, function, and secretion of gut microbiota-derived metabolites that modulate multiple metabolic and inflammatory pathways. Genetic studies [73] have highlighted the importance of host genotype in determining the relative numbers of certain microbiome groups but found that Bacteroidetes can be influenced by host genetics, meaning that most environmental factors (including diet) determine their relative numbers by epigenetic influence.

Hyperphagia is common in obese individuals and refers to excessive calorie intake compared to the energy needed to maintain body weight, and it has been suggested that Bacteroidetes numbers are sensitive to this condition. Jumpertz et al. conducted an inpatient study of obese and normal body weight subjects, who were randomly assigned to a diet to maintain weight or to a hypercaloric diet (2400 and 3400 kcal/day, respectively). In subjects with normal body weight, hypercaloric diet results in a decrease in the level of Bacteroidetes in fecal samples by 20% simultaneously with an increase in energy intake by approximately 150 kcal [74]. A similar observation was made in the Finnish monozygotic twin's study, where a hypercaloric diet was also associated with a decrease in the number of Bacteroides [75]. Interestingly, gastric bypass surgery results in an increase in Bacteroides that may be due to a reduction in caloric load rather than weight loss [76].

A diet high in refined and processed foods, red meat, and sugary drinks, combined with low fiber, fruit, and vegetable intake, correlates positively with the development of metabolic diseases, such as diabetes and obesity, both of which are associated with low-grade systemic inflammation and endotoxemia due to decreased commensal microbiota [77]. In obese people, a high-protein, low-carbohydrate diet combined with caloric restriction has been reported to result in increased quantities of branched-chain fatty acids, reduced butyrate, and reduced Roseburia/Eubacterium rectale [78]. On the other hand, a diet with a high percentage of fat and sucrose led to a decrease in the diversity of gut microbiota, metabolic dysfunction, and an increase in the number of opportunistic pathogens [79]. The study by de Wit et al. [80] showed that a diet high in fat (45% energy from fat) with palm oil resulted in reduced fat absorption and increased concentration of fat in the feces compared to a diet with the addition of olive or safflower oil. The increase in the concentration of fecal fat in the palm oil group was accompanied by a decrease in microbial diversity, an increase in the ratio of Firmicutes to Bacteroidetes, and an increase in the expression of lipid-related genes in the mucosa that can be considered a sign of dysbiosis [80].

Preclinical studies showed that a high-fat diet can increase the proportion of gram-negative bacteria while reducing the number of gram-positive E. rectale/Clostridium coccoides and Bifidobacterium [81]. There is evidence that the use of emulsifiers to improve the sensory properties of food has increased in the production of low-fat foods, in part due to innovations in specialized products for health-conscious consumers. It has been reported that emulsifiers can potentially increase virulence factors and thus the pro-inflammatory potential of the microbiota and contribute to low-grade inflammation, which may promote colon carcinogenesis [82]. According to epidemiological studies showing that high protein intake from plant sources and dairy products is associated with protection against obesity [83], rats fed dietary soya as a source of protein had a lower body weight than rats fed beef, pork, or turkey [84]. A recent review of human and animal studies examining the effects of soy feeding on the microbiome found that consumption of soy products increased the numbers of Bifidobacterium and Lactobacilli and altered the ratio between Firmicutes and Bacteroidetes [85]. A study of dietary interventions in obese and overweight individuals showed that a large number of gut microbiota taxa increased due to a high-fiber diet with a low content of animal fats that improved the clinical symptoms associated with obesity [86].

Similarly, in a recent randomized clinical trial, obese individuals that were randomly assigned to a Mediterranean diet for a 2-year period displayed an increase in the genera Bacteroides, Prevotella, and Faecalibacterium and the genera Roseburia, Ruminococcus as well as in Parabacteroides distasonis and Faecalibacterium, which are known for their saccharolytic activity and ability to metabolize carbohydrates to short-chain fatty acids [87]. In another study, adherence to a Mediterranean diet characterized by high consumption of vegetables, legumes, and fruits was associated with the enrichment of Bacteroidetes and increased levels of SCFAs in feces. In contrast, nonadherence to the Mediterranean diet was associated with an increase in Ruminococcus and Streptococcus, and higher concentrations of TMAO (trimethylamine N-oxide) [88]. Furthermore, a recent meta-analysis of 12 randomized controlled trials involving 609 overweight and obese adult participants showed that consumption of isolated soluble fiber resulted in a reduction in BMI, body weight by 2.52 kg, fat deposits by 0.41%, fasting glucose by 0.17 mmol/L, and fasting insulin by 15.88 pg./mL compared to placebo treatment [89]. Numerous clinical trials examining the effect of the Mediterranean diet pattern on metabolic syndrome as well as a meta-analysis of findings from eight studies of more than 10,000 participants and five studies have reported positive effects of the Mediterranean diet pattern [90]. Some of these benefits include decreased waist circumference (−0.42 cm), increased serum HDL cholesterol (1.17 mg/dL), decreased serum TGs (−6.14 mg/dL), decreased systolic (−2.35 mm Hg) and diastolic (−1.58 mm Hg) blood pressure, and decreased blood glucose (−3.89 mg/dL) in participants who were instructed to consume a Mediterranean diet pattern compared with those who were not given instructions to change their diet [91].

4. Health-enhancing physical exercise for the management of excessive body weight in middle-aged women

Solving the issue of overweight by workouts in gyms and fitness studios is complicated by periodic bans and quarantine restrictions on the operation of the latter, so the search for an alternative becomes particularly relevant. In light of the mentioned facts, designing independent preventive and health-enhancing workouts aimed at body weight management and their further implementation for middle-aged women is a full-fledged alternative for group exercise classes. The need for scientific substantiation of the criteria for assessing the effectiveness of independent workouts aimed at body weight management in middle-aged women determined the direction of our research.

The treatment of overweight in middle-aged women includes planning, managing, and controlling certain indicators to achieve the basic goal, that is, effective management of body weight. Body weight measurements are already criteria that allow for evaluation of the effectiveness of a body weight management program. However, our research allows us to suggest a more comprehensive approach to the organization of the management of excessive body weight using physical exercise [92]. We have identified and substantiated a list of indicators of physical condition, which, in our opinion, should serve as benchmarks in the planning, management, and control of excessive body weight in middle-aged women. Furthermore, we developed the recommendations that include the most effective parameters of physical exercise workouts aimed at body weight management in middle-aged women. Taken together, the proposed approach to planning, managing, and controlling excessive body weight can be seen as an original strategy for improving health in middle-aged women.

The following methods were used to address the objectives of the study—theoretical analysis of special scientific and methodological literature; anthropometric, physiological, and pedagogical methods; and mathematical statistics. The physiological research methods used were as follows—assessment of adaptation potential, assessment of the level of physical health using the Apanasenko technique, and measurement of vital capacity (VL) using ergospirometric system Oxycom Pro. Oxygen saturation was measured with a pulse oximeter Beurer PO 80 (Germany). To assess the level of physical fitness and evaluate the maximum oxygen consumption (VO2max) as well as the aerobic and anaerobic thresholds, cardiopulmonary exercise tests were performed with a treadmill (LE-200 CE, Jaeger, Germany). Pedagogical testing included performing several physical fitness tests from the Eurofit battery to determine the level of physical condition. The results of the study were subjected to statistical data analysis using conventional tools of Statistica 10.0 statistical software.

The data obtained during the study allowed to identify "problematic" indicators of physical and functional condition (such as signs of visceral obesity, risks of metabolic syndrome, hypertension, tachycardia, and an unsatisfactory level of adaptation potential) in overweight women. The identification of "problematic" indicators, in turn, allowed to provide recommendations on the most desirable profile of the organization of fitness classes for middle-aged women, that is, preventive and health-enhancing classes. Among the different variations of the means used in the modern fitness industry, the programs with preventive and health-enhancing goals are the most expedient in the framework of the management of excessive body weight. The validity of our recommendations was also confirmed by the results of our study of the motivational priorities of fitness classes in middle-aged women ($n = 105$). Good health was indicated as a priority motive for the participation in physical exercise classes by 82.7% of respondents. Moreover, a low level of quality of life in the parameter of health was observed in the studied contingent according to the Scale of Quality of Life (SF-36). Summing up, we can conclude that the most appropriate profile for organizations of fitness classes is preventive and health-enhancing classes.

Factor analysis was used to develop the most informative criteria for assessing the effectiveness of independent preventive and health-enhancing workouts for overweight middle-aged women. As a result of the analysis, four factors were identified that account for 81.4% of the total variance in the original data. We found that the largest factor loadings (42.1% of the total variance of the sample) had indicators that characterize physical development. This factor 1 included 14 indicators—chest circumference (CC) at inhalation ($r = 0.875$ at $p < 0.01$); chest circumference (CC) at exhalation ($r = 0.848$ at $p < 0.01$); relative muscle mass ($r = 0.777$ at $p < 0.01$); chest excursion ($r = 0.768$ at $p < 0.01$); and basal metabolic rate ($r = 0.711$ at $p < 0.01$). The following indicators had negative factor loading—abdomen circumference ($r = -0.927$ at $p < 0.01$); waist circumference ($r = -0.926$ at $p < 0.01$); waist-to-hip ratio (WHR) ($r = -0.922$ at $p < 0.01$); CC ($r = 0.893$ at $p < 0.01$); the waist-to-height ratio (WHtR) ($r = -0.884$ at $p < 0.01$); body weight ($r = -0.820$ at $p < 0.01$); BMI ($r = -0.807$ at $p < 0.01$); and hip circumference ($r = -0.732$ at $p < 0.01$). The second most important factor had a 21.2% contribution to the total variance, and identified 10 indicators that characterize the capacity of the aerobic energy supply and functional state. This factor showed a statistically significant direct correlation with the following indicators: VO_2max ($r = 0.945$ at $p < 0.01$); VC (mL) ($r = 0.791$ at $p < 0.01$); VC (mL/kg) ($r = 0.715$ at $p < 0.01$); and IPC ($r = 0.714$ at $p < 0.01$). The following indicators had negative factor loadings on the second factor: AP ($r = -0.936$ at $p < 0.01$); HR recovery time after 20 squats in 30 s (min) ($r = -0.837$ at $p < 0.01$); Robinson index ($r = -0.832$ at $p < 0.01$); BPsys ($r = -0.824$ at $p < 0.01$); Bayevsky's stress index ($r = -0.820$ at $p < 0.01$); resting heart rate ($r = -0.812$ at $p < 0.01$); and BPdia ($r = -0.806$ at $p< 0.01$). The third factor had a 9.8% contribution to the total variance and consisted of six indicators that characterize the endurance and strength abilities. The fourth factor, which had an 8.3% contribution to the total variance, was formed by the indicators that characterize coordination abilities.

Taking into account the specifics of the studied contingent and based on the data of factor analysis, we selected five indicators that are recommended to use for the assessment of the effectiveness of independent preventive and health-enhancing exercise workouts for middle-aged women—waist circumference, abdomen circumference, waist-to-hip ratio, adaptive potential, and maximum oxygen consumption. To assess the informativeness of the selected indicators, we performed a correlation analysis to identify significant relationships.

The waist circumference correlated with 28 of the studied parameters, and the correlation coefficients ranged from $r = 0.210$ at $p < 0.05$ to $r = 0.852$ at $p < 0.001$. The abdomen circumference correlated with 29 studied parameters, and the correlation coefficients ranged from $r = -0.211$ at $p < 0.05$ to $r = 0.852$ at $p < 0.001$. Waist-to-hip ratio (WHR) significantly correlated with 24 indicators of physical condition. The adaptation potential showed high correlations with 24 parameters and the correlations coefficients ranged from $r = 0.222$ at $p < 0.05$ to $r = 0.902$ at $p < 0.001$. Maximum oxygen consumption was significantly correlated with 18 parameters.

The indicators from the groups of the first and second factors had the highest loadings, so we consider them as criteria for effective planning, management, and control of body weight.

Furthermore, we experimentally substantiated methodological guidelines for the organization of fitness workouts for middle-aged women. We recommend doing 50–60 min of physical activity 3–4 times a week. Independent workouts should include exercise for the development of strength and general endurance with own body weight in the mode of alternating performance and aerobic exercise in the mode of continuous performance. Depending on the level of individual fitness, we recommend the percentage of special and general exercises ranged from 40–25% and 60 to 75%, respectively. The target heart rate zone for the aerobic part of workouts should be between 140 and 160 bpm for training activities and between 120 and 130 bpm for recovery activities. The intensity should range from 50–70% of VO_2max. Exercise load should be increased by increasing the coordination complexity of the exercises, the use of supersets of exercises, and circuit training.

We developed the plant for independent workouts that allowed to achieve a steady decrease in body weight and improved physical condition among the studied middle-aged women. After the study, we observed significant changes in the body weight, BMI, and body circumferences, as well as in the anthropometric measurements that indicate the harmony of the body: BMI decreased by 11.9%, waist circumference decreased by 12.1%, abdomen circumference decreased by 9.6%, and BW decreased by 10.6%. The data obtained showed the improvement of cardiopulmonary function

Hormonal changes	**High risk**	**leptin ↑, insulin ↑, GLP-1 ↓**
	Moderate risk	**IL-6 ↑, TNF-α ↑, OPG ↑, C-reactive protein ↑**
Genetic variants	High risk	*MC4R (rs17782313), BDNF (rs12291063), FTO (rs1558902), ADIPOQ (rs17300539, rs266729), PPARG (rs1801282)*
	Moderate risk	*ADCY3 (rs10182181), TCF7L2 (rs7903146, rs7901695), IRS1 (rs2943641), PPM1K (rs1440581), MTNR1B (rs10830963), PPARG (rs12629751, rs9833097), MTIF3 (rs1885988)*
Microbiome composition	High risk	Firmicutes/Bacteroidetes ↑
	Moderate risk	Decreased diversity (Bacteroides, Prevotella, Ruminococcus, Faecalibacterium, Roseburia, Bifidobacterium ↓)
Intestinal metabolite changes	High risk	SCFA ↓, deconjugated bile acids ↓
	Moderate risk	branched-chain fatty acids ↑, TMAO ↑

Table 3.
Risk factors in developing obesity and resistance to weight-loss intervention programs.

and increase in the body's adaptation potential, as well as the economization of cardiac pump function, which was evidenced by the changes in the heart rate, BPsys, and BPdia values. The risk of developing hypertension was reduced in the subjects as their BP values ranged from 90 to 130 mmHg for systolic pressure and from 65 to 80 mmHg for diastolic pressure. In women, there were observed statistically significant ($p < 0.05$; $p < 0.01$) improvements in lung vital capacity and heart rate recovery after dynamic exercise, which characterize the cardiopulmonary function. An increase of 10.8% in the mean group value of maximum oxygen consumption indicates an increase in the level of physical working capacity.

The results of the study demonstrate an example of an effective program for excessive body mass management in middle-aged women and allow to recommend a wider general use of the scientifically substantiated methodical guidelines for overweight management through health-enhancing physical activity for middle-aged women. Assessment of the obesity-related risks (**Table 3**) helps to establish a population that additionally benefits from the suggested weight-loss program. The annual blood check with selected hormone level determination and popularity of individual genetic tests may be practical tools for the advanced introduction of nutritional lifestyle changes and augmentation of physical activity. As well, specific identification of microbiome changes, shifts of its metabolite levels, and some genetic SNPs can be a basis of efficient individual dietary plan development.

5. Conclusions

One of the main ways of preventing the development of obesity, managing body weight, and improving the indicators of physical condition is properly organized physical activity and a balanced diet. The combination of a balanced diet with increased physical activity will reduce body weight, whereas a change in lifestyle will help to maintain the achieved result. Physical activity contributes not only to body weight normalization but also has positive effects on metabolic disorders characteristic of people with obesity and overweight. The effectiveness of physical activity can be significantly increased by taking into account a set of biochemical, genetic, and microbiome markers. The presented findings of clinical trials and meta-analyzes emphasize the complexity of interactions and the obvious relationships between genetic, epigenetic, metabolic factors and gut microbiota in the modulation of obesity and its complications. The application of a strategy of personalization of a highly effective health-enhancing exercise program, based on genetic, biochemical, and microbiome markers, will allow to achieve a high health-promoting effect and effectiveness of body weight management and prevent the development and progression of pathological conditions.

Author details

Svitlana Drozdovska[1*], Olena Andrieieva[1], Valeriya Orlenko[2], Igor Andrieiev[3], Victoriya Pastukhova[1], Iuliia Mazur[1], Olha Hurenko[1] and Anastasiia Nahorna[1]

1 National University of Ukraine on Physical Education and Sport, Ukraine

2 V.P. Komisarenko Institute Endocrinology and Metabolism of the National Academy of Medical Sciences of Ukraine, Ukraine

3 Institute of Molecular Biology and Genetics National Academy of Sciences of Ukraine, Ukraine

*Address all correspondence to: sdrozdovska@gmail.com

References

[1] Hruby A, Hu FB. The epidemiology of obesity: A big picture. Pharmaco Economics. 2015;**33**(7):673-689. DOI: 10.1007/s40273-014-0243-x

[2] Thyfault JP, Bergouignan A. Exercise and metabolic health: Beyond skeletal muscle. Diabetologia. 2020;**63**:1464-1474. DOI: 10.1007/s00125-020-05177-6

[3] Baud'huin M, Duplomb L, Teletchea S, Lamoureux F, Ruiz-Velasco C, Maillasson M, et al. Osteoprotegerin: Multiple partners for multiple functions. Cytokine & Growth Factor Reviews. 2013;**24**(5):401-409. DOI: 10.1016/j.cytogfr.2013.06.001

[4] Izquierdo AG, Crujeiras AB, Casanueva FF, Carreira MC. Leptin, obesity, and leptin resistance: Where are we 25 years later? Nutrients. 2019;**11**(11):2704. DOI: 10.3390/nu11112704

[5] Kotanidou EP, Kotanidis CP, Giza S, Serbis A, Tsinopoulou V-R, Karalazou P, et al. Osteoprotegerin increases parallel to insulin resistance in obese adolescents. Endocrine Research. 2018;**1-7**. DOI: 10.1080/07435800.2018.1480630

[6] DePaoli AM. 20 YEARS OF LEPTIN: Leptin in common obesity and associated disorders of metabolism. Journal of Endocrinology. 2014;**223**(1):T71-T81. Available from: https://joe.bioscientifica.com/view/journals/joe/223/1/T71.xml

[7] Wondmkun YT. Obesity, insulin resistance, and type 2 diabetes: Associations and therapeutic implications. Diabetes, Metabolic Syndrome and Obesity. 2020;**13**:3611-3616. DOI: 10.2147/DMSO.S27589

[8] Chia CW, Egan JM. Incretins in obesity and diabetes. Annals of the New York Academy of Sciences. 2020;**1461**(1):104-126. DOI: 10.1111/nyas.14211

[9] Michałowska J, Miller-Kasprzak E, Bogdański P. Incretin hormones in obesity and related Cardiometabolic disorders: The clinical perspective. Nutrients. 2021;**13**:351. DOI: 10.3390/nu13020351

[10] Colberg SR, Sigal RJ, Yardley JE, Riddell MC, Dunstan DW, Dempsey PC, et al. Physical activity/exercise and diabetes: A position statement of the American Diabetes Association. Diabetes Care. 2016;**39**(11):2065-2079. DOI: 10.2337/dc16-1728

[11] Eshghi SR, Fletcher K, Myette-Côté É, et al. Glycemic and metabolic effects of two long bouts of moderate-intensity exercise in men with Normal glucose tolerance or type 2 diabetes. Frontiers in Endocrinology. 2017;**8**:154

[12] Attarzadeh Hosseini SR, Mohammad Rahimi GR. Effect of aerobic training and diet on insulin resistance and quality of life in type II diabetic patients. The Horizon of Medical Sciences. 2016;**22**(1):57-64

[13] Golbidi S, Laher I. Exercise induced adipokine changes and the metabolic syndrome. Journal Diabetes Research. 2014;**2014**:726861. DOI: 10.1155/2014/726861

[14] Saeidi A, Soltani M, Daraei A, Nohbaradar H, Haghighi MM, Khosravi N, et al. The effects of aerobic-resistance training and broccoli supplementation on plasma Dectin-1 and insulin resistance in males with type 2 diabetes. Nutrients. 2021;**13**(9):3144. DOI: 10.3390/nu13093144

[15] Gonzalez-Gil AM, Elizondo-Montemayor L. The role of exercise in the interplay between Myokines, Hepatokines, Osteokines, Adipokines, and modulation of inflammation for energy substrate redistribution and fat mass loss: A review. Nutrients. 2020;**12**(6):1899. DOI: 10.3390/nu12061899

[16] Severinsen MCK, Pedersen BK. Muscle–organ crosstalk: The emerging roles of Myokines. Endocrine Reviews. 2020;**41**(4):594-609. DOI: 10.1210/endrev/bnaa016

[17] Pedersen BK. Anti-inflammatory effects of exercise: Role in diabetes and cardiovascular disease. European Journal of Clinical Investigation. 2017;**47**:600-611. DOI: 10.1111/eci.12781

[18] Chen X, Sun X, Wang C, He H. Effects of exercise on inflammatory cytokines in patients with type 2 diabetes: A Meta-analysis of randomized controlled trials. Oxidative Medicine and Cellular Longevity. 2020;**2020**:6660557. DOI: 10.1155/2020/6660557

[19] Fonseca TR, Mendes TT, Ramos GP, Cabido CET, Morandi RF, Ferraz FO, et al. Aerobic training modulates the increase in plasma concentrations of cytokines in response to a session of exercise. Journal of Environmental and Public Health. 2021;**2021**:1304139. DOI: 10.1155/2021/1304139

[20] Annibalini G, Lucertini F, Agostini D, Vallorani L, Gioacchini A, Barbieri E, et al. Concurrent aerobic and resistance training has anti-inflammatory effects and increases both plasma and leukocyte levels of IGF-1 in late middle-aged type 2 diabetic patients. Oxidative Medicine and Cellular Longevity. 2017;**2017**:3937842

[21] Simper TN, Morris C, Lynn A, O'Hagan C, Kilner K. Responses to oral glucose challenge differ by physical activity volume and intensity: A pilot study. Journal of Sport and Health Science. 2020;**9**(6):645-650. DOI: 10.1016/j.jshs.2017.04.010

[22] Sargeant JA, Gray LJ, Bodicoat DH, Willis SA, Stensel DJ, Nimmo MA, et al. The effect of exercise training on intrahepatic triglyceride and hepatic insulin sensitivity: A systematic review and meta-analysis. Obesity Reviews. 2018;**19**:1446-1459. DOI: 10.1111/obr.12719

[23] Locke AE, Kahali B, Berndt SI, et al. Genetic studies of body mass index yield new insights for obesity biology. Nature. 2015;**518**(7538):197-206. DOI: 10.1038/nature14177

[24] Williamson PJ, Atkinson G, Batterham AM. Inter-individual differences in weight change following exercise interventions: A systematic review and meta-analysis of randomized controlled trials. Obesity Reviews. 2019;**19**(7):960-975. DOI: 10.1111/obr.12682

[25] Casazza K, Brown A, Astrup A, et al. Weighing the evidence of common beliefs in obesity research. Critical Reviews in Food Science and Nutrition. 2015;**55**(14):2014-2053. DOI: 10.1080/10408398.2014.922044

[26] Farooqi S, O'Rahilly S. Genetics of obesity in humans. Endocrine Reviews. 2006;**27**(7):710-718. DOI: 10.1210/er.2006-0040

[27] Freire R. Scientific evidence of diets for weight loss: Different macronutrient composition, intermittent fasting, and popular diets. Nutrition. 2020;**69**:110549. DOI: 10.1016/j.nut.2019.07.001

[28] Sinha R, Kachru D, Ricchetti RR, et al. Leveraging genomic associations

in precision digital care for weight loss: Cohort study. Journal of Medical Internet Research. 2021;**23**(5):e25401. DOI: 10.2196/25401

[29] Benedict C, Axelsson T, Söderberg S, et al. Fat mass and obesity-associated gene (FTO) is linked to higher plasma levels of the hunger hormone ghrelin and lower serum levels of the satiety hormone leptin in older adults. Diabetes. 2014;**63**(11):3955-3959. DOI: 10.2337/db14-0470

[30] Merritt DC, Jamnik J, El-Sohemy A. FTO genotype, dietary protein intake, and body weight in a multiethnic population of young adults: A cross-sectional study. Genes & Nutrition. 2018;**13**:4. DOI: 10.1186/s12263-018-0593-7

[31] Zheng Y, Huang T, Zhang X, et al. Dietary fat modifies the effects of FTO genotype on changes in insulin sensitivity. The Journal of Nutrition. 2015;**145**(5):977-982. DOI: 10.3945/jn.115.210005

[32] Bayer S, Winkler V, Hauner H, Holzapfel C. Associations between genotype-diet interactions and weight loss-a systematic review. Nutrients. 2020;**12**(9):2891. DOI: 10.3390/nu12092891

[33] Ravaut G, Légiot A, Bergeron KF, Mounier C. Monounsaturated fatty acids in obesity-related inflammation. International Journal of Molecular Sciences. 2020;**22**(1):330. DOI: 10.3390/ijms22010330

[34] Goni L, Riezu-Boj JI, Milagro FI, et al. Interaction between an ADCY3 genetic variant and two weight-lowering diets affecting body fatness and body composition outcomes depending on macronutrient distribution: A randomized trial. Nutrients. 2018;**10**(6):789. DOI: 10.3390/nu10060789

[35] Celis-Morales C, Livingstone KM, Marsaux CF, et al. Food4Me study. Effect of personalized nutrition on health-related behaviour change: Evidence from the Food4Me European randomized controlled trial. International Journal of Epidemiology. 2017;**46**(2):578-588. DOI: 10.1093/ije/dyw186

[36] Bauer W, Adamska-Patruno E, Krasowska U, et al. Dietary macronutrient intake may influence the effects of TCF7L2 rs7901695 genetic variants on glucose homeostasis and obesity-related parameters: A cross-sectional population-based study. Nutrients. 2021;**13**(6):1936. DOI: 10.3390/nu13061936

[37] Goni L, Sun D, Heianza Y, et al. A circadian rhythm-related MTNR1B genetic variant modulates the effect of weight-loss diets on changes in adiposity and body composition: The POUNDS lost trial. European Journal of Nutrition. 2019;**58**(4):1381-1389. DOI: 10.1007/s00394-018-1660-y

[38] Qi Q, Bray GA, Smith SR, et al. Insulin receptor substrate 1 gene variation modifies insulin resistance response to weight-loss diets in a 2-year randomized trial: The preventing overweight using novel dietary strategies (POUNDS LOST) trial. Circulation. 2011;**124**(5):563-571. DOI: 10.1161/CIRCULATIONAHA.111.025767

[39] Garaulet M, Smith CE, Hernández-González T, et al. PPARγ Pro12Ala interacts with fat intake for obesity and weight loss in a behavioural treatment based on the Mediterranean diet. Molecular Nutrition & Food Research. 2011;**55**(12):1771-1779. DOI: 10.1002/mnfr.201100437

[40] Xu M, Qi Q, Liang J, et al. Genetic determinant for amino acid

metabolites and changes in body weight and insulin resistance in response to weight-loss diets: The preventing overweight using novel dietary strategies (POUNDS LOST) trial. Circulation. 2013;**127**(12):1283-1289. DOI: 10.1161/CIRCULATIONAHA.112.000586

[41] de Luis DA, Primo D, Izaola O, Aller R. Adiponectin gene variant rs266729 interacts with different macronutrient distribution of two different hypocaloric diets. Lifestyle Genomics. 2020;**13**(1):20-27. DOI: 10.1159/000503863

[42] de Luis D, Primo Martín D, Izaola O. Adiponectin gene variant rs266729 interacts with different macronutrient distributions of two different hypocaloric diets during nine months. Nutrición Hospitalaria. 2021;**38**(2):274-280. DOI: 10.20960/nh.03423

[43] Hu C, Jia W. Linking MTNR1B variants to diabetes: The role of circadian rhythms. Diabetes. 2016;**65**(6):1490-1492. DOI: 10.2337/dbi16-0012

[44] Garaulet M, Esteban Tardido A, Lee YC, et al. SIRT1 and CLOCK 3111T> C combined genotype is associated with evening preference and weight loss resistance in a behavioral therapy treatment for obesity. International Journal of Obesity. 2012;**36**(11):1436-1441. DOI: 10.1038/ijo.2011.270

[45] Mazur II, Drozdovska S, Andrieieva O, et al. PPARGC1A gene polymorphism is associated with exercise-induced fat loss. Molecular Biology Reports. 2020;**47**(10):7451-7457. DOI: 10.1007/s11033-020-05801-z

[46] Cardoso GA, Persuhn DC, Ribeiro MD, et al. Pro12Ala polymorphism on the PPARγ2 gene and weight loss after aerobic training: A randomized controlled trial. Frontiers in Physiology. 2020;**11**:385. DOI: 10.3389/fphys.2020.00385

[47] Leońska-Duniec A, Cieszczyk P, Jastrzębski Z, et al. The polymorphisms of the PPARD gene modify post-training body mass and biochemical parameter changes in women. PLoS One. 2018;**13**(8):e0202557. DOI: 10.1371/journal.pone.0202557

[48] Maciejewska-Karlowska A, Sawczuk M, Cieszczyk P, et al. Association between the Pro12Ala polymorphism of the peroxisome proliferator-activated receptor gamma gene and strength athlete status. PLoS One. 2013;**8**(6):e67172. DOI: 10.1371/journal.pone.0067172

[49] Papandonatos GD, Pan Q, Pajewski NM, et al. Genetic predisposition to weight loss and regain with lifestyle intervention: Analyses from the diabetes prevention program and the look AHEAD randomized controlled trials. Diabetes. 2015;**64**(12):4312-4321. DOI: 10.2337/db15-0441

[50] Cai G, Cole SA, Butte N, et al. A quantitative trait locus on chromosome 18q for physical activity and dietary intake in Hispanic children. Obesity. 2006;**14**(9):1596-1604. DOI: 10.1038/oby.2006.184

[51] Herring MP, Sailors MH, Bray MS. Genetic factors in exercise adoption, adherence and obesity. Obesity Reviews. 2014;**15**(1):29-39. DOI: 10.1111/obr.12089

[52] Drozdovska SB, Andrieieva OV, Yarmak OM, Blagii OL. Personalization of health-promoting fitness programs for young women based on genetic factors. Journal of Physical Education and Sport. 2020;**20**(S1):331-337. DOI: 10.7752/jpes.2020.s1046

[53] Turnbaugh PJ, Ley RE, Mahowald MA, Magrini V, Mardis ER, Gordon JI. An obesity-associated gut microbiome with increased

capacity for energy harvest. Nature. 2006;**444**(7122):1027-1031. DOI: 10.1038/nature05414

[54] Sheveleva SA, Kuvaeva IB, Efimochkina NR, Markova YM, Prosyannikov MY. Mikrobiom kishechnika: ot etalona normy k patologii. Voprosy Pitaniya. 2020;**89**(4):35-51

[55] Ursell LK, Haiser HJ, Van Treuren W, Garg N, Reddivari L, Vanamala J, et al. The intestinal metabolome: An intersection between microbiota and host. Gastroenterology. 2014;**146**(6): 1470-1476. DOI: 10.1053/j.gastro

[56] Zhang P, Meng X, Li D, Calderone R, Mao D, Sui B. Commensal homeostasis of gut microbiota-host for the impact of obesity. Frontiers in Physiology. 2017;**8**:1122. DOI: 10.3389/fphys.2017.01122

[57] Duncan SH, Lobley GE, Holtrop G, Ince J, Johnstone AM, Louis P, et al. Human colonic microbiota associated with diet, obesity and weight loss. International Journal of Obesity. 2008;**32**(11):1720-1724. DOI: 10.1038/ijo.2008.155

[58] Kravchuk EN, Nejmark AE, Grineva EN, Galagudza MM. Regulyaciya metabolicheskih processov, oposredovannaya kishechnoj mikrofloroj. Saharnyj Diabetes. 2016;**19**(4):280-285

[59] Schwiertz A, Taras D, Schäfer K, Beijer S, Bos NA, Donus C, et al. Microbiota and SCFA in lean and overweight healthy subjects. Obesity. 2010;**18**(1):190-195. DOI: 10.1038/oby.2009.167

[60] Ley RE, Turnbaugh PJ, Klein S, Gordon JI. Microbial ecology: Human gut microbes associated with obesity. Nature. 2006;**444**(7122):1022-1023. DOI: 10.1038/4441022a

[61] Castaner O, Goday A, Park Y-M, Lee S-H, Magkos F, Shiow S-ATE, et al. The gut microbiome profile in obesity: A systematic review. Int. The Journal of Endocrinology. 2018;**2018**:1-9. DOI: 10.1155/2018/4095789

[62] Marteau P. Microbiote intestinal en 20 questions. EMC-Gastro-Enterologie. 2013;**8**(2):1-8

[63] Vrieze A, Holleman F, Zoetendal EG, de Vos WM, Hoekstra JB, Nieuwdorp M. Diabetologia 2010; 53(4): 606-13 the environment within: How gut microbiota may influence metabolism and body composition. Diabetologia. 2010;**53**(4):606-613. DOI: 10.1007/s00125-010-1662-7

[64] Lin HV, Frassetto A, Kowalik EJ Jr, Nawrocki AR, Lu MM, Kosinski JR, et al. Butyrate and propionate protect against diet-induced obesity and regulate gut hormones via free fatty acid receptor 3-independent mechanisms. PLoS One. 2012;**7**(4):e35240. DOI: 10.1371/journal.pone.0035240

[65] Rovella V, Rodia G, Di Daniele F, Cardillo C, Campia U, Noce A, et al. Association of gut hormones and microbiota with vascular dysfunction in obesity. Nutrients. 2021;**13**(2):613. DOI: 10.3390/nu13020613

[66] Duttaroy AK. Role of gut microbiota and their metabolites on atherosclerosis, hypertension and human blood platelet function: A review. Nutrients. 2021;**13**(1):144. DOI: 10.3390/nu13010144

[67] Boets E, Gomand SV, Deroover L, Preston T, Vermeulen K, De Preter V, et al. Systemic availability and metabolism of colonic-derived

short-chain fatty acids in healthy subjects: A stable isotope study: Short-chain fatty acid systemic availability and metabolism in humans. The Journal of Physiology. 2017;**595**(2):541-555. DOI: 10.1113/JP272613

[68] Topping DL, Clifton PM. Short-chain fatty acids and human colonic function: Roles of resistant starch and nonstarch polysaccharides. Physiological Reviews. 2001;**81**(3):1031-1064. DOI: 10.1152/physrev.2001.81.3.1031

[69] Macfarlane S, Macfarlane GT. Regulation of short-chain fatty acid production. The Proceedings of the Nutrition Society. 2003;**62**(1):67-72. DOI: 10.1079/PNS2002207

[70] Den Besten G, van Eunen K, Groen AK, Venema K, Reijngoud D-J, Bakker BM. The role of short-chain fatty acids in the interplay between diet, gut microbiota, and host energy metabolism. Journal of Lipid Research. 2013;**54**(9):2325-2340. DOI: 10.1194/jlr.R036012

[71] De Vadder F, Kovatcheva-Datchary P, Goncalves D, Vinera J, Zitoun C, Duchampt A, et al. Microbiota-generated metabolites promote metabolic benefits via gut-brain neural circuits. Cell. 2014;**156**(1-2):84-96. DOI: 10.1016/j.cell.2013.12.016

[72] Kashtanova DA, Tkacheva ON, Bojcov SA. Mikrobiota kishechnika i faktory kardiovaskulyarnogo riska. CHast' 2. Mikrobiota kishechnika i ozhirenie. Kardiovaskulyarnaya terapiya i profilaktika. 2015;**14**(5):83-86

[73] Blekhman R, Goodrich JK, Huang K, Sun Q, Bukowski R, Bell JT, et al. Host genetic variation impacts microbiome composition across human body sites. Genome Biology. 2015;**16**(1). DOI: 10.1186/s13059-015-0759-1

[74] Jumpertz R, Le DS, Turnbaugh PJ, Trinidad C, Bogardus C, Gordon JI, et al. Energy-balance studies reveal associations between gut microbes, caloric load, and nutrient absorption in humans. The American Journal of Clinical Nutrition. 2011;**94**(1):58-65. DOI: 10.3945/ajcn.110.010132

[75] Simões CD, Maukonen J, Kaprio J, Rissanen A, Pietiläinen KH, Saarela M. Habitual dietary intake is associated with stool microbiota composition in monozygotic twins. The Journal of Nutrition. 2013;**143**(4):417-423. DOI: 10.3945/jn.112.166322

[76] Furet J-P, Kong L-C, Tap J, Poitou C, et al. Differential adaptation of human gut microbiota to bariatric surgery-induced weight loss: Links with metabolic and low-grade inflammation markers. Diabetes. 2010;**59**(12):3049-3057. DOI: 10.2337/db10-0253

[77] Statovci D, Aguilera M, MacSharry J, Melgar S. The impact of western diet and nutrients on the microbiota and immune response at mucosal interfaces. Frontiers in Immunology. 2017;**8**:838. DOI: 10.3389/fimmu.2017.00838

[78] Russell WR, Gratz SW, Duncan SH, Holtrop G, Ince J, Scobbie L, et al. High-protein, reduced-carbohydrate weight-loss diets promote metabolite profiles likely to be detrimental to colonic health. The American Journal of Clinical Nutrition. 2011;**93**(5):1062-1072. DOI: 10.3945/ajcn.110.002188

[79] Zhang C, Zhang M, Pang X, Zhao Y, Wang L, Zhao L. Structural resilience of the gut microbiota in adult mice under high-fat dietary perturbations. The ISME Journal. 2012;**6**(10):1848-1857. DOI: 10.1038/ismej.2012.27

[80] de Wit N, Derrien M, Bosch-Vermeulen H, Oosterink E, Keshtkar S, Duval C, et al. Saturated fat stimulates

obesity and hepatic steatosis and affects gut microbiota composition by an enhanced overflow of dietary fat to the distal intestine. American Journal of Physiology. Gastrointestinal and Liver Physiology. 2012;**303**(5):G589-G599. DOI: 10.1152/ajpgi.00488.2011

[81] Begley M, Gahan CGM, Hill C. The interaction between bacteria and bile. FEMS Microbiology Reviews. 2005;**29**(4):625-651. DOI: 10.1016/j.femsre.2004.09.003

[82] Viennois E, Merlin D, Gewirtz AT, Chassaing B. Dietary emulsifier–induced low-grade inflammation promotes colon carcinogenesis. Cancer Research. 2017;**77**(1):27-40. DOI: 10.1158/0008-5472.CAN-16-1359

[83] Fogelholm M, Anderssen S, Gunnarsdottir I, Lahti-Koski M. Dietary macronutrients and food consumption as determinants of long-term weight change in adult populations: A systematic literature review. Food & Nutrition Research. 2012;**56**(1):19103. DOI: 10.3402/fnr.v56i0.19103

[84] Brandsch C, Shukla A, Hirche F, Stangl GI, Eder K. Effect of proteins from beef, pork, and Turkey meat on plasma and liver lipids of rats compared with casein and soy protein. Nutrition. 2006;**22**(11-12):1162-1170. DOI: 10.1016/j.nut.2006.06.009

[85] Huang H, Krishnan HB, Pham Q, Yu LL, Wang TTY. Soy and gut microbiota: Interaction and implication for human health. Journal of Agricultural and Food Chemistry. 2016;**64**(46):8695-8709. DOI: 10.1021/acs.jafc.6b03725

[86] Cotillard A, Kennedy SP, Kong LC, Prifti E, Pons N, Le Chatelier E, et al. Erratum: Corrigendum: Dietary intervention impact on gut microbial gene richness. Nature. 2013;**502**(7472):580-580. DOI: 10.3945/an.114.005835

[87] Haro C, García-Carpintero S, Rangel-Zúñiga OA, Alcalá-Díaz JF, Landa BB, Clemente JC, et al. Consumption of two healthy dietary patterns restored microbiota dysbiosis in obese patients with metabolic dysfunction. Molecular Nutrition & Food Research. 2017;**61**(12). DOI: 10.1002/mnfr.201700300

[88] De Filippis F, Pellegrini N, Vannini L, Jeffery IB, La Storia A, Laghi L, et al. High-level adherence to a Mediterranean diet beneficially impacts the gut microbiota and associated metabolome. Gut. 2016;**65**(11):1812-1821. DOI: 10.1136/gutjnl-2015-309957

[89] Tosti V, Bertozzi B, Fontana L. Health benefits of the Mediterranean diet: Metabolic and molecular mechanisms. The Journals of Gerontology. Series A, Biological Sciences and Medical Sciences. 2018;**73**(3):318-326. DOI: 10.1093/gerona/glx227

[90] Kastorini C-M, Milionis HJ, Esposito K, Giugliano D, Goudevenos JA, Panagiotakos DB. The effect of Mediterranean diet on metabolic syndrome and its components: A meta-analysis of 50 studies and 534,906 individuals. Journal of the American College of Cardiology. 2011;**57**(11):1299-1313. DOI: 10.1016/j.jacc.2010.09.073

[91] Bailey MA, Holscher HD. Microbiome-mediated effects of the Mediterranean diet on inflammation. Advances in Nutrition. 2018;**9**(3):193-206. DOI: 10.1093/advances/nmy013

[92] Andrieieva OM, Nahorna A, Yarmak OM, Yerakova L, Kyrychenko V, Drozdovska SB, et al. Identification of informative physical condition indicators for self-training exercise programs Design for Middle-Aged Overweight and Obese Women. Sport Mont. 2021;**19**(S2):75-81

Chapter 7

Medical Weight Management: A Multidisciplinary Approach

Wahiba Elhag and Walid El Ansari

Abstract

A wide and interacting range of individual, environmental and socioeconomic factors contribute to obesity. As a consequence, weight management strategies almost always comprise a mixture of several parallel approaches, each with its challenges and unique goals. Broadly, weight management strategies comprise of two main strands. The non-pharmacotherapy approach includes various lifestyle modifications in terms of dietary therapy, exercise, and behavioral modifications, including the prevention of possible relapses. Pharmacotherapy, on the other hand, involves several anti-obesity medications, employed as single or combination therapy. Generally, the goals of weight management should be realistic and individualized to patient's experiences, abilities, and risks in order to maximize the likelihood of success. This chapter tackles these weight management strategies in turn, explaining each, as well as highlighting their distinctive features and challenges, effectiveness and safety, requisites, and where appropriate, indications and contraindications.

Keywords: obesity, weight management, dietary therapy, behavioral therapy, physical activity, exercise, anti-obesity medications, pharmacotherapy

1. Introduction

Obesity has significantly increased over the last years. Obesity is defined as excessive fat accumulation that adversely affects health, caused by consuming excess energy in relation to energy expenditure. Its etiology is complex and includes genetic, physiologic, environmental, lifestyle, psychological, social, economic, and political factors that interact to cause obesity (**Table 1**) [1–7]. Obesity is diagnosed using body mass index (BMI, kg/m^2), weight in kilogram divided by the height in meters squared. Obesity is defined as BMI ≥ 30 kg/m^2 while having a BMI 25.0–29.9 kg/m^2 is considered as overweight.

Obesity increases the probability of many ailments, with increased morbidity/mortality and decreased quality of life. It is implicated in many health problems and complications e.g., hypertension, type 2 diabetes (T2DM), hyperlipidemia, cardiovascular conditions, obstructive sleep apnea, metabolic syndrome, chronic kidney disease (CKD), nonalcoholic fatty liver disease (NAFLD), osteoarthritis, depression and some cancers [8]. These are mainly a consequence of the increased

Factors	
Individual	
Genetic predisposition	Monogenic single gene mutation: deficiency of melanocortin-4 receptor (MC4R), leptin, or proopiomelanocortin (POMC). Polygenic obesity: contribution of many genes. Syndromic obesity: Prader-Willi syndrome
Epigenetic modifications	DNA methylation: metabolic status of mother can influence DNA methylation of leptin at birth causing obesity. Adiponectin epigenetic status related to obesity
Prenatal	Maternal obesity, high weight gain during gestation, gestational diabetes
Neonatal	Prematurity
Post-natal	Formula versus breast feeding, infant overfeeding
Family history	Parental obesity: 3 fold increase risk in offspring if 1 parent is obese and 10 fold increase if 2 parents.
Excessive energy intake	High calorie diet rich in processed fat and carbohydrates
Physical inactivity	Sedentary lifestyle: prolonged screen time, sitting at home or work
Sleep deprivation associated with obesity	Due to imbalance of hormones, impaired glucose tolerance, increased nocturnal cortisol
Psychological	Depression, anxiety, stress
Drug-induced	Steroids, insulin, antidepressants (amitriptyline), antipsychotics (clozapine, quetiapine)
Gut microbiomes	Alteration causes changes in host weight and metabolism leading to obesity
Environmental	
Obesogenic environment	Easily accessible fast food/ high calorie diets, affordability of food
Built environment	Few sidewalks/green spaces, low access to recreational resources
Transport/technology	Utilization of cars for transport, less manual jobs
Socioeconomic	
Demographic	Age, ethnicity (black, Hispanic), menopause
Socioeconomic	Low income and educational level

Table 1.
Factors contributing to obesity.

body fat, which result in endocrine and metabolic disturbances as well as increased mechanical pressure on various organs [9].

Obesity is a chronic disease given its multifaceted etiology and complex pathophysiologies. It has characteristic signs and symptoms consistent with anatomical changes across various organs (cardiovascular, endocrine, immunological functions) and results in complications. Hence, it needs treatment for life; and because it is a heterogeneous condition, individual assessment, risk stratification, and management are necessary [9].

At the societal level, existing weight loss (WL) therapies are not likely to reduce the obesity epidemic, however, at the individual level, they can be useful in reducing the morbidity and mortality associated with obesity [10]. Current treatment guidelines for overweight and obesity recommend diet, exercise, and behavior modification for individuals whose BMI is ≥ 30 and those with BMI > 27 in addition to two weight-related comorbidities [11].

2. Goals of treatment

Management targets should be realistic and individualized according to the person's experience, ability, and risks [9]. This is specially important as the long-term treatment success is subject to the person agreement to change the daily lifestyle and to follow the suggested recommendations. Although improvements in cardiovascular (CV) risk factors are observed with as little as 2–3% WL, the existing guidelines propose ≥5–10% (clinically significant WL) during a range of 6 months such WL leads to greater improvement in CV risk [12]. Therefore, the aim is long-term weight reduction is to achieve WL target of >5% of baseline weight for BMI 25–35 kg/m^2, WL target of >10% of baseline weight for BMI > 35 kg/m^2; improvement in obesity-associated risk factors; eduction in obesity-related comorbidities; lowering early mortality risk; prevention of work disability and early retirement; as well as improving the quality of life improved quality of life [9].

3. Weight loss strategies

3.1 Lifestyle modification

Lifestyle modification program requires holistic approach and the plan of care should involve multidisciplinary team of interventionists including physician, dietitian, psychologist, exercise physiologist, health care professionals. In this program, patients should be followed every week (30–90 minutes) for 16–26 weeks to ensure compliance, then every other week for 6–12 months for weight maintenance [9]. Treatment plan includes counseling individuals regarding proper balanced nutrition, appropriate physical activity, and long-term weight control strategies.

Lifestyle modification programs can be implemented in many venues e.g., specialized obesity clinics, primary care, commercial, private dietetics practice or academic medical centers [13–16]. Typically, these programs induce modest WL that results in significant improvement in obesity-associated health conditions (sleep apnea, T2D, hypertension, hyperlipidemia) as well as positive psycho-social effects (mood, quality of life, body image) [17, 18]. Several studies have demonstrated the efficacy of life style modification in promoting WL and improving obesity-associated comorbidities. We outline two examples of lifestyle modification interventions that validate that WL and long-term health advances that can be accomplished via lifestyle modification.

The Diabetes Prevention Program (DPP) randomized more than 3200 participants with overweight/obesity and impaired glucose tolerance to placebo, metformin, or intensive lifestyle intervention, aiming for 7% WL [19]. Dietitians counseled the lifestyle intervention group for 16 individual sessions in the initial 24 weeks, followed by ≥1 interaction every other month for the rest of the study [19]. The participants were advised to reduce their caloric intake and to follow low fat diet, and to perform 150 minutes of physical activity per week [19]. After an average of 2.8 years, the mean weight loss in the lifestyle intervention group was 5.6 kg vs. 0.1 and 2.1 kg in the placebo and metformin groups, respectively [19]. This 5.6 kg WL was equivalent to 58% relative decrease in the likelihood of developing T2DM [19]. Ten years after the start of the study, the lifestyle intervention group had regained most of the weight they lost, although their T2DM incidence stayed 34% below that of the placebo group [19].

The Look AHEAD Study (Action for Health in Diabetes) enrolled >5100 overweight/obese persons with T2DM [20, 21]. Participants were randomized to diabetes support and education group (3 group-education meetings per year for the first 4 years) or an intensive lifestyle intervention group (weekly group treatment sessions, monthly individual visit, meal replacement with liquid supplement and 1200–1800 kcal/day dietary plan individualized by weight) [20]. After 1 year, the lifestyle intervention group lost 8.6% of their weight vs. 0.6% for the diabetes support and education group; at the fourth year, average WL was 4.7% vs. 1.1%, respectively [20]. The WL was maintained at 8 years (4.7%) for the lifestyle intervention group vs. 2.1% for the diabetes support and education participants [22]. In addition, the lifestyle intervention participants exhibited significantly lower HbA1C (glycated hemoglobin) and showed improvements in CV risk factors including reduced systolic, diastolic pressure and triglycerides [22, 23]. Moreover, the lifestyle intervention group consumed less diabetes, hypertension, and lipid-lowering medications and had remissions or decreased in the severity of obstructive sleep apnea as well as improved depression symptoms [22, 23].

3.2 Dietary therapy

Several dietary approaches are utilized to achieve WL among overweight and obese adults (**Table 2**). Individuals with obesity should receive personalized nutritional plans in line with their therapeutic goals and risk in order to achieve sustainable and healthy weight. The choice of a diet should address their preferences to facilitate compliance with the dietary plans. Dietary therapy involves individual or group nutritional counseling. Group sessions are usually more effective. Weight management recommendations include healthy eating that emphasize reducing intake of energy dense food, portion control, and improving diet quality leading to energy deficit that results on WL on the long term without impairing health [24]. For instance, energy deficit of 500–600 kcal/day permits about 0.5 kg/week WL over 12 weeks, up to a maximum of 24 weeks [25]. To achieve WL, various nutrition strategies are employed, and because all the diets assessed below have near equivalent short and long-term safety, the selection can be driven by the required control of comorbidities such as T2DM and hypertension (HTN).

3.2.1 Low carbohydrate diet (LCD)

LCD provides 20–120 g carbohydrates/day [26] and is used as treatment for obesity, T2DM and other obesity-related conditions, with good short and medium-term WL as well as cardiometabolic control [27, 28]. Reported WL with LCD was 11% at 1 year and 7% at 2 years [29]. At the first 6 months, LCD reduces diastolic blood pressure (DBP), triglyceride (TG), very-low-density lipoprotein cholesterol (VLDL), along with improvement in high density lipoprotein cholesterol and to a lesser extend in the low density lipoprotein cholesterol (LDL) [27, 29].

3.2.2 Low fat diet

Comprises 10–30% of total calorie intake from fat [11]. At 2 years, mean weight and BMI changes were -3.3 ± 4.1 kg and -1.0 ± 1.4 kg/m^2 respectively [27]. Low fat diet also results in significant improvement in the CV risk including reduction in waist circumference (-2.8 ± 4.3 cm), systolic blood pressure (SBP), total cholesterol (TC), LDL, fasting glucose and insulin levels [27, 30, 31].

3.2.3 Low-carbohydrate versus low-fat diets

Several studies compared low-carbohydrate to low-fat diets. A study found that, at 6 months, participants assigned to LCD lost significantly more weight than those

Weight loss strategies	Summary
Lifestyle modification	
Dietary therapy	
Low carbohydrate diet	Restrict carbohydrates to 20–120 g per day
Low fat diet	10–30% total calorie intake from fat
High protein diet	25% of total calorie from protein
Mediterranean diet	35–40% fat, rich in omega-3, whole grains, fruits, vegetables, legumes, nuts, fish
Low calorie diet	Energy deficit of 500–800 kcal/day
Ketogenic diet	Reduced carbohydrates (<50 g/day), rich in protein
Very low-calorie ketogenic Diet	Energy intake < 800 calories, protein 1.2–1.5 g/kg of ideal body weight, fat 15–30 g/day, carbohydrates < 30 g/day
Meal replacements	Liquid formula or bars
Exercise	
Aerobic	Important during weight loss phase
Resistance	Increase muscle mass, for weight maintenance
Behavioral modifications	
Behavioral skills	
Self-monitoring	Weight, food record, exercise minutes
Goal-setting	Weight, calorie intake, exercise
Stimulus control	Keep tempting foods out of sight
Behavioral substitution	Relaxation techniques
Cognitive skills	
Problem-solving	Tactics to deal with weight-related health behaviors (social eating)
Cognitive restructuring	Identify/modify maladaptive thoughts contributing to overeating/physical inactivity
Relapse prevention	Learn to get back on track, maintain long term motivation, stress management
Pharmacotherapy	Single/combination anti-obesity medications

Table 2.
Summary of weight loss strategies.

on a low-calorie and low-fat regimen [32, 33]. However, the WL was not different at 12 months (−5.1 vs. −3.1 kg) [32, 33]. In another study, participants were assigned to LCD or low fat diet in combination with lifestyle modification and both groups lost 11% and 7% of their TW at 1 and 2 years respectively with no significant difference between the two group [29]. Hence, successful WL can be accomplished with LCD or low-fat diet in conjunction with behavioral therapy. Furthermore, lifestyle modification that enables adherence to the proposed calorie goals is more critical for WL than the macronutrient constituents per se [29, 34, 35].

3.2.4 High protein diet

In this diet, 25%, 30% and 45% of the total calories are from protein, fat, and carbohydrate respectively, whilst providing foods that achieve energy deficit [11]. Expected WL is −3.5 kg at 6 months and may achieve 15% TWL% at 1 year [36, 37]. High protein diet could result in significant reduction in BP, fasting glucose and insulin level as well as significant improvement in lipid profile including LDL, TC, TG and HDL [36, 37].

3.2.5 Mediterranean diet

It has moderate amount of fat (35–40%) and is rich in Omega-3, where the primary fat source is extra virgin olive oil. Mediterranean diet has more whole grains, fruits, vegetables, legumes, nuts, fish and seafood, with limited poultry, dairy, red meat and usually prescribed with energy restriction to achieve WL [11, 27]. Reported WL at 2 years is −3.4 kg (−5.1 to −3.0). In addition, it decreases waist circumference, improves SBP, HDL and glucose levels [27].

3.2.6 Low calorie diet

Low calorie diet is based on balanced nutrition where 45 – 55% of intake is from carbohydrates, 15–25% is from proteins, and 25–30% is from fat [38]. It must be tailored to individual energy requirements, sex, age, and physical activity [38]. The diet's composition should be modified to minimize comorbidities e.g., T2DM, HTN, hyperlipidemia [38]. This diet is should be designed to result in energy deficit of 500–800 kcal/d. Therefore, women can be prescribed 1200–1500 kcal/d and men 1500–1800 kcal/d. Low calorie diet with relatively high protein contents facilitates WL and prevents weight regain due to the greater satiety and energy expenditure through diet-induced thermogenesis and preservation of lean muscle mass. Studies reported weight loss of 11 kg at 26 weeks [39]. In addition, significant improvement in CV risk factors was observed with this diet such as BP, waist circumference, glucose, insulin level and lipid profile (TC, TG) [40–42].

3.2.7 Ketogenic diet

This diet has been utilized since 1920s as treatment for epilepsy and has been shown in some case to reduce or eliminate the need for epilepsy medications for epilepsy drugs. It became a common method for obesity treatment since the 1960s. This diet has therapeutic potential in many obesity-associated conditions, e.g., T2DM, polycystic ovary syndrome, acne, and cancer [43]. Ketogenic diets comprise reduced carbohydrates (<50 g/day) with an increase in protein and fat [43].

3.2.8 Very low-calorie ketogenic diet (VLCKD)

This provides energy intake of <800 calories/day, protein 1.2–1.5 g/kg of ideal body weight, carbohydrates of <30 g/day and 15–30 g of fat/day [26, 44, 45]. The low carbohydrate stimulates lipolysis of stored fat and synthesis of ketone bodies utilized as fuel by extrahepatic tissues. Ketosis associated with VLCKD is always moderate (ketonemia never >3 mmol/L) and is different than diabetic ketoacidosis [45]. WL (0.5–2.0 kg/week) is achieved as a result of the proteins' satiety effect on appetite hormones, appetite-suppressant actions of ketone bodies and also due to the decrease in diminished lipogenesis along with increase in lipolysis [46].

VLCKD is delivered through a mix of meal replacements that include protein (milk, peas, whey, soy) and natural food to improve patient compliance. Daily vitamins and minerals are also provided [45]. VLCKD is advised for BMI ≥30 kg/m^2 for a maximum of 12 weeks. This diet should be under medical supervision as there is increased risk of side effects such as dehydration, nausea, diarrhea, constipation, hyperuricemia, gallstones, and vitamin/microelement deficiencies [45]. Studies have shown that at 4 weeks, VLCKD resulted in significant WL (6–37% TWL%), improvement in BMI (−5.3 kg/m^2), SBP, DBP, insulin resistance (HOMA-IR) and lipids (TG, TC, HDL) [47–49]. Similar findings were also reported among obese diabetic patients, where VLCKD achieved significant WL at 3 months (8.5%) and 12 months (11.5%) and improvement in blood glucose [50]. Moreover, 26.6% of the patients who completed the study were able to stop all antidiabetic medications, while 73.3% took metformin only [50].

3.2.9 Meal replacements

Meal placements is produced in different forms such as drink, bars or soup to substitute solid food. They have controlled calories and nutrient contents and are commonly used in energy restricted diet to facilitate WL. It also contains the necessary vitamins and minerals. Many studies reported the effectiveness of utilizing meal replacements as dietary intervention for weight management [51–53]. Participants who replaced two meals and two snacks per day with liquid shakes and meal bars lost 7.1 kg in 3 months compared to 1.3 kg for individuals on conventional foods with the same calories (1200–1500 kcal/d) [54]. Moreover, those who substitute 1 meal and 1 snack a day during follow-up maintained a WL of 10.4 kg at 27 months [54]. Similarly, the use of meal replacement in patients with T2DM resulted in significant WL at 12 months compared to conventional diet (−4.4 vs. −2.4 kg, P = 0.07), with significant glycemic (HbA1c) improvement and reduced medications [52].

3.3 Exercise

Exercise improves body composition and CV health independent of WL [55, 56]. In the absence of significant WL, aerobic exercise improves blood pressure (BP), lipids, and visceral fat [57–61]. The reduced visceral fat improves glucose tolerance and insulin sensitivity in nondiabetic individuals as well as glycemic control in diabetic patients [62, 63]. Exercise also leads to positive changes in quality of life, vitality and mental health [56]. Therefore, individuals with obesity should be encouraged to exercise to improve their CV health, rather than lose weight only [34, 64].

Guidelines for care of patients with obesity include recommendations for "aerobic training of ≥150 min/week of moderate intensity, with better outcomes with increasing amounts and intensity of exercise" [12]. However, PA alone induces limited WL [65], unless it is accompanied by energy restriction. For instance, losing 0.45 kg/week, requires high PA is (e.g., walking 35 miles/week), but is feasible to be accomplished by decreasing food intake by 500 kcal/day. Hence, effective WL requires exercise >150 min/week with 1200–1800 kcal/week energy consumption [65]. Exercise combined with decrease caloric intake produces greater WL than exercise or caloric restriction alone. Hence, PA should be paired with adjusted caloric intake to achieve optimal WL and body composition. Physical activity should be prescribed according to patient's ability, preference. It is also important to ascertain that there are no contraindications to physical activity particularly in individuals with BMI of 35 kg/m^2 or higher.

3.3.1 Aerobic exercise

Aerobic exercise is essential for weight management. It facilitates weight loss and improves body composition by inducing fat and visceral fat loss [66]. One study found that supervised exercise with 400 or 600 kcal/session five days/week for 10 months resulted in 3.9 ± 4.9 and 5.2 ± 5.6 kg among overweight or obese individuals respectively compared with weight gain (0.5 ± 3.5 kg) for controls [67]. Aerobic exercise intensity also influences WL. Among sedentary college students with obesity, 12 weeks of high and moderate intensity training led to significant reduction in body weight, BMI, waist circumference, and body fat percentage than light intensity training [68]. Likewise, the time of the session is essential for body weight outcomes, where early-exercise (50% of sessions between 7 and 11.59 am) led to significantly more weight loss compared to late-exercise (>50% of sessions between 3 and 7 pm) [69]. In contrast, there is no significant difference in terms of weight loss between continuous and intermittent exercise. For example a study compared the effect of 18 months of continuous (3 times/wk, 30 min/session) versus intermittent (5 times/wk, 15 min/session) aerobic exercise in overweight and obese individuals and found small reductions in weight (2.0%) in the continuous training group with no significant change in intermittent groups [70].

3.3.2 Resistance exercise

This type of exercise may not result in WL if performed alone because it does not generate enough negative energy balance to achieve clinically significant weight loss when compared with aerobic exercises [71]. Aerobic exercises have superior total energy expenditure when compared to resistance exercises [72]. Combinations of aerobic and resistance exercise provide greater benefits for WL, fat loss and cardiorespiratory fitness than aerobic or resistance exercise alone [73]. Resistance training might support negative energy balance by augmenting the lean mass, resting metabolic rate, and the oxidation of fat and may assist with weight maintenance [65, 72].

3.4 Behavioral modifications

The cornerstone treatment of obesity is a lifestyle modification program that consist of diet, exercise, and behavior therapy. Psychotherapists use group or individual behavior therapy to provide principles, techniques and skills to alter the eating and exercise patterns and to facilitate achievement of energy intake and expenditure goals [10]. When overweight/obesity is accompanied with serious symptoms (e.g., depression, eating disorders, and lack of motivation), then psychiatrists should be involved in the care patients [74]. Various strategies should be adapted to the individual situation and the patient's needs [75]. Typical behavioral WL programs include 60–90 min weekly sittings for 6 months followed by maintenance gatherings every other week through another 12 months to prevent weight regain [34].

3.4.1 Behavioral skills

3.4.1.1 Self-monitoring

Teaching participants to self-monitor their eating, PA and progress is a behavioral therapy technique known as self-monitoring. It is a key strategy in behavioral therapy of obesity. Self-Monitoring increases self-awareness of personal behaviors as it slows down the decision-making processes, allowing individuals to make healthier choices [76]. Although self-monitoring of food and energy is considered the most important skill in behavior therapy, however it can be difficult to implement. For example, reporting the lack of ability to lose weight underestimated their food consumption by 50% [77]. Hence, patients require education on using measurement tools, nutrition labels, and calorie guides. They should also be encouraged to make note of the time, amount, preparation, and calorie of foods and beverages and bring their records to group meetings for feedback.

PA is also important to be monitored in behavior therapy. Participants are instructed to record the type and amount of their PA. Pedometers provide immediate feedback, encouraging participants to gradually increase their energy expenditure and the number of steps reach the target of 10,000 steps per day [78]. Self-monitoring should be daily for the first 6 months and then intermittently during maintenance. Participants are instructed to record their intake and PA daily and bring their books to individual or group meetings. Research demonstrated strong associations between adherence to self monitoring of dietary consumption, self-weighing, and PA and WL where greater frequency and more days of self-monitoring corresponded to greater monthly WL [79, 80].

3.4.1.2 Goal-setting

Setting personal targets is an important behavioral element in weight management. To modify behavior, participants need to set specific quantifiable achievable PA and dietary goals (e.g., consume ≤1200 kcal) [76]. Setting weight management goals is better when tied to health benefits such as better blood pressure control or improved lipid profile to increase motivation and adherence [76]. Similarly, short-term goals are more effective than longer-term goals. More importantly, goals need to be realistic, yet challenging. Deciding on reasonable, achievable goals supports long-term success. Therefore, is better to set easier goals initially and increase them gradually as the participant progresses to facilitate adherence and increase the sense of accomplishment [81, 82]. Patients frequently assume they need to lose much weight to be successful. Helping patients choose an achievable WL goal (e.g., 5% WL) strengthens adherence. Studies have shown that participants who set targets were 10.3 times more likely to accomplish WL ≥10% at 1 year was compared to those who did not [81]. Goal setting related to diet or PA was found to be more predictive of adherence to dietary and physical activity strategies than goal setting related to weight loss [82].

3.4.1.3 Stimulus control

Stimulus control strategies focus on changing an individual's environment to reinforce healthy changes [76]. Behavioral treatment teaches participants to reorganize their environment in order to lessen the cues for inappropriate food consumption, and increase those for appropriate diet or physical activity [83]. For instance, if a person frequently snacks on the couch or while watching television, the act of sitting on the sofa or watching television becomes a cue to future snacking. To modify this, participants need to confine their meals to the dining room to decrease the cues associated with eating [84]. Likewise, individuals may keep tempting food out of sight or remove them from home to limit consumption. Similarly, individuals are encouraged to buy more fruits and vegetables and make them more visible by storing in obvious places. A reminder notes about healthy eating and exercise on the refrigerator or bathroom mirror could also be a useful strategy to alter the home environment and promote healthy habits.

3.4.1.4 Behavioral substitution

Many individuals eat as a reaction to emotional stimuli (e.g., anger, boredom, stress, anxiety, frustration), with has substantial impacts on weight and health. Self-monitoring assists individuals in behavior therapy to recognize non-hunger cues to snack and replace eating with different behaviors. Individuals and their relatives need to find other means to deal with negative feelings [76]. If a person eats when anxious, practicing relaxation techniques or alternative activities such as writing, knitting, housekeeping, and exercising in response to anxieties could be more useful as these activities hinder eating.

3.4.2 Cognitive skills

Cognitive approaches to behavior change are also utilized in the behavioral treatment of obesity. The two most commonly taught skills are problem-solving and cognitive restructuring.

3.4.2.1 Problem-solving

Individuals may face obstacles when attempting to make lifestyle changes [76]. In order to support participants during this process, it is important to train them in problem-solving skills. This problem solving tactics help patients explore their weight-related health behaviors. Using a multistep interactive behavioral strategy, they identify a problem that hinders their WL, contemplate outcomes associated with different choices, choose the healthiest, implement a specific plan, assess the success of the selected solution and repeat the problem-solving process if necessary [74, 76]. Group visits is useful in helping participants to engage in problem solving of a given health aspect, learn from the way other people solved similar problems and creating solutions specific to their situation [76]. A 6-month lifestyle intervention for obesity involving problem-solving skills resulted in 8.8% reduction in body weight [85]. Weight change was associated with increased problem-solving skills and higher adherence to treatment [85]. Moreover, participants with WL > 10% had greater problem-solving skills than those with <5% reduction [85].

3.4.2.2 Cognitive restructuring

Behavior therapy trains individuals to observe the thoughts that hinder their capacity to achieve behavioral targets, recognize distortions in those thoughts, and exchange dysfunctional thoughts with more rational ones. Cognitive restructuring identifies and modifies maladaptive thoughts that promote overeating and lack of exercise. Such thoughts can be dichotomous thinking ("As I am unable to exercise for 30 minutes, I might then not exercise at all") and rationalization ("I had a stressful day, this justifies a portion of cake"). Participants are unaware of the effect of these thoughts on behavior. With cognitive restructuring participants learn how to develop a positive self statement to facilitate behavioral modifications [86].

3.4.3 Cognitive behavioral therapy

Behavior therapy include cognitive strategies to modify eating and activity behaviors [87]. It focuses on altering the cognitive and behavioral mechanisms that causes the problem behavior, and utilize cognitive and behavioral strategies to make positive changes in such behavior. Cognitive behavioral therapy resulted in significant improvement in anthropometric profile, eating behaviors, quality of life across physical, psychological, social, environmental domains, as well as reduced depression [88].

3.4.4 Relapse prevention

Assisting individuals to prepare and plan for relapse prevention includes educating them to foresee challenging situations that could result in overeating, and to utilize strategies to overcome such intervals. Individuals are motivated to plan so that one overeating mistake does not become a full-scale relapse [89]. A WL maintenance program, implemented via telephone that addressed outcome satisfaction, relapse-prevention planning, self-monitoring, and social support found that at 56 weeks, there was statistically significantly less weight regain in the intervention group (0.75 kg) than those receiving usual care [89].

As for the technology use for lifestyle modification: Behavioral treatment improves adherence to lifestyle intervention, but face-to-face delivery is time and resource intensive and travel time is costly and inconvenient. Using the telephone or internet provide cost-effective delivery of lifestyle interventions to many individuals [84, 90]. A study compared the efficacy of phone versus face-to-face clinic approach to achieve 10% WL found that WL at 12 weeks was 10.4% for phone, 13.7% for clinic visits, and both were significantly more than the control group (0.24%) [91]. Individual telephone counseling to provide extended care for obesity management in rural communities diminished the weight regain and increased the proportion of participants who maintained clinically significant WL [92]. Likewise, evidence indicates that Internet-based interventions are better when compared to no or minimal intervention but are less efficacious than in-person treatment [93] . An Internet behavioral WL program resulted in 8 kg, 5.5 kg and 6 kg WL for in person, internet, and hybrid respectively ($p < 0.01$), suggesting that internet is a viable alternative for delivery and dissemination of behavioral weight-control interventions [93]. Smart-phone applications are recently gaining popularity for weight management but its effectiveness has not been proven in the long term. A randomized controlled trial among overweight/obese young adults reported that at 6 months, individuals who received personal coaching enhanced by self-monitoring using a smartphone lost significantly more weight than the controls, but not at 12 or 24 months [94]. Moreover, WL loss outcomes in the group who received lifestyle intervention through interactive smartphone application only was not superior to control in WL [94].

4. Pharmacotherapy

Pharmacotherapy can counteract the increase in appetite the decrease in energy expenditure that occur as an adaptive mechanism to weight loss which, improve adherence to lifestyle modifications. Pharmacotherapy is indicated for BMI ≥30 or BMI ≥27 with obesity-associated conditions [95]. It is prescribed together with comprehensive diet, physical activity and behavioral therapy to achieve adequate WL, and should result in clinically significant WL (≥5% mean TWL%). Anti-obesity medications are prescribed according to their efficacy and safety, the type of obesity associated comorbidities. Several medications are approved for obesity management (**Table 3**).

	Mode of action	Dose	Side effect/s	Contraindication/s
Single drug				
Phentermine* Schedule IV controlled substance	Sympathomimetic amine Adrenergic agonist	8 mg, 15 mg capsule, 37.5 mg tablet	Dry mouth, insomnia, agitation, constipation, tachycardia	G, severe HTN, CV disease, history of drug/alcohol abuse, pregnancy, MOI, selective serotonin reuptake inhibitor use
Orlistat	Pancreatic and gastric lipase inhibitor	60 mg OTC, 120 mg TID	Steatorrhea, oily spotting, flatulence/discharge, fecal incontinence, fat soluble vitamins deficiencies, malabsorption	P, malabsorption syndromes/GI conditions that predispose to GI upset/diarrhea
Liraglutide	GLP-1 agonist	3.0 mg daily	Nausea, vomiting, diarrhea, constipation. Rarely pancreatitis, cholecystitis	Severe renal/hepatic insufficiency, pregnancy, Personal/family history of MTC or MEN2 and major depression/psychiatric disorder
Semaglutide	GLP-1 agonist	2.4 mg weekly	Nausea, vomiting, diarrhea, constipation, headache rarely pancreatitis, cholecystitis	Severe renal/hepatic insufficiency, pregnancy, personal/family history of MTC or MEN2. Past history of P + major depression or psychiatric disorder
Combination				
Phentermine-Topiramate. Schedule IV controlled substance	Sympatho-mimetic amine, anorectic, extended-release anti-epileptic drug	3.75/23 mg, 7.5/46 mg, 11.25/69 mg, 15/92 mg	Paraesthesia, dry mouth, constipation, insomnia, dizziness, altered taste sensation, cognitive effects Rare: closed angle glaucoma, depression, suicidal ideation	G, renal stones, pregnancy (when utilized for WL)
Naltrexone-Bupropion	Opioid receptor antagonist, inhibits dopamine/ norepinephrine reuptake	8/90 mg daily to 16/180 mg BID Tablet	Nausea, vomiting, constipation, dizziness, insomnia, headache, dry mouth	Pregnancy, uncontrolled HTN, uncontrolled pain, recent MOI use, history of seizures/conditions that predispose to seizure e.g., anorexia/BN, abrupt discontinuation of alcohol, benzodiazepines, barbiturates or antiepileptic drugs

**Approved for short-term use; MEN2multiple endocrine neoplasia syndrome type 2; MTC, medullary thyroid carcinoma, BN bulimia nervosa, CV cardiovascular, HTN hypertension, MOI monoamine oxidase inhibitors*

Table 3.
Pharmacotherapy: anti-obesity medications.

4.1 Single medication

4.1.1 Phentermine

Phentermine is a sympathomimetic amine approved in 1959. It increases hypothalamic catecholamine secretion and resting energy expenditure to suppresses appetite. Phentermine is the most frequently used obesity medication in the USA [96]. It is indicated for short-term (3 months), as no long-term safety research exists, but it was approved in combination with topiramate extended release (ER) for long-term therapy. However, many obesity physicians prescribe it for >3 months as off-label therapy for weight management [96]. It is available in 8, 15, 30 and 37.5 mg (single dose early in the day to prevent insomnia). Side effects are mild and due to sympathomimetic effects e.g., dry mouth, insomnia, agitation, constipation and tachycardia. Administering the lowest effective dose decreases the side effects. Phentermine is a schedule IV-controlled substance, and it is contraindicated in patients with history of cardiovascular disease, anxiety, hyperthyroidism, drug or alcohol abuse/dependence. Other contraindications include concomitant treatment with monoamine oxidase inhibitors, pregnancy and breastfeeding [97]. Expected WL with phentermine is 3.6 kg at 6 months [98]. After 6 months, phentermine 15 mg induced a WL of 4.5 kg over placebo [99]. Forty-six percent of participants on phentermine lost ≥5% of their weight, while 20.8% lost ≥10% [99].

4.1.2 Liraglutide

Liraglutide 3 mg is an FDA-approved injectable GLP-1 agonist. A gut-derived incretin hormone, it stimulates the GLP-1 receptor in the pancreatic islets, increases the delivery of insulin and lowers glucagon secretion [100]. It mediates WL through peripheral and CNS pathways, inhibits gastric emptying, promotes satiety and reduces hunger thereby decreasing food intake. The most common side effects encountered with liraglutide are nausea, vomiting, diarrhea, constipation and dyspepsia. These symptoms are usually mild and improve within days or weeks with continuation of treatment and gradual dose titration of the dose. WL with liraglutide may also increase the risk of symptomatic gallstones, and in rare cases may cause pancreatitis. Liraglutide is contraindicated in severe renal/hepatic insufficiency, pregnancy, history of pancreatitis or major psychiatric disorder [101]. In terms weight loss, liraglutide resulted in 5.4% weight loss at one year in large RCT [102]. A total 63.2% of the participants in the liraglutide group lost at least 5% of their weight compared with 27.1% in the placebo group (P<0.001) [102]. Likewise, 33.1% of liraglutide group lost more than 10% of their body weight versus 10.6% in the control group(P<0.001) [102]. Moreover, cardiometabolic risk, inflammatory markers, glycaemic parameters, blood pressure and lipids also improved [102]. For weight maintenance, the SCALE study found that among individuals who lost 5% of their initial body weight on a low-calorie diet, liraglutide added another 6.2% TWL% vs. 0.2% in the placebo group [103].

4.1.3 Semaglutide

Approved in 2019, semaglutide is a long-acting GLP-1 analogue that mimics the effects of native GLP-1, stimulating WL by decreasing the energy intake and hunger, increasing satiety, and enhancing glycemic control [104]. It is approved for treatment of T2D using ≤1.0 mg once weekly subcutaneously or as tablets at a dosage of up to 14 mg. Side effects and contraindications are similar to liraglutide (**Table 3**). In STEP 1 trail, semaglutide 2.4 mg resulted in significant TWL% at 68 weeks compared to placebo (−14.9% vs. − 2.4%) [105]. More participants on semaglutide than placebo achieved ≥5% TWL% (86.4% vs. 31.5%), ≥10% (69.1% vs. 12.0%), and ≥ 15% (50.5% vs. 4.9%) [105]. Moreover, semaglutide led to more improvement in cardiometabolic risk and physical functioning than placebo [105]. In the STEP 4 trial, individuals completing a 20-week run-in period with semaglutide 2.4 mg once per week, maintenance with semaglutide resulted in continuous WL over the next 48 weeks compared to switching to placebo (−7.9% vs. +6.9%) [106].

4.1.4 Orlistat

Approved in 1999, orlistat is the single anti-obesity medication that does not function via the CNS pathway. Instead, it inhibits pancreatic and gastric lipases, reducing absorption of 25–30% of ingested fat [101]. The recommended dose is 120 mg three times per day up to 1 hour after food intake. Side effects are related to fat malabsorption and include steatorrhea, oily spotting, flatulence, and fecal incontinence. The gastrointestinal symptoms can be reduced by a low-fat diet and increasing intake the dietary fiber [107]. Multivitamin supplementation is essential, as orlistat decreases absorption of fat-soluble vitamins (A, D, E, K). Orlistat resulted in a mean 2.9–3.4% weight loss at one year [107]. Long term WL (4 years) can reach 5.8 kg, where 53% of participants lost ≥5% of their weight, and 26.2% lost ≥10% of their weight [108]. Orlistat also reduces the serum glucose levels and increases insulin sensitivity. Individuals with T2DM prescribed orlistat 120 mg exhibited significantly more reduction in fasting blood glucose and HbA1c compared to placebo [109].

4.2 Combination medications

4.2.1 Phentermine-topiramate ER

This long-acting combination was approved in 2012. Phentermine is a short-term appetite suppressant; topiramate is an antiepileptic and migraine medication [107]. The mechanisms of appetite suppression is not well understood, perhaps vis modulation of gamma-aminobutyric acid receptors [110]. Because of its anorexigenic properties, it is used off-label for obesity and binge eating, alone or combined with phentermine. Phentermine/topiramate ER is available as 4 doses daily (**Table 2**), taken in the morning, titrated every 2 weeks and stopped if 5% WL is not accomplished within 12 weeks on maximum daily dose 15/92 mg [111]. Phentermine/topiramate ER, a schedule IV controlled substance. The FDA (Food and drug administration) requires a Risk Evaluation and Mitigation Strategy to inform physicians and women of reproductive age about potential increased likelihood of orofacial clefts in infants exposed to phentermine/topiramate ER during the first trimester of pregnancy [97]. The side effects are those of phentermine and topiramate. Topiramate has dose-dependent side effects and this include cognitive side effects such as psychomotor slowing, diminished concentration, memory impairment and language difficulties (**Table 3**) [111]. Many side effects of topiramate are due to the inhibition of carbonic anhydrase activity, such as metabolic acidosis, hypokalemia, renal stones, angle-closure glaucoma, myopia, and anhidrosis. Therefore, topiramate should not be given with other medications that inhibit carbonic anhydrase [111]. Rare side effects also include increased suicidal thoughts or ideations, where the drug should be stopped immediately.

Phentermine/topiramate ER resulted in significantly greater WL compared to placebo where participants in the 3.75/23, and 15/92 groups lost 5.1%, and 10.9% of their baseline weight, respectively compared with 1.6% in the placebo group [112]. Moreover, 44.9% of 3.75/23 group, and 66.7% of 15/92 group, lost ≥5% of their weight after 56 weeks of treatment compared to 17.3% of the placebo group ($p<0.0001$) [112]. Phentermine/topiramate ER for 52 weeks also resulted in 76% reduction in the progression to diabetes in participants receiving 15/92 mg and a 54% reduction in participants receiving 7.5/46 mg compared with placebo [113].

4.2.2 Naltrexone-bupropion sustained release (SR)

A combination approved in 2014, bupropion (dopamine and norepinephrine reuptake inhibitor) is used for depression and smoking cessation treatment while naltrexone is an opioid antagonist [97, 111]. Their combined use has synergistic effect on appetite suppression [111, 114]. Bupropion inhibits food consumption and increases energy expenditure by stimulating the neuropeptide pro-opiomelanocortin (POMC) and supplementing dopamine activation, which is lower among obese individuals [111]. Naltrexone is used for treating opioid and alcohol dependence [97]. It inhibits the appetite-enhancing influence of beta-endorphin caused by cannabinoid-1 receptor stimulation.

Starting with one tablet (8 mg ER naltrexone and 90 mg ER bupropion) daily, the dose is increased by one tablet per week to a therapeutic dosage of two tablets two times per day (32/360 mg). The medication should be discontinued if WL ≥ 5% is not achieved at 16 weeks [97]. The most common side effects are highlighted in **Table 3**. The medication is contraindicated with monoamine oxidase inhibitors and chronic opioids. It is also contraindicated in patients with uncontrolled HTN, and history of seizures. Bupropion increases the risk of suicidality in patients younger 24 years and therefore they need to be observed closely for mood changes [97].

Studies have shown that patients on naltrexone/bupropion 360/32 mg had a mean 6.1% WL in comparison to 1.3% for those on placebo; and 48% of naltrexone/bupropion individuals lost >5% body weight compared to 16% of placebo patients [114]. Others reported that 44.5% of patients on naltrexone/bupropion lost ≥5% of their body weight after 56 weeks vs. 18.9% on placebo [115]. Furthermore, the medication resulted in better glycemic control and improvements in triglycerides and HDL cholesterol when compared to those on placebo [115].

5. Conclusions

Obesity is a chronic condition with considerably increased morbidity and mortality. Obesity has complex genetic, physiological, behavioral, sociocultural, and environmental etiologies. Hence, a multi-pronged and comprehensive strategy is critical. Lifestyle and behavioral modifications are key in the treatment of obesity, combined with diet, exercise, and behavioral therapy to achieve adequate WL. Pharmacology should be considered for individuals not responding to lifestyle modifications or those who have difficulty maintaining the weight loss initial achieved by lifestyle modifications.

Acronyms and abbreviations

BMI	body mass index
T2DM	type 2 diabetes
CKD	chronic kidney disease
NAFLD	nonalcoholic fatty liver disease
WL	weight loss
CV	cardiovascular
vs	versus
HbA1c	glycosylated hemoglobin refers to glucose and hemoglobin joined together (the hemoglobin is 'glycated') and the normal range for the HbA1c level is between 4% and 5.6%
BP	blood pressure
SBP	systolic blood pressure
DBP	diastolic blood pressure
TG	triglyceride
VLDL	very-low-density lipoprotein
LDL	low-density lipoprotein
HDL	high-density lipoprotein
TW	total weight
TWL%	total WL percentage
TC	total cholesterol
HTN	hypertension refers to high blood pressure defined as systolic 140 mm Hg or higher and diastolic: 90 mm Hg or higher
VLCKD	very low-calorie ketogenic diet
HOMA-IR	homeostasis model assessment-insulin resistance
PA	physical activity
ER	extended release
SR	sustained release
POMC	pro-opiomelanocortin

Author details

Wahiba Elhag[1] and Walid El Ansari[2,3,4*]

1 Bariatric and Metabolic Surgery Section, Hamad Medical Corporation, Doha, Qatar

2 Department of Surgery, Hamad General Hospital, Hamad Medical Corporation, Doha, Qatar

3 College of Medicine, Qatar University, Doha, Qatar

4 Weill Cornell Medicine—Qatar, Doha, Qatar

*Address all correspondence to: welansari9@gmail.com

References

[1] Singh RK, Kumar P, Mahalingam K. Molecular genetics of human obesity: A comprehensive review. Comptes Rendus Biologies. 2017;**340**:87-108

[2] Sadeghirad B, Duhaney T, Motaghipisheh S, Campbell NRC, Johnston BC. Influence of unhealthy food and beverage marketing on children's dietary intake and preference: A systematic review and meta-analysis of randomized trials. Obesity Reviews. 2016;**17**:945-959

[3] Lin X, Li H. Obesity: Epidemiology. Pathophysiology, and Therapeutics: Front Endocrinology. 2021;**12**:706978

[4] Ben Slama F, Achour A, Belhadj O, Hsairi M, Oueslati M, Achour N. Obesity and life style in a population of male school children aged 6 to 10 years in Ariana (Tunisia). La Tunisie Médicale. 2002;**80**:542-547

[5] Duffey KJ, Gordon-Larsen P, Jacobs DR, Williams OD, Popkin BM. Differential associations of fast food and restaurant food consumption with 3-y change in body mass index: The Coronary Artery Risk Development in Young Adults Study. The American Journal of Clinical Nutrition. 2007;**85**:201-208

[6] Corica D, Aversa T, Valenzise M, et al. Does family history of obesity, cardiovascular, and metabolic diseases influence onset and severity of childhood obesity? Frontiers in Endocrinology. 2018;**9**:187

[7] Wright SM, Aronne LJ. Causes of obesity. Abdominal Radiology. 2012;**37**:730-732

[8] Swinburn BA, Sacks G, Hall KD, et al. The global obesity pandemic: Shaped by global drivers and local environments. The Lancet London England. 2011;**378**:804-814

[9] Wirth A, Wabitsch M, Hauner H. The prevention and treatment of obesity. Dtsch Ärztebl International. 2014;**111**:705-713

[10] Fabricatore AN. Behavior therapy and cognitive-behavioral therapy of obesity: Is there a difference? Journal of the American Dietetic Association. 2007;**107**:92-99

[11] Jensen MD, Ryan DH, Apovian CM, et al. 2013 AHA/ACC/TOS guideline for the management of overweight and obesity in adults: A report of the American college of cardiology/American heart association task force on practice guidelines and the obesity society. Circulation. 2014;**129**:S102-S138

[12] Garvey WT, Mechanick JI, Brett EM, et al. American association of clinical endocrinologists and American college of endocrinology comprehensive clinical practice guidelines for medical care of patients with obesity. ***Endocr Pract Off J Am Coll Endocrinol The American Association Of Clinical Endocrinologists. 2016;**22**(Suppl. 3):1-203

[13] Grant P, Piya M, McGowan B, Taheri S. The bariatric physician. Clinical Medicine (London, England). 2014;**14**:30-33

[14] Forgione N, Deed G, Kilov G, Rigas G. Managing obesity in primary care: Breaking down the barriers. Advances in Therapy. 2018;**35**:191-198

[15] Gudzune KA, Doshi RS, Mehta AK, et al. Efficacy of commercial weight loss programs: An updated systematic review. Annals of Internal Medicine. 2015;**162**:501-512

[16] Willaing I, Ladelund S, Jørgensen T, Simonsen T, Nielsen LM. Nutritional counselling in primary health care: A randomized comparison of an intervention by general practitioner or dietician. European Journal of Cardiovascular Prevention and Rehabilitation. 2004;**11**:513-520

[17] Franz MJ, Boucher JL, Rutten-Ramos S, VanWormer JJ. Lifestyle weight-loss intervention outcomes in overweight and obese adults with type 2 diabetes: A systematic review and meta-analysis of randomized clinical trials. Journal of the Academy of Nutrition and Dietetics. 2015;**115**:1447-1463

[18] de Lannoy L, Cowan T, Fernandez A, Ross R. Physical activity, diet, and weight loss in patients recruited from primary care settings: An update on obesity management interventions. Obesity Science and Practice. 2021;7:619-628

[19] Knowler WC, Barrett-Connor E, et al. Reduction in the incidence of type 2 diabetes with lifestyle intervention or metformin. The New England Journal of Medicine. 2002;**346**:393-403

[20] Look AHEAD Research Group, Wing RR, Bolin P, Brancati, et al. Cardiovascular effects of intensive lifestyle intervention in type 2 diabetes. The New England Journal of Medicine. 2013;**369**:145-154

[21] Wing RR, Lang W, Wadden TA, et al. Benefits of modest weight loss in improving cardiovascular risk factors in overweight and obese individuals with type 2 diabetes. Diabetes Care. 2011;**34**:1481-1486

[22] Look AHEAD Research Group. Eight-year weight losses with an intensive lifestyle intervention: the look AHEAD study. Obesity (Silver Spring, Md.). 2014;**22**:5-13

[23] Kuna ST, Reboussin DM, Strotmeyer ES, et al. Effects of weight loss on obstructive sleep apnea severity. Ten-year results of the sleep AHEAD study. American Journal of Respiratory and Critical Care Medicine. 2021;**203**:221-229

[24] Smethers AD, Rolls BJ. Dietary management of obesity: Cornerstones of healthy eating patterns. The Medical Clinics of North America. 2018;**102**:107-124

[25] Witham MD, Avenell A. Interventions to achieve long-term weight loss in obese older people: A systematic review and meta-analysis. Age and Ageing. 2010;**39**:176-184

[26] Sukkar SG, Muscaritoli M. A clinical perspective of low carbohydrate ketogenic diets: A narrative review. Frontiers in Nutrition. 2021;**8**:642628

[27] Shai I, Schwarzfuchs D, Henkin Y, et al. Weight loss with a low-carbohydrate, Mediterranean, or low-fat diet. The New England Journal of Medicine. 2008;**359**:229-241

[28] Brehm BJ, Seeley RJ, Daniels SR, D'Alessio DA. A randomized trial comparing a very low carbohydrate diet and a calorie-restricted low fat diet on body weight and cardiovascular risk factors in healthy women. The Journal of Clinical Endocrinology and Metabolism. 2003;**88**:1617-1623

[29] Foster GD, Wyatt HR, Hill JO, et al. Weight and metabolic outcomes after 2 years on a low-carbohydrate versus low-fat diet. Annals of Internal Medicine. 2010;**153**:147-157

[30] Schwingshackl L, Hoffmann G. Comparison of effects of long-term low-fat vs high-fat diets on blood lipid

levels in overweight or obese patients: A systematic review and meta-analysis. Journal of the Academy of Nutrition and Dietetics. 2013;**113**:1640-1661

[31] Mansoor N, Vinknes KJ, Veierød MB, Retterstøl K. Effects of low-carbohydrate diets v. low-fat diets on body weight and cardiovascular risk factors: A meta-analysis of randomised controlled trials. The British Journal of Nutrition. 2016;**115**:466-479

[32] Stern L, Iqbal N, Seshadri P, et al. The effects of low-carbohydrate versus conventional weight loss diets in severely obese adults: One-year follow-up of a randomized trial. Annals of Internal Medicine American College of Physicians. 2004;**140**:778-785

[33] Samaha FF, Iqbal N, Seshadri P, et al. A low-carbohydrate as compared with a low-fat diet in severe obesity. The New England Journal of Medicine. 2003;**348**:2074-2081

[34] Wadden TA, Webb VL, Moran CH, Bailer BA. Lifestyle modification for obesity. Circulation. American Heart Association. 2012;**125**:1157-1170

[35] Gardner CD, Trepanowski JF, Del Gobbo LC, et al. Effect of low-fat vs low-carbohydrate diet on 12-month weight loss in overweight adults and the association with genotype pattern or insulin secretion: The DIETFITS randomized clinical trial. Journal of the American Medical Association. 2018;**319**:667-679

[36] Sacks FM, Bray GA, Carey VJ, et al. Comparison of weight-loss diets with different compositions of fat, protein, and carbohydrates. The New England Journal of Medicine. 2009;**360**:859-873

[37] Dalle Grave R, Calugi S, Gavasso I, El Ghoch M, Marchesini G. A: randomized trial of energy-restricted high-protein versus high-carbohydrate, low-fat diet in morbid obesity. Obesity. 2013;**21**:1774-1781

[38] Zubrzycki A, Cierpka-Kmiec K, Kmiec Z, Wronska A. The role of low-calorie diets and intermittent fasting in the treatment of obesity and type-2 diabetes. Journal of Physiology and Pharmacology. 2018;**69**

[39] Larsen JK, van Ramshorst B, Geenen R, et al. Binge eating and its relationship to outcome after laparoscopic adjustable gastric banding. Obesity Surgery. 2004;**14**:1111-1117

[40] Ghachem A, Prud'homme D, Rabasa-Lhoret R, Brochu M. Effects of a 6-month caloric restriction induced-weight loss program in obese postmenopausal women with and without the metabolic syndrome: A MONET study. Menopause N Y N. 2017;**24**:908-915

[41] Ruggenenti P, Abbate M, Ruggiero B, et al. Renal and systemic effects of calorie restriction in patients with type 2 diabetes with abdominal obesity: A randomized controlled trial. Diabetes. 2017;**66**:75-86

[42] Nicoll R, Henein MY. Caloric restriction and its effect on blood pressure, heart rate variability and arterial stiffness and dilatation: A review of the evidence. International Journal of Molecular Sciences. 2018;**19**:751

[43] Paoli A, Rubini A, Volek JS, Grimaldi KA. Beyond weight loss: A review of the therapeutic uses of very-low-carbohydrate (ketogenic) diets. European Journal of Clinical Nutrition. 2013;**67**:789-796

[44] Caprio M, Infante M, Moriconi E, et al. Very-low-calorie ketogenic diet (VLCKD) in the management of

metabolic diseases: Aystematic review and consensus statement from the Italian Society of Endocrinology (SIE). Journal of Endocrinological Investigation. 2019;**42**:1365-1386

[45] Muscogiuri G, El Ghoch M, Colao A, et al. European guidelines for obesity management in adults with a very low-calorie ketogenic diet: A systematic review and meta-analysis. Obesity Facts. 2021;**14**:222-245

[46] Veldhorst M, Smeets A, Soenen S, et al. Protein-induced satiety: Effects and mechanisms of different proteins. Physiology & Behavior. 2008;**94**:300-307

[47] Castellana M, Conte E, Cignarelli A, et al. Efficacy and safety of very low calorie ketogenic diet (VLCKD) in patients with overweight and obesity: A systematic review and meta-analysis. Reviews in Endocrine & Metabolic Disorders. 2020;**21**:5-16

[48] Bueno NB, Melo ISV d, Oliveira SL d, Ataide T d R. Very-low-carbohydrate ketogenic diet v. low-fat diet for long-term weight loss: A meta-analysis of randomised controlled trials. British Journal of Nutrition. 2013;**110**:1178-1187

[49] Tragni E, Vigna L, Ruscica M, et al. Reduction of cardio-metabolic risk and body weight through a multiphasic very-low calorie ketogenic diet program in women with overweight/obesity: A study in a real-world setting. Nutrients. 2021;**13**:1804

[50] Moriconi E, Camajani E, Fabbri A, Lenzi A, Caprio M. Very-low-calorie ketogenic diet as a safe and valuable tool for long-term glycemic management in patients with obesity and type 2 diabetes. Nutrients. 2021;**13**:758

[51] Min J, Kim S-Y, Shin I-S, Park Y-B, Lim Y-W. The effect of meal replacement on weight loss according to calorie-restriction type and proportion of energy intake: A systematic review and meta-analysis of randomized controlled trials. Journal of the Academy of Nutrition and Dietetics. 2021;**121**:1551-1564.e3

[52] Li Z, Hong K, Saltsman P, et al. Long-term efficacy of soy-based meal replacements vs an individualized diet plan in obese type II DM patients: Relative effects on weight loss, metabolic parameters, and C-reactive protein. European Journal of Clinical Nutrition. Nature Publishing Group. 2005;**59**:411-418

[53] Heymsfield SB, van MC, van der KH, Heo M, Frier HI. Weight management using a meal replacement strategy: Meta and pooling analysis from six studies [Internet]. Database Abstr. Rev. Eff. DARE Qual.-Assess. Rev. Internet. Centre for Reviews and Dissemination (UK). 2003. Available from: https://www.ncbi.nlm.nih.gov/books/NBK69881/

[54] Ditschuneit HH, Flechtner-Mors M, Johnson TD, Adler G. Metabolic and weight-loss effects of a long-term dietary intervention in obese patients. The American Journal of Clinical Nutrition. 1999;**69**:198-204

[55] Gaesser GA, Angadi SS. Obesity treatment: Weight loss versus increasing fitness and physical activity for reducing health risks. iScience. 2021;**24**:102995

[56] Carraça E, Encantado J, Battista F, et al. Effective behavior change techniques to promote physical activity in adults with overweight or obesity: A systematic review and meta-analysis. Obesity Reviews. 2021;**22**:e13258

[57] Wen H, Wang L. Reducing effect of aerobic exercise on blood pressure of essential hypertensive patients. Medicine (Baltimore). 2017;**96**:e6150

[58] Whelton SP, Chin A, Xin X, He J. Effect of aerobic exercise on blood pressure: A meta-analysis of randomized, controlled trials. Database Abstr. Rev. Eff. DARE Qual.-Assess. Rev. Internet. Centre for Reviews and Dissemination (UK). 2002. Available from: https://www.ncbi.nlm.nih.gov/books/NBK69571/

[59] Kannan U, Vasudevan K, Balasubramaniam K, Yerrabelli D, Shanmugavel K, John NA. Effect of exercise intensity on lipid profile in sedentary obese adults. Journal of Clinical and Diagnostic Research for Doctors JCDR. 2014;**8**:BC08-BC10

[60] Ross R, Janssen I, Dawson J, et al. Exercise-induced reduction in obesity and insulin resistance in women: A randomized controlled trial. Obesity Research. 2004;**12**:789-798

[61] Vissers D, Hens W, Taeymans J, Baeyens J-P, Poortmans J, Van Gaal L. The effect of exercise on visceral adipose tissue in overweight adults: A systematic review and meta-analysis. PLoS One. 2013;**8**:e56415

[62] Hayes C, Kriska A. Role of physical activity in diabetes management and prevention. Journal of the American Dietetic Association. 2008;**108**:S19-S23

[63] Sigal RJ, Kenny GP, Wasserman DH, Castaneda-Sceppa C, White RD. Physical activity/exercise and type 2 diabetes: A consensus statement from the American diabetes association. Diabetes Care. American Diabetes Association. 2006;**29**:1433-1438

[64] Shaw KA. Exercise for overweight or obesity. Cochrane Library. 2006. Available from: https://www.cochranelibrary.com/cdsr/doi/10.1002/14651858.CD003817.pub3/abstract

[65] Donnelly JE, Blair SN, Jakicic JM, et al. American college of sports medicine position Stand. Appropriate physical activity intervention strategies for weight loss and prevention of weight regain for adults. Medicine and Science in Sports and Exercise. 2009;**41**:459-471

[66] Bellicha A, van Baak MA, Battista F, et al. Effect of exercise training on weight loss, body composition changes, and weight maintenance in adults with overweight or obesity: An overview of 12 systematic reviews and 149 studies. Obesity Reviews. 2021;**22**(Suppl 4):e13256

[67] Donnelly JE, Honas JJ, Smith BK, Mayo, et al. Aerobic exercise alone results in clinically significant weight loss for men and women: Midwest exercise trial 2. Obesity Silver Spring, Md. 2013;**21**:E219-E228

[68] Chiu C-H, Ko M-C, Wu L-S, et al. Benefits of different intensity of aerobic exercise in modulating body composition among obese young adults: A pilot randomized controlled trial. Health and Quality of Life Outcomes. 2017;**15**:168

[69] Willis EA, Creasy SA, Honas JJ, Melanson EL, Donnelly JE. The effects of exercise session timing on weight loss and components of energy balance: Midwest exercise trial 2. International Journal of Obesity. 2020;**44**:114-124

[70] Donnelly JE, Jacobsen DJ, Heelan KS, Seip R, Smith S. The effects of 18 months of intermittent vs. continuous exercise on aerobic capacity, body weight and composition, and metabolic fitness in previously sedentary, moderately obese females. International Journal of Obesity and Related Metabolic Disorders. 2000;**24**:566-572

[71] Willis LH, Slentz CA, Bateman LA, et al. Effects of aerobic and/or resistance

training on body mass and fat mass in overweight or obese adults. Journal of Applied Physiology. 1985;**2012**(113):1831-1837

[72] Swift DL, Johannsen NM, Lavie CJ, Earnest CP, Blair SN, Church TS. Effects of clinically significant weight loss with exercise training on insulin resistance and cardiometabolic adaptations. Obesity Silver Spring Md. 2016;**24**:812-819

[73] Ho SS, Dhaliwal SS, Hills AP, Pal S. The effect of 12 weeks of aerobic, resistance or combination exercise training on cardiovascular risk factors in the overweight and obese in a randomized trial. BMC Public Health. 2012;**12**:704

[74] Anderson JW, Reynolds LR, Bush HM, Rinsky JL, Washnock C. Effect of a behavioral/nutritional intervention program on weight loss in obese adults: A randomized controlled trial. Postgraduate Medicine. 2011;**123**:205-213

[75] Juchacz K, Kłos P, Dziedziejko V, Wójciak RW. The effectiveness of supportive psychotherapy in weight loss in a group of young overweight and obese women. Nutrients. 2021;**13**:532

[76] Kelley CP, Sbrocco G, Sbrocco T. Behavioral modification for the management of obesity. Primary Care. 2016;**43**:159-175

[77] Lichtman SW, Pisarska K, Berman ER, et al. Discrepancy between self-reported and actual caloric intake and exercise in obese subjects. The New England Journal of Medicine. 1992;**327**:1893-1898

[78] Tudor-Locke C, Bassett DR. How many steps/day are enough? Preliminary pedometer indices for public health. Sports Medicine Auckl NZ. 2004;**34**:1-8

[79] Goldstein SP, Goldstein CM, Bond DS, Raynor HA, Wing RR, Thomas JG. Associations between self-monitoring and weight change in behavioral weight loss interventions. Health Psychology. 2019;**38**:1128-1136

[80] Ross KM, Qiu P, You L, Wing RR. Week-to-week predictors of weight loss and regain. Health Psychology. 2019;**38**:1150-1158

[81] Avery A, Langley-Evans SC, Harrington M, Swift JA. Setting targets leads to greater long-term weight losses and 'unrealistic' targets increase the effect in a large community-based commercial weight management group. Journal of Human Nutrition and Dietetics. 2016;**29**:687-696

[82] Nothwehr F, Yang J. Goal setting frequency and the use of behavioral strategies related to diet and physical activity. Health Education Research. 2007;**22**:532-538

[83] Watson P, Wiers RW, Hommel B, Gerdes VEA, de Wit S. Stimulus control over action for food in obese versus healthy-weight individuals. Frontiers in Psychology. 2017;**8**:580

[84] Mb NA, Tronieri JS, Wadden T. Behavioral approaches to obesity management. In: Feingold KR, Anawalt B, Boyce A, et al., editors. Endotext [Internet]. South Dartmouth (MA): MDText.com, Inc.; 2000. Available from: http://www.ncbi.nlm.nih.gov/books/NBK278952/

[85] Murawski ME, Milsom VA, Ross KM, et al. Problem solving, treatment adherence, and weight-loss outcome among women participating in lifestyle treatment for obesity. Eating Behaviors. 2009;**10**:146-151

[86] Wing RR, Gorin A, Tate D. Strategies for Changing Eating and Exercise Behavior

[87] Castelnuovo G, Pietrabissa G, Manzoni GM, et al. Cognitive behavioral therapy to aid weight loss in obese patients: Current perspectives. In: Psychol Res Behav Manag. New Zealand: Dove Medical Press Ltd.; 2017. p. 10

[88] Moraes A d S, Padovani R d C, La Scala Teixeira CV, et al. Cognitive behavioral approach to treat obesity: A randomized clinical trial. Frontiers in Nutrition. 2021;**8**:14

[89] Voils CI, Olsen MK, Gierisch JM, et al. Maintenance of weight loss after initiation of nutrition training: A randomized trial. Annals of Internal Medicine. 2017;**166**:463-471

[90] Driscoll S, Meyerowitz-Katz G, Ahlenstiel G, Reynolds T, Reid K, Bishay RH. Efficacy of telephone health coaching integration with standard multidisciplinary care for adults with obesity attending a weight management service: A pilot study. Nutrients. 2021;**13**:4078

[91] Donnelly JE, Smith BK, Dunn L, et al. Comparison of a phone vs clinic approach to achieve 10% weight loss. International Journal of Obesity. 2005;**2007**(31):1270-1276

[92] Perri MG, Shankar MN, Daniels MJ, et al. Effect of telehealth extended care for maintenance of weight loss in rural us communities: A randomized clinical trial. JAMA Network Open. 2020;**3**:e206764

[93] Harvey-Berino J, West D, Krukowski R, et al. Internet delivered behavioral obesity treatment. Preventive Medicine. 2010;**51**:123-128

[94] Svetkey LP, Batch BC, Lin P-H, et al. Cell phone intervention for you (CITY): A randomized, controlled trial of behavioral weight loss intervention for young adults using mobile technology. Obesity Silver Spring Md. 2015;**23**:2133-2141

[95] Telles S, Gangadhar BN, Chandwani KD. Lifestyle modification in the prevention and management of obesity. Journal of Obesity. 2016;**2016**:5818601

[96] Patel D. Pharmacotherapy for the management of obesity. Metabolism. 2015;**64**:1376-1385

[97] Saunders KH, Umashanker D, Igel LI, Kumar RB, Aronne LJ. Obesity pharmacotherapy. The Medical Clinics of North America. 2018;**102**:135-148

[98] Li Z, Maglione M, Tu W, et al. Meta-analysis: Pharmacologic treatment of obesity. Annals of Internal Medicine. 2005;**142**:532-546

[99] Aronne LJ, Wadden TA, Peterson C, Winslow D, Odeh S, Gadde KM. Evaluation of phentermine and topiramate versus phentermine/topiramate extended-release in obese adults. Obesity Silver Spring Md. 2013;**21**:2163-2171

[100] Astrup A, Carraro R, Finer N, et al. Safety, tolerability and sustained weight loss over 2 years with the once-daily human GLP-1 analog, liraglutide. International Journal of Obesity. 2005;**2012**(36):843-854

[101] Lee PC, Dixon J. Pharmacotherapy for obesity. Australian Family Physician. 2017;**46**:472-477

[102] Pi-Sunyer X, Astrup A, Fujioka K, et al. A randomized, controlled trial of 3.0 mg of liraglutide in weight management. The New England Journal of Medicine. 2015;**373**:11-22

[103] Wadden TA, Hollander P, Klein S, et al. Weight maintenance and additional

weight loss with liraglutide after low-calorie-diet-induced weight loss: The SCALE Maintenance randomized study. International Journal of Obesity. 2005;**2013**(37):1443-1451

[104] Kushner RF, Calanna S, Davies M, et al. Semaglutide 2.4 mg for the treatment of obesity: Key elements of the step trials 1 to 5. Obesity Silver Spring Md. 2020;**28**:1050-1061

[105] Wilding JPH, Batterham RL, Calanna S, et al. Once-weekly semaglutide in adults with overweight or obesity. The New England Journal of Medicine. 2021;**384**:989

[106] Rubino D, Abrahamsson N, Davies M, et al. Effect of continued weekly subcutaneous semaglutide vs placebo on weight loss maintenance in adults with overweight or obesity: The step 4 randomized clinical trial. Journal of the American Medical Association. 2021;**325**:1414-1425

[107] Apovian CM, Aronne LJ, Bessesen DH, et al. Pharmacological management of obesity: An endocrine Society clinical practice guideline. The Journal of Clinical Endocrinology and Metabolism. 2015;**100**:342-362

[108] Torgerson JS, Hauptman J, Boldrin MN, Sjöström L. XENical in the Prevention of Diabetes in Obese Subjects (XENDOS) Study: A randomized study of orlistat as an adjunct to lifestyle changes for the prevention of type 2 diabetes in obese patients. Diabetes Care. American Diabetes Association. 2004;**27**:155-161

[109] Jacob S, Rabbia M, Meier MK, Hauptman J. Orlistat 120 mg improves glycaemic control in type 2 diabetic patients with or without concurrent weight loss. Diabetes, Obesity & Metabolism. 2009;**11**:361-371

[110] Kushner RF. Weight loss strategies for treatment of obesity. Progress in Cardiovascular Diseases. 2014;**56**:465-472

[111] Son JW, Kim S. Comprehensive review of current and upcoming anti-obesity drugs. Diabetes and Metabolism Journal. 2020;**44**:802-818

[112] Allison DB, Gadde KM, Garvey WT, et al. Controlled-release phentermine/topiramate in severely obese adults: A randomized controlled trial (EQUIP). Obesity Silver Spring Md. 2012;**20**:330-342

[113] Garvey WT, Ryan DH, Look M, et al. Two-year sustained weight loss and metabolic benefits with controlled-release phentermine/topiramate in obese and overweight adults (SEQUEL): A randomized, placebo-controlled, phase 3 extension study. The American Journal of Clinical Nutrition. 2012;**95**:297-308

[114] Greenway FL, Fujioka K, Plodkowski RA, et al. Effect of naltrexone plus bupropion on weight loss in overweight and obese adults (COR-I): A multicentre, randomised, double-blind, placebo-controlled, phase 3 trial. The Lancet. 2010;**376**:595-605

[115] Hollander P, Gupta AK, Plodkowski R, et al. Effects of naltrexone sustained-release/bupropion sustained-release combination therapy on body weight and glycemic parameters in overweight and obese patients with type 2 diabetes. Diabetes Care. American Diabetes Association. 2013;**36**:4022-4029

Chapter 8

Resistance Training and Weight Management: Rationale and Efficacy

Ina Shaw, Travis Triplett and Brandon S. Shaw

Abstract

In addition to the impact of normal ageing on body composition, increasing levels of sedentariness reduce an individual's ability to mobilise fat, resulting in an altered body composition characterised by increased fat mass, and more specifically an increased total and abdominal fat, and reduced muscle mass. While exercise, and aerobic exercise in general, has been promoted as a means to maintaining an appropriate body weight, aerobic exercise should not be considered as the golden standard to do so. This is because resistance training (RT) has an unsurpassed ability to improve lean mass along with other simultaneous improvements in multiple body composition parameters. An increased muscle mass is essential in that it is the amount of exercising muscle that determines the magnitude of lipolysis (fatty acid release from adipocytes) during exercise. In addition, an increased muscle mass results in an elevated basal metabolic rate (BMR) and resting metabolic rate (RMR), effectively increasing the amount of energy or calories utilised even at rest. RT is especially useful in the general population for weight management in that the ideal form of RT required for improvements in body composition is of moderate intensity, which reduces the risk of injury and improves adherence.

Keywords: body composition, kinanthropometry, obesity, overweight, resistance exercise, strength training, weight training

1. Introduction

Overweight and obesity are global health problems affecting more than 1.1 billion adults [1]. This is problematic in that overweight and obesity are prominent risk factors for the development of numerous conditions and diseases, including cardiovascular, pulmonary and metabolic diseases, such as diabetes mellitus [1, 2]. Consequently, overweight and obesity then result in enormous burdens on the healthcare system and burgeoning healthcare costs [3]. In weight loss regimes, it is important to note that the use of the term "overweight" is a misnomer, since overweight and obesity are situations of an individual being "overfat" and not just having a high weight [4].

Weight loss is a common aim for athletes, obese, overweight and even normal weight individuals. However, an optimal weight loss programme should

IntechOpen

concomitantly reduce body fat while maintaining lean mass [5]. As such, the relative effect of various interventions should be assessed on how they impact body composition, rather than weight loss. In this regard, body composition is the amount or percentage of tissues within in the body, primarily including body fluids, bone, fat and muscle tissue an individual has. Typically, body composition is defined as the distribution of the body tissues into extracellular water, fat-free mass/lean mass and fat mass [6]. In this regard, two individuals of the same gender, height and weight can look completely different because of differences in body composition.

Further, in addition to total fatness, fat topography or distribution in the body has been found to be even more important for health promotion and disease prevention [7, 8]. This is so since abdominal visceral fat deposition is especially associated with an increased risk for a variety of health problems and metabolic disturbances such as "syndrome x" [9]. An increased intra-abdominal visceral fat even in the absence of a high body mass index (BMI) or generalised obesity can increase mortality and morbidity from chronic diseases and health conditions such as heart disease, hypertension and diabetes mellitus [7].

2. Exercise as an adjunct weight loss strategy

The most common strategy employed globally for weight loss is the use of dietary intervention or the cutting of calories [10]. This strategy is based on the "calories in versus calories out" model and maintains that you will lose weight if you take in less calories than you use. Problematically, the human body is more complex than that. Human bodies are not static and have a multitude of fluctuations in energy needs, such as stress and activity levels. Further, even the timing and composition of meals will affect nutrient intake, such as the thermic effect of food [11].

Further reasons against the use of caloric restriction strategies for weight loss arise from research findings that treatments relying only on energy restriction commonly cause substantial loss of lean mass [12]. Further, severe caloric restriction is also associated with impairment of muscle dysfunction and aerobic capacity, which is especially detrimental for athletes [13].

Thankfully, the addition of exercise, has frequently been shown to mitigate this loss in lean mass and physiological impairments [12], and potentially offset athletic performance decrements. Exercise is especially useful with weight loss in that it acutely increases energy and lipid utilisation and contributes to increases in lean mass and metabolic rate, which indirectly aids weight loss [14]. It is for this reason that exercise is considered an important component of weight loss and perhaps the best predictor of weight maintenance [15]. Specifically, at least 30 min a day of moderate intensity aerobic exercise per day is recommended for weight loss and maintenance but greater amounts appear to increase the magnitude of weight loss and maintenance [15].

3. Resistance training as an adjunct weight loss strategy

It is critical to note that many weight loss programmes incorporating diet-only and/or even aerobic-only exercise results in weight loss as a result of a deleterious reduction in muscle mass [16], sometimes even without a decrease in fat mass [16]. When it comes to weight loss, it is clear that a combination of interventions is more effective than a single intervention strategy [17]. Thus, it is critical for clients and health professionals alike to emphasis body recomposition, rather than weight loss, since it focuses on the process of changing the ratio of fat and lean mass, with a focus on losing fat mass while gaining muscle mass. In this regard, research indicates that resistance training (RT) as an exercise modality is most effective at increasing lean mass [8]. RT, also known as strength training or weight training, is any type of exercise in which a muscle or muscle group has to overcome some sort of external resistance. This can be achieved through a variety of techniques, including incremental weight increases, the use of a variety of exercises and types of equipment to target specific muscles or muscle groups. As such, RT can also incorporate a variety of training techniques, such as callisthenics, Pilates, yoga, free weights, weight machines, resistance bands, isometrics, high-intensity interval training (HITT) and plyometrics.

Problematically, a challenge to body recomposition and RT's unpopularity in weight management is that this loss in fat mass coupled with an increase in fat mass results in a relatively stable weight, that is undesirable by those engaged in "weight loss". In addition, due to this stigma of an increased muscle mass following RT, many individual engaging in a weight management programme fail to engage in RT [18].

RT results in a plethora of physiological changes and adaptions that are well suited to weight loss and body recomposition. In this regard, a unique feature of RT is its ability to maintain or increase muscle mass. It is this increase in muscle mass that not only offsets declines in performance and health, but also increases metabolic rate. In this regard, while aerobic exercise may burn slightly more calories per hour than RT (i.e. running at five miles per hour burns approximately 606 calories per hour for a 73 kg individual versus a general resistance training session for 1 h that burns an average of 448 calories per hour for a 70 kg individual), each kg of muscle burns off around 13 calories per day [19]. As such, even a modest 5 kg increase in muscle mass will result in an additional 65 calories being burnt daily. Further, research has demonstrated that while caloric expenditure of RT is only slightly less than aerobic exercise, excess post-exercise oxygen consumption (EPOC) and post-exercise caloric expenditure are higher following RT (even when matched for oxygen consumption and equal durations) [20] and this may have an additional favourable consequence on weight management programmes.

Physiologists may be interested in the effect of exercise on basal metabolic.

rate, fat size and distribution, and dietary-induced thermogenesis, whereas other scientists, such as nutritionists and psychologists may be concerned about the possible effect of exercise on other factors, such as habitual nutrient intake, and effect on body image and self-concept, feelings of well-being and adherence, respectively. In this regard, the addition (but not sole use) of RT to aerobic training can reduce the amount of total calories, carbohydrates, proteins and fats consumed and as such promotes a favourable improvement in self-reported dietary intake [21].

4. Common myths about resistance training and weight loss

While greater amounts of exercise appear to increase the magnitude of weight loss and maintenance [15], it must be noted that too much exercising actually prevents body fat loss due to increases in cortisol. In fact, research suggests this raised cortisol leads to overeating, weight gain and an increase in abdominal fat [22].

Further, many individuals engaging in a weight loss programme fail to utilise RT for fear of "bulking up", "looking manly", or "becoming muscle-bound". While it is true that RT is the exercise of choice for bodybuilders, many individuals, and females in general, lack the hormonal and genetic profile to develop overly large muscles [23].

A particular problem amongst children and health professionals working with children is the erroneous belief that all RT results in damage to the epiphyseal or growth plates [24]. Despite the need for RT in supporting neural adaptation during normal physiological maturation, RT has proven effective at weight loss and body recomposition in children and adolescents [25, 26]. While literature and research indicate that some risk of injury from RT does exist, this is comparable to that of sports children are already participating in and that risk for injury in children is not dramatically elevated by RT and can be minimised by effective programme design (i.e. appropriate programme development) and education (i.e. on lifting technique) [24, 27].

While the term spot reduction or spot training (the localised loss of fat as a result of exercising a particular part of the body), is commonly practiced using RT, research in this area is still contradictory [28]. In this regard, the present body of knowledge is insufficient about the plastic heterogeneity of regional body tissues when a localised RT programme is applied [28].

A common prevailing myth is the belief that fat can be turned into muscle. However, this is not a physiological probability since skeletal muscle consists of numerous protein muscle fibres, which in turn, are comprised of a number of myofibrils containing multiple myofilaments [29]. On the contrary, body fat, which is known as adipose tissue consists of triglycerides, which consist of glycerol and three fatty acid chains. Fat is exclusively made up of numerous carbon, hydrogen, and oxygen atoms [30]. As such, due to this differentiation in muscle and fat cell chemical composition, neither can be converted into the other [31].

5. Resistance training programme design for body recomposition and weight Loss

The majority of exercise recommendations for weight loss endorse aerobic-type activities with a focus on a significant caloric expenditure during the exercise session [10]. In this regard, the American College of Sports Medicine (ACSM) emphasises diet restriction and aerobic exercise, while not assigning RT a major role in weight maintenance and weight loss, due to insufficient evidence. This is problematic in that RT has a multitude of health benefits and has proven effective in the short-term for modestly decreasing body fat, especially in conjunction with dietary interventions [32]. More importantly, research suggests that RT can also play a vital role in long-term weight management, especially in that it utilises additional mechanisms to that of aerobic exercise [33].

However, for any exercise programme to be effective at weight management, continuous adjustments need to be made to the programme design variables, namely; choice of exercises, order of exercises, frequency, load (weight), volume, rest periods, variation and progression [34].

5.1 Resistance training choice and order exercises for weight management

While almost any RT exercise will have a positive impact on health promotion and weight management, RT exercises for weight management should focus on large muscle groups and those exercises utilising compound movements, such Olympic lifts, deadlifts and squats. Since these compound exercises require an elevated oxygen use and hormonal response and result in high-calorie-expenditure. These compound exercises should be prioritised in an effective RT programme for weight management. In addition, training the larger muscle groups will also result in an enhanced hypertrophy and increased basal metabolic rate (BMR) (i.e. minimum number of calories required for basic functions at rest) and resting metabolic rate (RMR) (i.e. the number of calories the body burns while at rest) in the long-term [35].

Further, although many programme designs exist or RT sessions, recommendations for weight loss suggest progressing from multi-joint to single-joint exercises in RT sessions. This may be especially important from a safety standpoint to prevent any undue consequences of muscle fatigue at the end of a workout [35].

5.2 Resistance training load (weight) and volume for weight management

Since the principal determinant of BMR is body mass, and more specifically lean mass [36], RT has important long-term implications for successful weight management. This is because RT is the primary exercise intervention for increasing muscle mass [37]. When it comes to hypertrophy, recent research indicates a dose-response relationship between the total number of weekly sets and increases in muscle growth [38]. In this regard, health professionals should consider all aspects related to increasing training volume, such as the total number of sets, reps or time under tension, and resistance (weight) utilised during a training day, month or other block of training time. Thankfully, this increased volume of training serves a dual purpose as it is also deemed high-caloric expenditure in nature. Specifically, moderate loads for hypertrophy correspond to approximately 8–15 of one-repetition maximum (1-RM) [39] and should be performed for three to five sets per exercise to increase volume [37, 40].

5.3 Resistance training frequency for weight management

As the outcome of RT is the same as for that of aerobic exercise interventions for weight loss, it important to note that research indicates a graded dose-response relationship whereby increases in RT volume (i.e. increased number of weekly sets) produce greater gains in muscle hypertrophy [37]. This increase in RT dose also results in an increased caloric expenditure and improves the prognosis not only for hypertrophy but also for weight loss. As for any exercise intervention (whether RT or aerobic), cognisance should be taken of the training status of the individual, with beginners training less frequently and well-trained individuals training more frequently. RT is especially useful in this area of programme design in that it allows for split routines, whereby upper-body and lower-body can be trained on alternate days to facilitate and enhance recovery.

5.4 Resistance training rest periods for weight management

While 3–5 min rest periods are advocated between RT sets for multiple sets per exercise [40], well-trained individuals can consider exercise sets with minimal rest periods for optimising weight loss [41]. This is because decreasing rest periods or making use of super sets has been demonstrated to increase training intensity [40]. Problematically, while RT with minimal rest periods is considered as most effective for weight and fat loss, it can cause significant central nervous system fatigue and eventual overtraining [42].

Frequency	Intensity	Repetitions	Sets	Type
3 or more days/week; aim to increase volume and caloric expenditure; split routines can be utilised to enhance recovery; beginners: train less frequently; well-trained: train more frequently	Moderate loads for hypertrophy	8–15 of 1-RM; emphasis is on volume	3–5 per exercise; with minimal duration rest intervals; emphasis is on volume	Multi-joint/compound exercise utilising more than one muscle or muscle group

Table 1.
Guidelines for resistance training programme design for body recomposition and weight loss.

5.5 Resistance training progression for weight management

While it is important to keep the exercises used in a programme fairly consistent for weeks or months in a particular training period to prevent overuse, health professionals must allow for new ways to stimulate muscle growth and fat utilisation. For example; this could be accomplished by manipulating the number of sets, the number or repetitions, the weight utilised during exercises or additional training days could be added as well to increase overall volume. In turn, when training at a specific repetition maximum (RM) load, it is recommended that a 2–10% increase in load be applied when the individual can perform the current workload for one to two repetitions over the desired number [40]. Progressive increases in volume should be observed for a particular training block of weeks or months, followed by a period of decreased volume. This aids in preventing training plateaus, injury and boredom [40]. **Table 1** provides guidelines on the approaches for the implementation of resistance training in weight management.

6. Conclusions

Despite the credible evidence that exists to suggest that RT can play an important role in a comprehensive weight loss programme, RT is not promoted as widely as aerobic interventions. Problematically, while the inclusion of RT may not optimally enhance short-term weight loss in all populations, the integration of RT with dietary interventions could facilitate long-term fat loss, while preserving lean mass while increasing RMR and BMR. This is in addition to the significant and unique health and functional benefits that RT provides. However, in order to stimulate adaptation toward weight loss and body recomposition, specific progressive RT protocols are necessary that focus on caloric expenditure through high volume training (s with other modes of exercise) and hypertrophy.

Acknowledgements

The authors would like to acknowledge the contributions made by the Non-Communicable Disease Intervention Research Unit (NCDIRU).

Conflict of interest

The authors declare no conflict of interest.

Author details

Ina Shaw[1,2], Travis Triplett[3] and Brandon S. Shaw[1,2*]

1 School of Sport, Rehabilitation and Exercise Sciences, University of Essex, Wivenhoe Park, Colchester, Essex, United Kingdom

2 Department of Human Movement Science, University of Zululand, Kwadlangezwa, South Africa

3 Department of Health and Exercise Science, Appalachian State University, Boone, United States of America

*Address all correspondence to: shawb@unizulu.ac.za

References

[1] Elagizi A, Kachur S, Lavie CJ, Carbone S, Pandey A, Ortega FB, et al. An overview and update on obesity and the obesity paradox in cardiovascular diseases. Progress in Cardiovascular Diseases. 2018;**61**(2):142-150. DOI: 10.1016/j.pcad.2018.07.003

[2] Shaw I, Shaw BS. Relationship between resistance training and lipoprotein profiles in sedentary male smokers. Cardiovascular Journal of Africa. 2008;**19**(4):194-197

[3] American Diabetes Association. Economic costs of diabetes in the U.S. in 2017. Diabetes Care. 2018;**41**:917-928. DOI: 10.2337/dci18-0007

[4] Shaw BS, Shaw I. Resistance training as a countermeasure for key non-communicable diseases in low-resource settings: A review. Asian Journal of Sports Medicine. 2021;**12**(1):1-8, e106588. DOI: 10.5812/asjsm.106588

[5] Walberg JL. Aerobic exercise and resistance weight-training during weight reduction. Sports Medicine. 1989;7: 343-356. DOI: 10.2165/00007256-198907060-00001

[6] Spano M. Nutrition strategies for maximizing performance. In: Haff GG, Triplett NT, editors. Essentials of Strength Training and Conditioning. 4th ed. Champaign, Illinois: Human Kinetics; 2015

[7] Chartterjee D, Ghosh JR, Chanda S, Bandyopadhyay AR. Relationship between anthropometric measurements and body composition among Santal girls aged between 6-18 years of Galudih, Jharkhand, India. Anthropologist. 2006;**8**(4):241-243. DOI: 10.1080/09720073.2006.11890970

[8] Shaw BS, Shaw I, Mamen A. Contrasting effects in body composition following endurance, resistance and concurrent endurance and resistance training. Journal of Sports Medicine and Physical Fitness. 2012;**50**(2):207-213

[9] Sientz CA, Aiken LB, Houmard JA, Bales CW, Johnson JL, Tanner CJ, et al. Inactivity, exercise, and visceral fat. STRRIDE: A randomized, controlled study of exercise intensity and amount. Journal of Applied Physiology. 2005;**99**(4):1613-1618. DOI: 10.1152/japplphysiol.00124.2005

[10] Sword D. O. Exercise as a management strategy for the overweight and obese. Where does resistance exercise fit in? Strength and Conditioning Journal. 2012;**34**(5):47-55. DOI: 10.1519/SSC.0b013e31826d9403

[11] University of Hawai'i at Mānoa Food Science and Human Nutrition Program. Human Nutrition: 2020 Edition. University of Hawai'i at Mānoa; 2020

[12] Shaw BS, Shaw I, Brown GA. Self-reported dietary intake following endurance, resistance and concurrent endurance and resistance training. Journal of Sports Science and Medicine. 2008;7(2):255-259

[13] Ross R, Dagnone D, Jones PJH, Smith H, Paddags A, Hudson R, et al. Reduction in obesity and related comorbid conditions after diet-induced weight loss or exercise-induced weight loss in men: A randomized, controlled trial. Annals of Internal Medicine. 2000;**133**(2):92-103. DOI: 10.7326/0003-4819-133-2-200007180-00008

[14] Shaw BS, Dullabh M, Forbes G, Brandkamp J, Shaw I. Analysis of

physiological determinants during a single bout of crossfit. International Journal of Performance Analysis in Sport. 2015;**15**:809-815. DOI: 10.1080/24748668.2015.11868832

[15] Joseph E, Donnelly EDD, Smith B, Jacobsen DJ, Kirk E, DuBose K, et al. The role of exercise for weight loss and maintenance. Best Practice & Research Clinical Gastroenterology. 2004;**18**(6):1009-1029. DOI: 10.1016/j.bpg.2004.06.022

[16] Bryner RW, Ullrich IH, Sauers J, Donley D, Hornsby G, Kolar M, et al. Effects of resistance vs. aerobic training combined with an 800 calorie liquid diet on lean body mass and resting metabolic rate. Journal of the American College of Nutrition. 1999;**18**(2):115-121. DOI: 10.1080/07315724.1999.10718838

[17] Avila JJ, Gutierres JA, Sheehy ME, Lofgren IE, Delmonico MJ. Effect of moderate intensity resistance training during weight loss on body composition and physical performance in overweight older adults. European Journal of Applied Physiology. 2010;**109**(3):517-525. DOI: 10.1007/s00421-010-1387-9

[18] Shaw BS, Brown GA, Shaw I. Importance of resistance training in the management of cardiovascular disease risk. In: Chahine J, editor. Cardiovascular risk factors. London, United Kingdom: IntechOpen Publishers; 2021. ISBN: 978-1-83968-709-9

[19] Ainsworth BE et al. Compendium of physical activities: A second update of codes and MET values. Medicine & Science in Sports & Exercise. 2011;**43**:1575. DOI: 10.1249/MSS.0b013e31821ece12

[20] Burleson MA Jr, O'Bryant HS, Stone MH, Collins MA, Triplett McBride T. Effect of weight training exercise and treadmill exercise on post-exercise oxygen consumption. Medicine & Science in Sports & Exercise. 1998;**30**(4):518-522. DOI: 10.1097/00005768-199804000-00008

[21] Shaw BS, Shaw I, Brown GA. Relationship between resistance training and self-reported habitual nutrient intake. South African Journal for Research in Sport, Physical Education and Recreation. 2010;**32**(2):109-116. DOI: 10.4314/sajrs.v32i2.59300

[22] Herhaus B, Ullmann E, Chrousos G, Petrowski K. High/low cortisol reactivity and food intake in people with obesity and healthy weight. Translational Psychiatry. 2020;**10**(1):40. DOI: 10.1038/s41398-020-0729-6

[23] Shaw BS, Shaw I, Brown GA. Resistance exercise is medicine: Strength training in health promotion and rehabilitation. International Journal of Therapy and Rehabilitation. 2015;**22**(8): 385-389. DOI: 10.12968/ijtr.2015.22.8.385

[24] Myers AM, Beam NW, Fakhoury JD. Resistance training for children and adolescents. Translational Pediatrics. 2017;**6**(3):137-143. DOI: 10.21037/tp.2017.04.01

[25] Shaw BS, Shaw I, Brown GA. Effect of resistance training on total, central and abdominal adiposity. South African Journal for Research in Sport, Physical Education and Recreation. 2009;**31**(2):97-108. DOI: 10.4314/sajrs.v31i2.46331

[26] Shaw I, Shaw BS, Goon DT, Erasmus S. Total and abdominal adiposity changes in response to upper body resistance training. African Journal for Physical, Health Education, Recreation and Dance. 2011;**2**(Suppl. 2:2):51-59

[27] Faigenbaum AD, Myer GD. Pediatric resistance training: Benefits, concerns,

and program design considerations. Current Sports Medicine Reports. 2010;**9**(3):161-168. DOI: 10.1249/JSR.0b013e3181de1214

[28] Ramírez-Campillo R, Andrade DC, Campos-Jara C, Henríquez-Olguín C, Alvarez-Lepín C, Izquierdo M. Regional fat changes induced by localized muscle endurance resistance training. Journal of Strength and Conditioning Research. 2013;**27**(8):2219-2224. DOI: 10.1519/JSC.0b013e31827e8681

[29] Goodman CA, Hornberger TA, Robling AG. Bone and skeletal muscle: Key players in mechanotransduction and potential overlapping mechanisms. Bone. 2015;**80**:24-36. DOI: 10.1016/j.bone.2015.04.014

[30] Cohen P, Spiegelman BM. Cell biology of fat storage. Molecular Biology of the Cell. 2016;**27**(16):2523-2527. DOI: 10.1091/mbc.E15-10-0749

[31] Pedersen BK. Muscle-to-fat interaction: A two-way street. Journal of Physiology. 2016;**588**(Pt 1):21. DOI: 10.1113/jphysiol.2009.184747

[32] Shaw BS, Shaw I, Brown GA. Comparison of resistance and concurrent resistance and endurance training regimes in the development of strength. Journal of Strength and Conditioning Research. 2009;**23**(9):2507-2514. DOI: 10.1519/JSC.0b013e3181bc191e

[33] Fourie M, Gildenhuys GM, Shaw I, Shaw BS, Toriola AL, Goon DT. Effects of a mat Pilates programme on muscular strength and endurance in elderly women. African Journal for Physical, Health Education, Recreation and Dance. 2012;**18**(2):296-304

[34] Shaw BS, Gouveia M, McIntyre S, Shaw I. Anthropometric and cardiovascular responses to hypertrophic resistance training in postmenopausal women. Menopause. 2016;**23**(11):1176-1181. DOI: 10.1097/GME.0000000000000687

[35] Simao R, de Salles BF, Figueiredo T, Dias I, Willardson JM. Exercise order in resistance training. Sports Medicine. 2012;**42**(3):251-265. DOI: 10.2165/11597240-000000000-00000

[36] McNab BK. What determines the basal rate of metabolism? Journal of Experimental Biology. 2019;**222**(Pt 15): jeb205591. DOI: 10.1242/jeb.205591

[37] Schoenfeld BJ, Contreras B, Krieger J, Grgic J, Delcastillo K, Belliard R, et al. Resistance training volume enhances muscle hypertrophy but not strength in trained men. Medicine and Science in Sports and Exercise. 2019;**51**(1):94-103. DOI: 10.1249/MSS.0000000000001764

[38] Peterson MD, Rhea MR, Alvar BA. Applications of the dose–response for muscular strength development: A review of meta-analytic efficacy and reliability for designing training prescription. Journal of Strength and Conditioning Research. 2005;**19**(4): 950-958. DOI: 10.1519/R-16874.1

[39] Bird SP, Tarpenning KM, Marino FE. Programmes to enhance muscular fitness. a review of the acute programme variables. Sports Medicine. 2005;**35**(10):841-851. DOI: 10.2165/00007256-200535100-00002

[40] American College of Sports Medicine (ACSM). American College of Sports Medicine position stand. Progression models in resistance training for healthy adults. Medicine and Science in Sports and Exercise. 2009;**41**(3):687-708. DOI: 10.1249/MSS.0b013e3181915670

[41] Donnelly JE, Blair SN, Jakicic JM, Manore MM, Rankin JW,

Smith BK. Appropriate physical activity intervention strategies for weight loss and prevention of weight regain for adults. Medicine and Science in Sports and Exercise. 2009;**41**(2):459-471. DOI: 10.1249/MSS.0b013e3181949333

[42] Shaw I, Shaw BS, Brown GA. Concurrent training and pulmonary function in smokers. International Journal of Sports Medicine. 2011;**32**:776-780. DOI: 10.1055/s-0031-1277214

Chapter 9

The Potential of Precision Probiotic *Hafnia alvei* HA4597 to Support Weight Loss

Nina Vinot, Emma Baghtchedjian, Clémentine Picolo and Grégory Lambert

Abstract

Hafnia alvei HA4597® is a novel probiotic strain producing an anorexigenic mimetic protein. This report summarizes the innovative approach leading to the discovery of the precision probiotic *H. alvei* HA4597® and its benefits on body weight and metabolic parameters. *H. alvei* HA4597® has been identified after the striking findings on the effects of the bacterial metabolite ClpB (Caseinolytic peptidase B) on appetite regulation, through a screening of ClpB-producing strains. Its efficacy in humans has been validated by a multicentric, double-blind, randomized placebo-controlled trial including 236 overweight adults. The successful results on body weight loss of the clinical study support the use of *H. alvei* HA4597® in the global management of excess weight.

Keywords: *Hafnia alvei* HA4597®, precision probiotic, mimetic, body weight management, appetite

1. Introduction

With the growing obesity epidemic and its associated comorbidities including cardiovascular diseases, diabetes, musculoskeletal disorders, cancer [1], depression [2, 3], and now even Covid-19 [4, 5], there is an urgent need to address this public health issue. As highlighted by the World Health Organization (WHO), obesity is preventable.

The understanding of the physiopathology of obesity started to shift back in 2006 when a publication in Nature highlighted that the microbiota of obese individuals differed from that of lean individuals. In addition, when this microbiota was transplanted into mice, propensity to gain weight was transmitted as well [6].

Since the discovery of the roles of the microbiota in metabolism, Pr. Sergueï Fetissov, neuroendocrinologist and professor of physiology, investigated extensively the roles of the gut microbiota in host appetite control. As early as 2002, he identified human autoantibodies reacting with the key hormone of satiety alpha-melanocyte stimulating hormone (alpha-MSH). He discovered an anorexigenic peptide produced by the microbiota with a homology of sequence with alpha-MSH [7]. In a review published in *Nature Reviews Endocrinology*, he demonstrated that metabolites produced by the microbiota can regulate food intake, and more specifically identified a bacterial protein called caseinolytic peptidase B (ClpB), a conformational antigen mimetic of alpha-MSH (**Figure 1**) [8, 9].

Observations showed that ClpB levels in human fecal or serum samples negatively associated with Body Mass Index (BMI) [10]. Pr. Sergueï Fetissov and Pr. Pierre Déchelotte, gastroenterologist, professor in human nutrition and director of the Gut Brain Axis Laboratory at the French National Institute of Health and Medical Research (Inserm), carried on their investigations to better understand and describe the cause-and-effect relationship, demonstrate the proof of concept on animal models and translate the discovery into a lever of action in the battle against obesity.

2. From amino acid sequence homology to functional mimicry of the anorexigenic pathway

In the beginning, the bacterium encountered to study ClpB was *E. coli* K12, the standard model used in biotechnology. *In silico* sequence alignments allowed to identify a 6-amino acid sequence homology between a bacterial protein, *E. coli* K12 ClpB, and alpha-MSH [11]. The properties of the *E. coli* K12 ClpB sequence explain its folded shape, exposing the epitope and thus making it a specific conformational mimetic of alpha-MSH [9, 11].

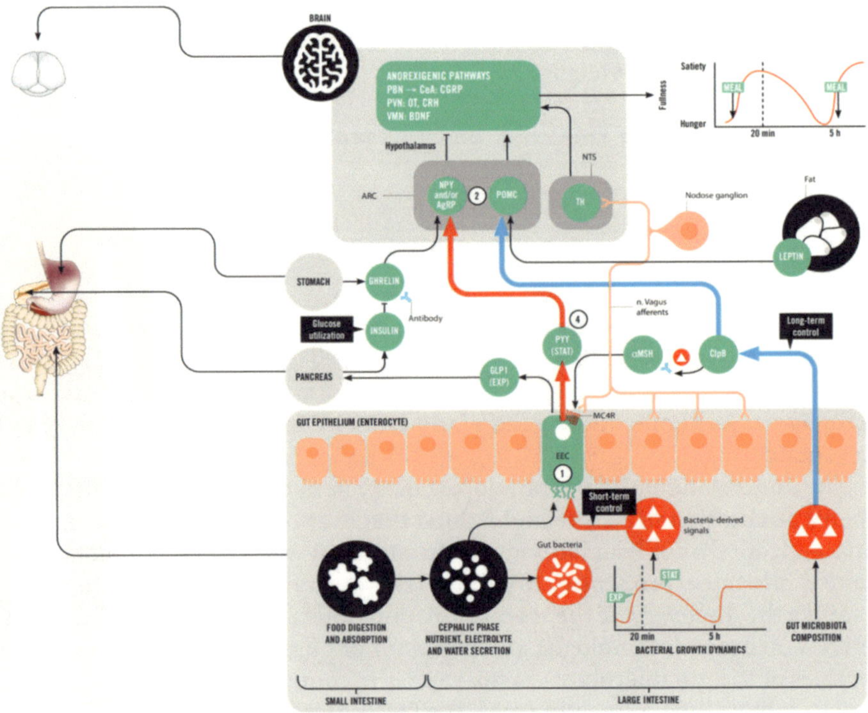

Figure 1.
Adapted from Sergueï Fetissov, nature reviews *2016*.

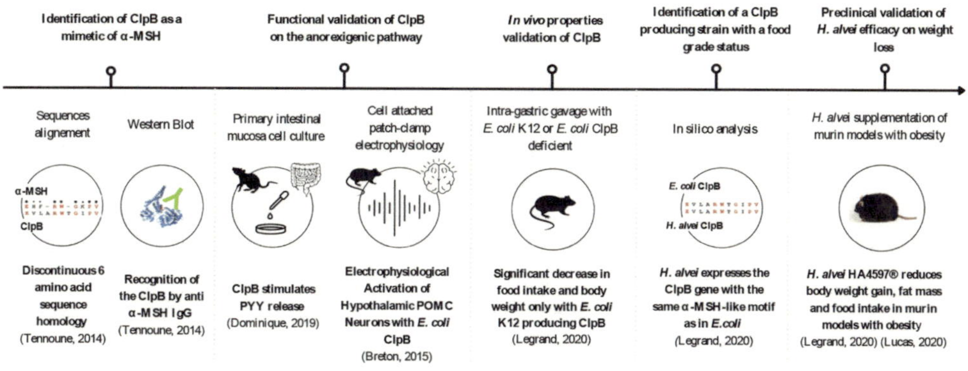

Figure 2.
From in vitro identification of ClpB to in vivo proof of concept.

The functional mimetic properties of *E. coli* K12 ClpB were first confirmed with a proteomic approach. ClpB was identified after Western Blot analysis of *E. coli* K12 stationary phase total protein extract of *E. coli* K12 using anti alpha-MSH IgG [9]. Then, two pathways used by the ClpB to regulate satiety were identified with preliminary protocols in mice:

- Both ClpB protein (recombinant) and *E. coli* K12 total stationary phase protein extract act locally in the gut by stimulating peptide YY (PYY) secretion by L-cells [12–14]. In addition, colonic infusion of *E. coli* K12 stationary phase protein extract on rats increases plasma PYY levels [13].

- ClpB also circulates in the blood and can stimulate the anorexigenic pathways in the hypothalamus by activating POMC neurons [13].

Anorexigenic properties of *E. coli* K12 ClpB were then confirmed *in vivo* on mice. Oral gavage of mice with *E. coli* K12 triggers a decrease of the food intake and body weight that wasn't shown with ClpB-deficient strains [14].

The alpha-MSH mimetic properties of bacterial *E. coli* ClpB made it a good candidate to develop an anti-obesity solution, but to develop a product with unquestionable safety, the team looked for a ClpB-producing strain with a food grade status. *Hafnia alvei,* a starter culture used in cheese production, in particular the Normandy traditional cheeses Camembert and Brie, was identified thanks to *in silico* approach [14]. *H. alvei* is a commensal bacterium from the *Enterobacteriaceae* family, naturally present in cheese [15, 16] and in the human gut [14], and thus benefitting from a long history of safe use.

The summary of these steps of discovery and development are exposed in **Figure 2** hereunder.

3. *Hafnia alvei* HA4597® reduces body weight gain, fat mass and food intake in murine models of obesity

The first preclinical study was conducted to validate *H. alvei* and its production of ClpB, as a potential probiotic and its postbiotic for appetite and body weight management in overweight and obesity. Legrand *et al.* [14] tested *H. alvei* HA4597® on two mouse models of obesity: genetic, leptin deficient ob/ob mice (a model of hyperphagia) and nutritional, High-Fat Diet (HFD)-induced obesity.

This study confirmed that *H. alvei* HA4597® significantly reduces body weight gain and fat mass in both models of obese mice (**Figure 3a-d**). In the hyperphagic ob/ob model, *H. alvei* HA4597® treatment significantly reduces food intake with a 20.8% decrease (vs placebo) in total intake measured after 18 days ($p < 0.001$), the difference becoming significant from day 8 (**Figure 3e**) and was accompanied by a higher level of phosphorylated hormone-sensitive lipase in fat tissues ($p < 0.01$) (**Figure 3g**).

The effect of *H. alvei* on food intake was not observed in mice on HFD, considering that HFD models tend to hypophagia because mice are not attracted to fat (**Figure 3f**).

Thus, *H. alvei* HA4597® exhibits the desired probiotic properties of an appetite and body weight management supplement i.e., it triggers anorexigenic and lipolytic effects in hyperphagic mice resulting in decreased body weight gain and fat mass.

A second trial conducted by Lucas *et al.* [17] evaluated the efficacy of *Hafnia* on another animal model of obesity based on a combined model of both HFD-fed and genetic ob/ob mice that may represent most closely hyperphagia and diet-induced obesity in humans (compulsive eating behavior combined with hypercaloric diet and accompanied by functional leptin resistance). This study also compares the efficacy of the strain to the drug Orlistat, a lipase inhibitor used in humans for the management of obesity.

A daily provision of 1.4×10^{10} Colony Forming Units (CFU) of *H. alvei* HA4597® in these mice significantly decreased the food intake, the body weight gain (**Figure 4A** and **B**) and total fat mass and preserved lean mass, resulting in an improved lean/fat mass ratio (**Figure 4C**). On top of that, other metabolic parameters were improved with the *H. alvei* treatment, including glycemia, total cholesterol and hepatic alanine aminotransferase (ALAT) (**Figure 4E**).

Although Orlistat is effective for weight loss, in contrast to *H. alvei* HA4597®, it is accompanied in this study by a strong hyperphagic effect which may be the cause of the increased glycemia observed for this group (**Figure 4D**).

After *H. alvei* proved successful in the regulation of appetite and weight in mice models, the next step was to evaluate efficacy in humans.

H. alvei HA4597® improves weight loss in a multicentric, double-blind, randomized placebo-controlled trial including 236 overweight adults.

To **investigate the clinical efficacy** of the strain, a 12-week prospective, double-blind, randomized study was realized on 236 overweight men and women (230 followed protocol and were analyzed in the per protocol results) [18]. All subjects were on a – 20% low-caloric diet and were asked to maintain their usual physical activity. Subjects received either 2 capsules per day providing 10^{11} bacteria of *H. alvei* HA4597® per day (HA) or a placebo (P).

The primary outcome was the percentage of subjects losing 3% or more of their body weight after 12 weeks. Indeed, **significantly more subjects (+38%) lost at least 3% of their initial weight** after 12 weeks than in the placebo group (57.7 vs. 41.7%, $p = 0.028$, Per Protocol results) (**Figure 5A**). 51% more participants also lost more than 4% of their body weight on HA than on placebo (46.2% vs. 30.6%, $p = 0.024$) (**Figure 5B**). The average weight loss observed in the treated group was 3.6% at 12 weeks, vs. 2.9% in the placebo group, a high figure linked to the strong effect of the hypocaloric diet.

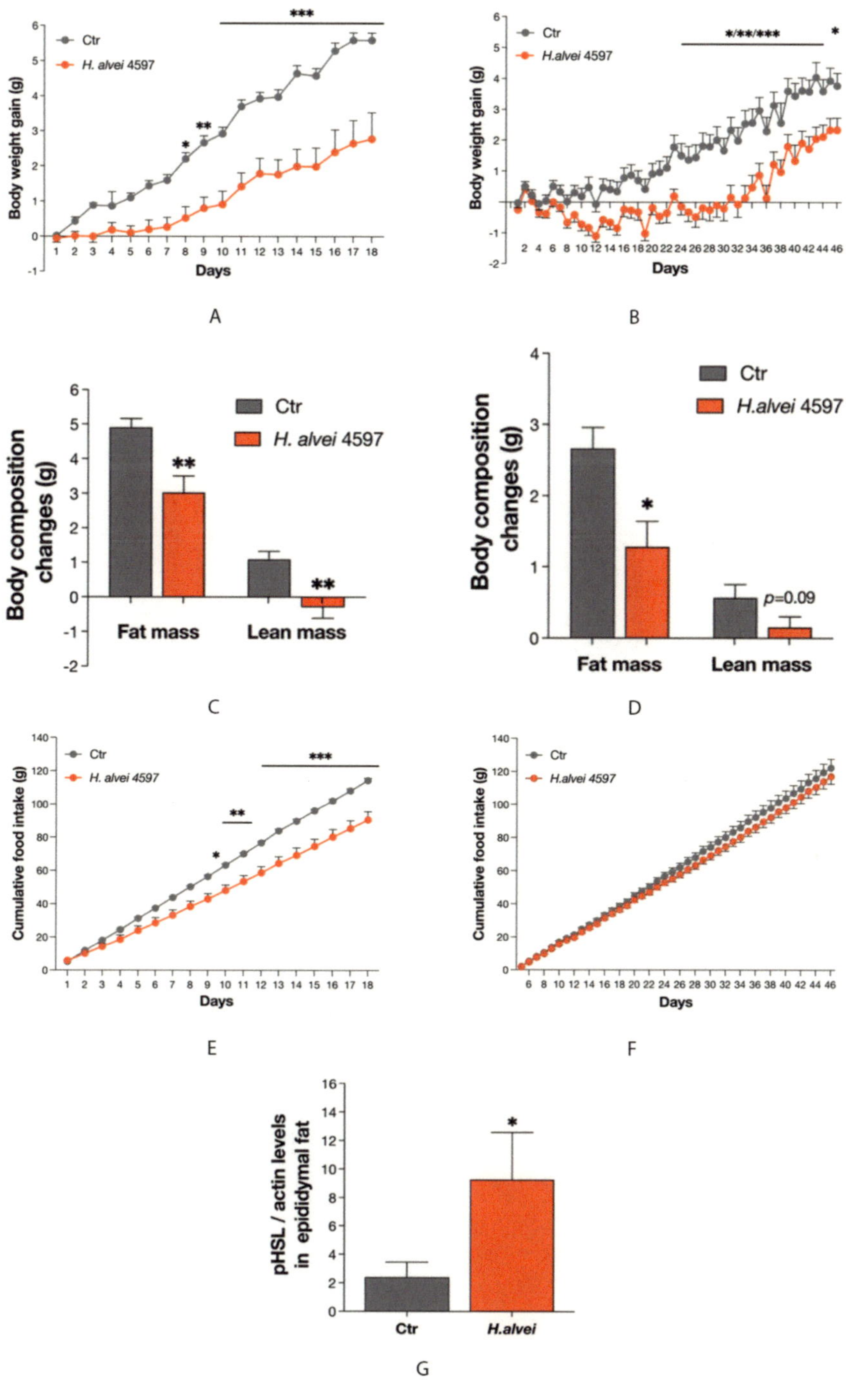

Figure 3.
Results of Hafnia alvei *HA4597® supplementation vs. control in Ob/Ob mice and HFD mice models of obesity (adapted from Legrand et al., 2020). Body weight dynamics in ob/ob (a) and in HFD-fed obese mice (b), Two-way RM ANOVA, $p < 0.001$, (b) *for days 23–25, 38, 41, and 47, **for days 26, 27, 30, 37, 39, 42, and 43, ***for days 28, 29, 31–36, and 40. Total fat and lean tissue mass in ob/ob (c) and in HFD-fed obese mice (d). Mann–Whitney tests, **$p < 0.01$, *$p < 0.05$. Cumulative food intake in ob/ob (e) and in HFD-fed obese mice (f), Two-way RM ANOVA, $p < 0.05$, Bonferroni post tests, ***$p < 0.001$, **$p < 0.01$, *$p < 0.05$. Actin-normalized pHSL levels in the epididymal fat tissue in ob/ob (g), Mann-Whitney tests, *$p<0.05$.*

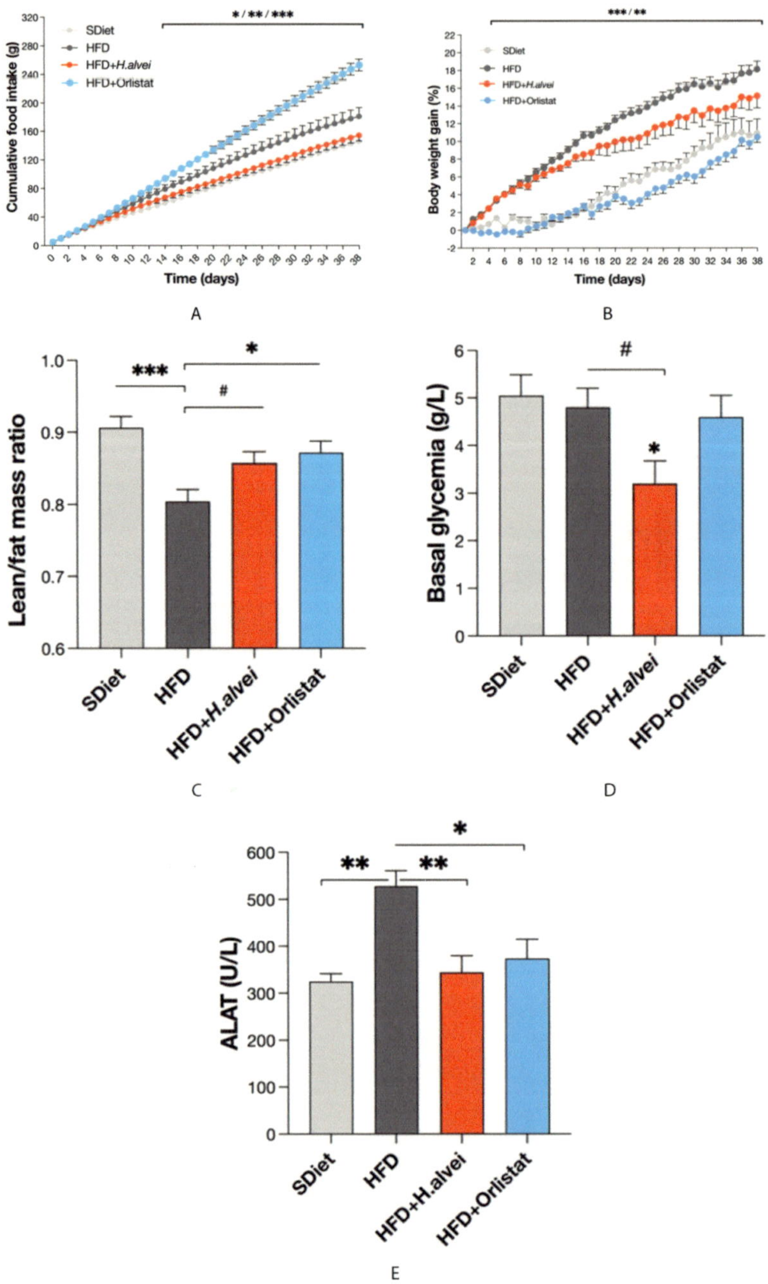

Figure 4.

Results on body weight gain and other parameters after 37 days of oral gavage with Hafnia alvei *HA4597® vs. orlistat in HFD Ob/Ob mice (adapted from Lucas et al., 2020). (A) Cumulative food intake (g). Two≃way RM ANOVA, $p < 0.0001$, Bonferroni's posttests, HFD vs. HFD + Orlistat. *** $p < 0.001$; ** $p < 0.01$ days 24,25; * $p < 0.05$ days 22,23. HFD + H. alvei vs. HFD + Orlistat. *** $p < 0.001$, ** $p < 0.01$, days 17,18; *$p < 0.05$ days 15,16. (B) Body weight gain (%). Two≃way RM ANOVA, $p < 0.0001$, Bonferroni's posttests, HFD vs. HFD + Orlistat, *** $p < 0.001$,** $p < 0.01$, * $p < 0.05$; C. ANOVA, $p < 0.0001$, Tukey's posttests avs. HFD and bvs. HFD + H. alvei, both *** $p < 0.001$, Student's t≃tests, * $p < 0.05$, (mean ± SEM; SDiet, $n = 16$, all other groups, $n = 24$). (C) Lean/fat mass ratio at the end of the treatment. Student's t≃tests, # $p < 0.05$, (mean ± SEM; SDiet, $n = 16$, all other groups, $n = 24$). (D) Basal glycemia at end of treatment (g/L). ANOVA $p < 0.05$, Tukey's posttest vs. SDiet * $p < 0.05$. Student's t≃test # $p < 0.05$. (E) Alanine transaminase (ALAT) levels at end of treatment (U/L). ANOVA $p = 0.0006$, Tukey's posttests ** $p < 0.01$, * $p < 0.05$, (mean ± SEM; SDiet, $n = 8$, all other groups $n = 12$).*

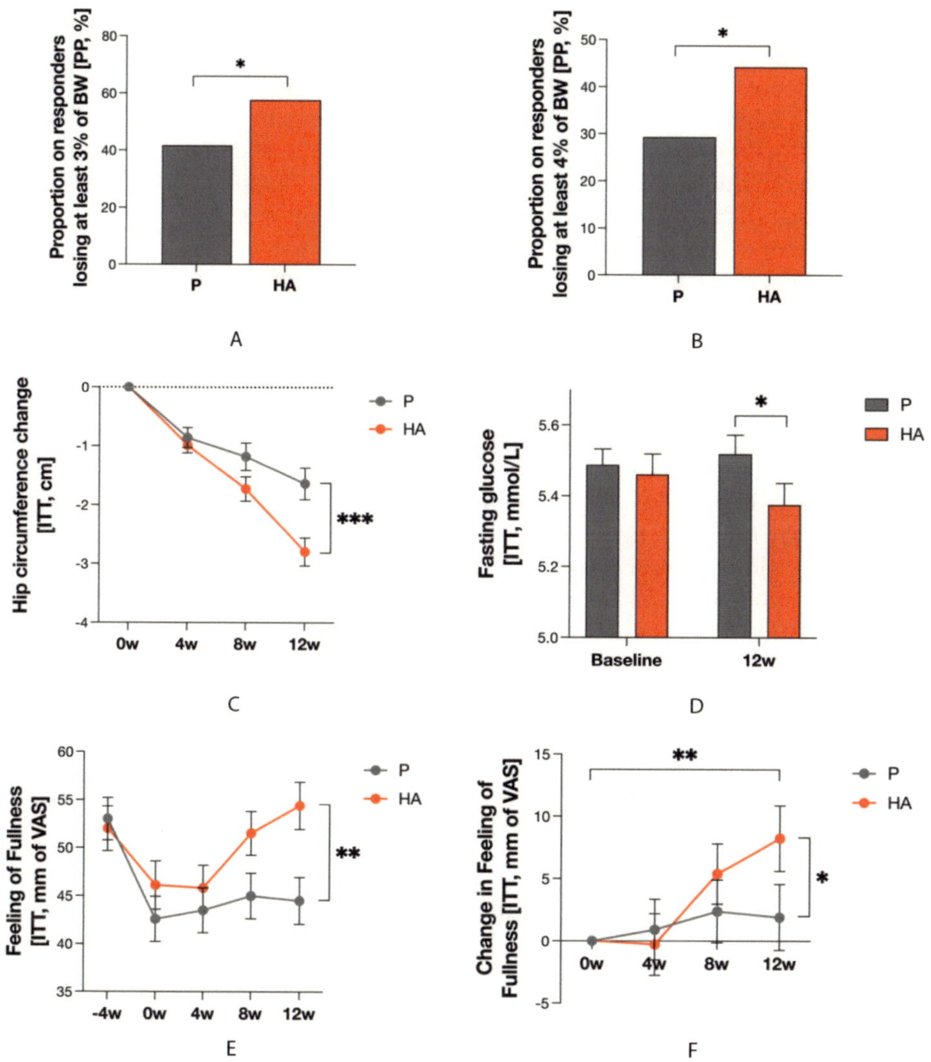

Figure 5.
Results of the clinical study with 12-week supplementation of overweight subjects with Hafnia alvei *HA4597® or placebo (adapted from Déchelotte et al., 2021, except* **Figure 5D**, *unpublished). (A) Proportion of subjects who lost at least 3% of body weight after 12 weeks PP population, Exact Fisher's test P. vs HA. *p≤0.05. (B) Proportion of subjects who lost at least 4% of body weight after 12 weeks PP population, Exact Fisher's test P. vs HA. *p≤0.05. (C) Hip circumference change vs. To ITT population, Mann-Whitney-U test (w12-w0) P. vs. (w12-w0) HA. *pU≤0.001. (D) Serum glucose concentration before and after supplementation ITT population, Mann-Whitney-U test (w12) P. vs. (w12) HA. *pU ≤ 0.05. (E) Feeling of fullness ITT population, Mann-Whitney-U test (w12) P. vs. (w12) HA.**pU ≤ 0.01. (F) Change in Feeling of fullness ITT population, Mann-Whitney-U test; (w12-w0)P. vs. (w12-w0)HA.* pU ≤ 0.05. Paired Wilcoxon test; HA(w0) vs. HA(w12).** pwi ≤ 0.01.*

Compared to the placebo group, the participants in the probiotic group saw a significant further 1.2 cm reduction in **hip circumference** ($p < 0.001$ at 12 weeks) as well as a significant decrease in **blood glucose** ($p = 0.027$ at 12 weeks) (**Figure 5C** and **D**). Furthermore, the HA group recorded a significant decrease of **cholesterol** compared to the beginning of the study ($p = 0.008$ for total cholesterol and $p = 0.028$ for LDL-cholesterol at 12 weeks) (unpublished).

Importantly, this study also revealed an **increased feeling of fullness** assessed by visual analog scale (VAS) ($p = 0.009$ at 8 weeks) in the HA group (**Figure 5F**). In the VAS, a score of 50 means that there is no feeling of hunger. Both groups were under a – 20% hypocaloric diet, but only the treated group led to feeling of fullness scores above 50 (**Figure 5E**). This confirms the mechanism of action of this precision probiotic through the regulation of appetite and this led, despite the constraints of the diet, to a significantly higher level of satisfaction of the subjects from the treated group, compared to the placebo group.

Indeed, in the HA group, benefit of treatment was rated as "very good" or "good" by 67.9% of subjects compared to 53.1% in the placebo group ($p = 0.019$). Only 5% of subjects in the probiotic group rated it as "poor", as opposed to 14.2% in the placebo group.

This level of satisfaction shows the users have a clear perception of efficacy, and the good appetite regulation during a diet makes it easier to keep compliant to the reduced caloric intake, without the difficulty and discomfort associated with hunger.

According to the official guidelines for the management of obesity, a 3 to 5% weight loss is the reference interval associated with meaningful clinical benefits: reductions in serum triglycerides concentrations, of blood glucose, HbA1C, and the risks of developing type 2 diabetes [19].

With clinically relevant efficacy as soon as in the first 12 weeks, excellent tolerability and no adverse events, **these results support the use of *H. alvei* HA4597® in the global management of excess weight.**

4. From the clinical setting to the market: benefits of *H. alvei* HA4597® for overweight to obese consumers

As previously described, *H. alvei* HA4597® through its production of ClpB, a mimetic of the anorexigenic hormone alpha-MSH, constitutes an innovative and effective solution for body weight management in overweight and obesity. The French biotech TargEDys, pioneer in microbiome-based solutions and grounded in 15 years of academic research in collaboration with the prestigious laboratories of Inserm (Institut national de la santé et de la recherche médicale) in Rouen, developed a food supplement with 100 billion cells of *H. alvei* HA4597® per daily dose. It is the first PreciBiomic Strain product on the market for body weight management combining efficacy with no side effects. During product development, TargEDys ensured that the strain produces ClpB during the fermentation process so that both the strain and its protein ClpB are present in the product.

A consumer study confirmed the efficacy of the product in overweight people, and even in people suffering from obesity, in real life conditions, i.e., without caloric restriction. Above all, this study confirmed that the extension of the program over time intensifies the body weight loss.

5. Conclusion

As concluded by the authors of the clinical trial, supplementation with the precision probiotic [20] *H. alvei* HA4597® represents an innovative and well-tolerated strategy to enhance the efficacy of dietary advice for the control of excess body weight; paving the way to precision nutrition thanks to a gut microbial-based personalized approach.

Acknowledgements

The authors join to thank all the people who made this research possible, from the researchers themselves, to the investors and funds, as well as all the people and institutions who contributed to all the articles cited in the list of references. They all participated to the development of this new solution, directly or indirectly.

Thank you most particularly to Pierre Déchelotte and Sergueï Fetissov who made the discovery of the conformational antigen ClpB and its role in appetite regulation and founded TargEDys to transpose this knowledge into a product and approach to safely help people regulate their hunger and weight.

Thank you to Manon Dominique, Marie Galmiche Nicolas Lucas et Romain Legrand for all their research work in investigating the precise mechanism of action of *H. alvei* and ClpB as Ph.D. students and TargEDys research team.

The authors also thank warmly all TargEDys employees and partners who worked together and enabled the development of processes and production of the strain, from fermentation to blending and encapsulation, all the suppliers who provide high-quality delivery systems and packaging, to optimize the protection of the bacteria and protein all the way to the gut as well as the product's stability, and all the regulatory advisers that made it possible to reach the market with this food grade strain that was never used as a probiotic before.

Conflict of interest

The co-authors are employees of TargEDys, the company producing and commercializing a food supplement based on *H. alvei* HA4597.

Author details

Nina Vinot*, Emma Baghtchedjian, Clémentine Picolo and Grégory Lambert
TargEDys SA, Longjumeau, France

*Address all correspondence to: nvinot@targedys.com

References

[1] https://www.who.int/news-room/fact-sheets/detail/obesity-and-overweight

[2] Milaneschi Y, Simmons WK, van Rossum E, et al. Depression and obesity: Evidence of shared biological mechanisms. Molecular Psychiatry. 2019;**24**(1):18-33

[3] Jantaratnotai N, Mosikanon K, Lee Y, et al. The interface of depression and obesity. Obesity Research & Clinical Practice. 2017;**11**(1):1-10

[4] Petrakis D, Margină D, Tsarouhas K, et al. Obesity - a risk factor for increased COVID-19 prevalence, severity and lethality (review). Molecular Medicine Reports. 2020;**22**(1):9-19

[5] Yang J, Hu J, Zhu C. Obesity aggravates COVID-19: A systematic review and meta-analysis. Journal of Medical Virology. 2021;**93**(1):257-261

[6] Turnbaugh PJ, Ley RE, Mahowald MA, Magrini V, et al. An obesity-associated gut microbiome with increased capacity for energy harvest. Nature. 2006;**444**(7122):1027-1031

[7] Fetissov SO, Harro J, Jaanisk M, et al. Autoantibodies against neuropeptides are associated with psychological traits in eating disorders. Proceedings of the National Academy of Sciences of the United States of America. 2005;**102**(41):14865-14870

[8] Fetissov SO. Role of the gut microbiota in host appetite control: Bacterial growth to animal feeding behaviour. Nature reviews. Endocrinology. 2017;**13**(1):11-25

[9] Tennoune N, Chan P, Breton J, et al. Bacterial ClpB heat-shock protein, an antigen-mimetic of the anorexigenic peptide α-MSH, at the origin of eating disorders. Translational Psychiatry. 2014;**4**(10):e458-e458

[10] Arnoriaga-Rodríguez M, Mayneris-Perxachs J, Burokas A. Gut bacterial ClpB-like gene function is associated with decreased body weight and a characteristic microbiota profile. Microbiome. 2020;**8**(1):59

[11] Fetissov SO, Legrand R, Lucas N. Bacterial protein mimetic of peptide hormone as a new class of protein- based drugs. Current Medicinal Chemistry. 2019;**26**(3):546-553

[12] Dominique M, Breton J, Guérin C, et al. Effects of macronutrients on the in vitro production of ClpB, a bacterial mimetic protein of α-MSH and its possible role in satiety signaling. Nutrients. 2019;**11**(9):2115

[13] Breton J, Tennoune N, Lucas N, et al. Gut commensal E. coli proteins activate host satiety pathways following nutrient-induced bacterial growth. Cell Metabolism. 2016;**23**(2):324-334

[14] Legrand R, Lucas N, Dominique M, et al. Commensal hafnia alvei strain reduces food intake and fat mass in obese mice-a new potential probiotic for appetite and body weight management. International Journal of Obesity. 2020;**44**(5):1041-1051

[15] Mourgues R, Vassal L, Auclair J, Mocquot G, Vandeweghe J. Origine et développement des bactéries coliformes dans les fromages à pâte molle. Le Lait. 1977;**57**(563-564):131-149

[16] Richard J, Zadi H. Inventaire de la flore bactérienne dominante des

Camemberts fabriqués avec du lait cru. INRA Ed. 1983;**63**(623-624):25-42

[17] Lucas N, Legrand R, Deroissart C, et al. Hafnia alvei ha4597 strain reduces food intake and body weight gain and improves body composition, glucose, and lipid metabolism in a mouse model of hyperphagic obesity. Microorganisms. 2020;**8**(1):35

[18] Déchelotte P, Breton J, Trotin-Picolo C, et al. The probiotic strain *hafnia alvei* HA4597® improves weight loss in overweight subjects under moderate hypocaloric diet: A proof-of-concept, multicenter randomized, double-blind placebo-controlled study. Nutrients. 2021;**13**:1902

[19] Jensen MD, Ryan DH, Donato KA, et al. Guidelines (2013) for managing overweight and obesity in adults. Obesity. 2014;**22**:S1-S410

[20] Veiga P, Suez J, Derrien M, et al. Moving from probiotics to precision probiotics. Nature Microbiology. 2020;**5**(7):878-880

Chapter 10

Inability to Understand the Complexity of Maintaining Weight Loss and the Complications

Anvi Rana

Abstract

Weight management can be aided by behavior management therapies, although weight is frequently regained. To avoid this, available interventions are necessary. Researchers did a comprehensive evaluation and integration of qualitative studies on people's weight control and sustaining perspectives. They looked for descriptive studies examining the reality of presently or formerly overweight individuals striving to sustain weight loss in bibliographic databases. Researchers developed the model of weight loss maintenance by thematically aggregating study data. There were 16 studies with 610 individuals from 5 nations. Because of the requirement to overcome established behaviors and the incompatibility of the new behaviors with the satisfaction of emotional factors, the model generated via our integration posits that implementing the action modifications essential for weight loss stability generates psychological "stress." This stress must be managed or resolved for successful maintenance. Self-regulation, motivation renewal, and regulating influences can all help with stress management, while it can take a lot of work. Changes in behavior, nonobesogenic means of fulfilling needs, and maybe a shift in self-concept can all help with recovery.

Keywords: maintenance of weight loss, behavioral modification, evidence synthesis, weight loss difficulties, stability

1. Introduction

Obesity growth follows a simple formula: energy intake exceeds energy expenditure. Overweight and obesity, on the other hand, are the result of a complex series of interactions among genetic, psychological, and environmental variables. Whereas the overweight public has been offered hundreds, if not thousands, of weight-loss strategies, diets, potions, and devices, the multi-factorial causative agents of overweight challenges practitioners, researchers, and the overweight themselves to identify permanent, efficacious weight-loss and maintenance strategies [1]. The number of people who effectively lose weight and keep it off has been reported to be as low as 1–3%. In the genesis of overweight and obesity, heredity plays a role. Genes, on the other hand, cannot explain the rise in overweight people [2]. Rather, the behavioral and environmental variables that cause people to engage in too little physical activity and consume too much food

 IntechOpen

about their energy expenditure must bear the brunt of the responsibility. These are the issues that weight-loss initiatives aim to address [3]. This chapter examines the effectiveness and safety of weight-reduction techniques, as well as the combos of approaches that exist for healthy weight loss [4].

A complicated combination of environmental, biochemical, social, and cognitive factors, which are only partially understood, makes weight reduction maintenance difficult. **Figure 1** illustrates their configuration; they react differently in different patients to an extent that is difficult to predict. This answers why many people regain most of the weight they lost following a successful diet plan. Nevertheless, a small percentage of people succeed in maintaining long-term weight loss, and research into this group, which achieves their aim despite significant urges to gain weight, may assist discover the variables that lead to this preferred result [5].

To increase patients' commitment to long-term weight control, the much more current advancements of comprehensive lifestyle modification plans integrate food and physical activity guidelines with particular behavioral and cognitive methods [6]. They show that a significant portion of treated individuals may sustain a healthy body weight decrease over time. These encouraging findings have prompted the formation of multidisciplinary lifestyle modification teams to provide patients with moment longer overweight therapy [7].

The goals of this narrative review are to [8]

1. Provide such a meaning of fat loss

2. Data sets on lengthy losing weight maintenance

3. Characterize the characteristics of people who achieve a lengthy losing weight

4. Evaluation of scientific proof initiatives to increase weight reduction maintenance

5. Identify a holistic approach based on lifestyle interventions aimed at giving clients with moment longer management of their diabetes.

The components of good weight control will also be investigated, as the difficulties in sustaining weight reduction may contribute to the overweight condition. There is also a brief discussion of public policy approaches that may help prevent obesity and support people who are seeking to reduce or manage weight reduction [9].

Many types of research have been successful in inducing weight reduction in individuals; nevertheless, weight loss management has proven to be far more challenging [10]. According to a recent comprehensive analysis, weight-reduction systems have been able to produce a 9.5% weight loss from starting body weight on aggregate; unfortunately, only 54% of this loss weight was sustained one year following the treatments [11]. As a consequence, scientific proof guidelines for weight loss and maintenance techniques that people may apply are needed. Approaches based on the notion of energy equation may base on energy consumption (i.e., food) or energy expended (i.e., physical activity), or on habits that encourage improvements in either caloric intake or energy expended (i.e., self-monitoring of dietary intake) [12].

A theoretical model was developed in which elements such as nutritional intake, physical activity, and attitude were investigated for their impact on reducing weight and management. Since it was anticipated that activities connected to the energy

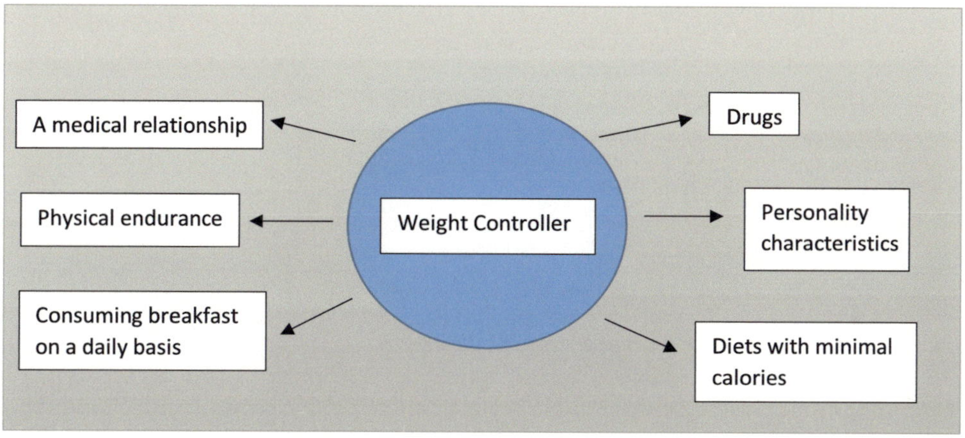

Figure 1.
In the overall population of obese patients enrolled in noninvasive weight reduction procedures, there are a number of characteristics linked to long-term weight loss stabilization.

equation would impact weight reduction differentially than weight control, losing weight and weight control were handled as separate events within the theoretical model [13]. The paradigm also depicts the idea of recurrence, which is prevalent in this group and may be linked to the characteristics described in the paradigm [14].

Postrach et al. (2008) stated that for weight control, the first weight-loss strategy should be very broad and that most of the information and abilities gained during the weight-loss phase may be transferred to the weight-control period.

2. The maintenance of a weight loss

Several criteria for "successful weight loss maintain" have been developed during the last 10 years. Successful weight loss managers, according to Avnell, are "persons who have consciously dropped at least 10% of their body weight and maintained it off for at least one year." A persistent weight reduction of roughly 5–10% of baseline body weight, according to Barners, indicates a high level of effectiveness. The 2013 American Heart Association (AHA), American College of Cardiology (ACC), and Term of Service (TOS) Guideline for the Management of Overweight and Obesity in Adults also recommends this aim as shown in **Figure 2** [15].

The preceding criteria all agree that good weight management does not need a huge weight decrease, but rather a modest 5–10% reduction. This level of weight reduction, from a clinical standpoint, dramatically lowers the risk of type 2 diabetes in susceptible people and removes the majority of the additional hazards linked to obesity [16]. Furthermore, even minor weight reduction has been shown to enhance mental wellbeing, including happiness, self-image, and bingeing [17].

Teixeria et al. [18] definition adds two more weight-maintenance markers. First and foremost, fat loss should be planned. Such a parameter is critical since various studies have found that inadvertent weight loss is widespread and might have unique causes and impacts than deliberate weight reduction. Weight loss must be sustained for at least one year. This criterion was established as an acceptable goal for study into the elements that enable people to sustain their weight loss. Nevertheless, the term "success" might imply a considerably extra duration of weight management, ideally throughout the rest of one's life [19].

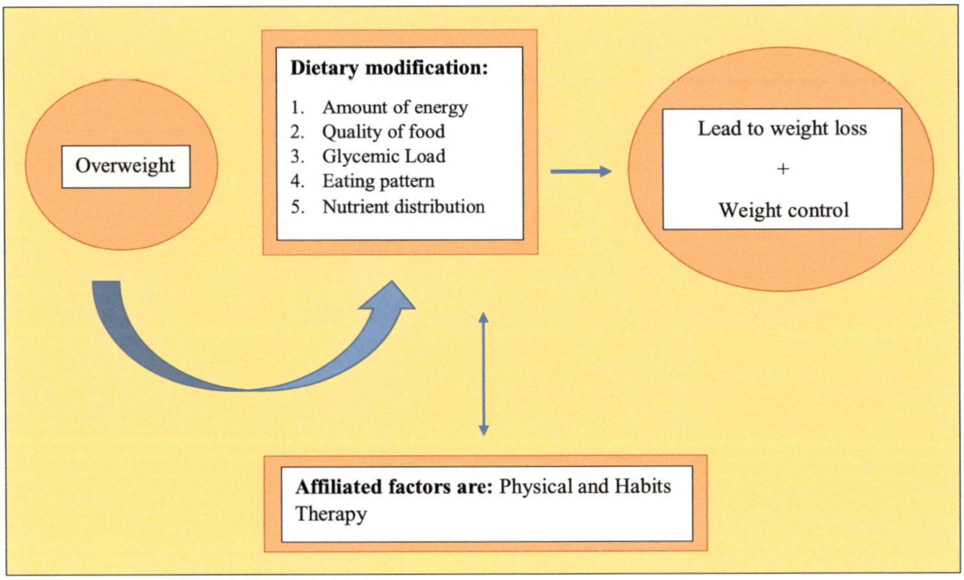

Figure 2.
Weight loss and weight control scope of the study Weight loss is attributed to a reduction of at minimum 10% of benchmark body mass, while weight stabilization is defined as maintaining a body mass of at minimum 10% less than initial body mass for at minimum one year.

2.1 Physical activity

The quantity of energy exerted vs the quantity of energy eaten influences weight fluctuations. As a result, weight gain will occur if the metabolic rate stays low but food levels of consumption are excessive. Some researchers suggest that decreases in regular exercise, both at work and in leisure, may have played a significant part in the rising obesity prevalence over the previous 30 years [20].

In addition, several epidemiological data imply that physical activity plays a key role in weight growth. Low levels of self-reported recreational physical activity were related to three-fold increased risk of substantial weight gain in males and even a four-fold larger hazard in women, according to [21] who used data from the National Health and Nutrition Examination Survey (NHANES) and he found that in a retrospective study of 34,079 middle-aged women (mean: 52.2 years), the chance of increased weight over three years was 11 percent higher in women who engaged in fewer than 7.5 metabolic equivalents (MET).

For overweight people who are healthful, enhanced physical activity and exercise are part of a complete weight-loss plan. The capacity to create and maintain an exercise regime is one of the strongest indicators of results of this case in the therapy of overweight [22]. Exercise and fitness regimens that are required to satisfy the forces' physical preparedness demands overall, and for weight management, in particular, can be boosted by the presence of engaging in physical activity in army facilities. The intensity, length, frequency, and kind of physical exercise for a specific individual will be determined by pre-existing medical issues, past activity levels, physical constraints, and personal preferences. Individuals who have more than one of the aforementioned mitigating situations may need to be referred for extra expert examination [23]. Physical activity has several advantages that can be experienced even if weight loss is not achieved. One of the advantages, an increase in high-density low-density lipoprotein, has been demonstrated to be achievable with a minimum of 10–11 h of cardiovascular exercise each month as shown below in **Figure 3** [24].

2.2 Alterations of habits and attitudes

By use of habit and varying levels of intensity in weight control is based on a weight of information indicating people develop or stay obese as a consequence of adjustable routines or activities, and that weight reduction and maintenance may be achieved by modifying those tendencies [25]. The main aim of psychological weight-control techniques is to promote a healthy lifestyle and reduce calorie intake via changing dietary patterns. Cognitive treatment can be given to a single person or a group of people. Individuals typically participate in 15–30 weekly sessions lasting 2–3 h each, with a weight-loss objective of 2–3 pounds each week. Behavioral techniques were formerly used as hold therapies to just change eating patterns and lower calorie intake. Nevertheless, these methods have lately been applied to induce weight reduction and as an element of routine maintenance in addition to low diets, nutritional support therapy, proper nutrition, fitness programs, supervision, pharmaceutical medications, and social protection as shown in **Figure 4** [26].

2.3 Input efforts and self-control

One of the pillars of behavioral interventions is the identity of nutritional intake and physical exercise, which allows the client to establish a sense of social responsibility. Participants are advised to keep a usual dietary diary in which participants note what they did eat, how very much patients did eat, where and when they did

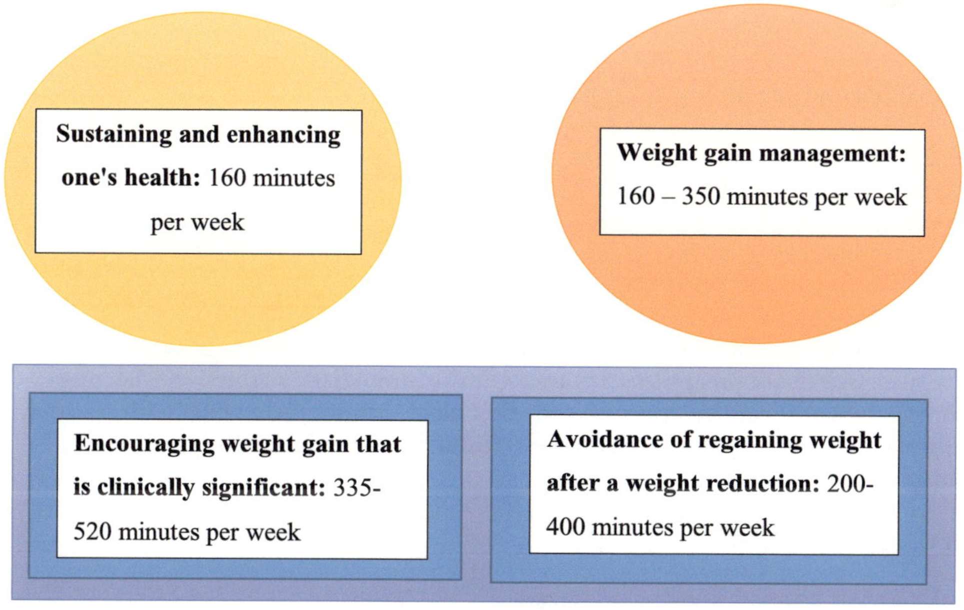

Figure 3.
Physical activity guideline.

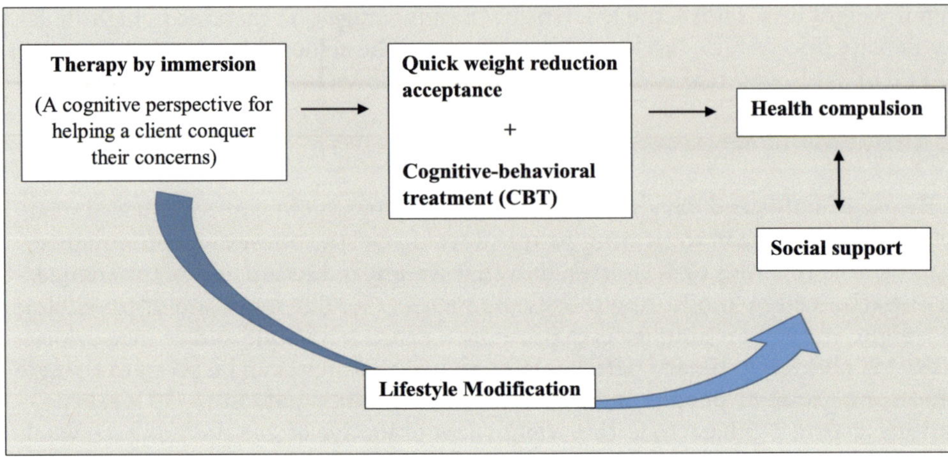

Figure 4.
Engagement in a new way of life.

eat it, and the environment in which they started eating it. Individuals may also be required to keep a log sheet of their physical activity. Self-monitoring of food intake is frequently linked to a rapid decrease in energy consumption and, as a result, losing weight. This decrease in food intake is thought to be the consequence of greater food consciousness and/or fear of what the nutritionist or nutritional therapist may say about the participant's eating habits. Food diaries are also used to discover internal and social variables that lead to excess eating, as well as to choose and implement appropriate weight-loss techniques for the person [27].

The same might be said for regular exercise tracking, even though the little study has been done in this area. Self-control also allows therapists and clients to assess which approaches are effective and how changes in sleep and eating habits or exercise affect weight reduction [28].

2.4 Additional psychological approaches

Eating only prescheduled meals; just doing nothing while choosing to eat; ingesting meals only in one location and having left the table after consuming; buying groceries only from a list, and buying on an empty stomach are some of the additional techniques included in psychosocial therapeutic interventions. Motivational strategies are also used in the psychological treatment of overweight and fat people. Respondents may choose a strongly rewarding experience, such as engaging in a particularly pleasurable activity or acquiring a special item after achieving a goal. Overweight behavioral approaches are typically immediately effective. The long-term success of these therapies, on the other hand, is more debatable, with research indicating that many people regain their original body weight within 4–6 years of finishing therapy [29].

Among the strategies for enhancing the long-term advantages of cognitive behavior therapy are the following: [30].

1. Improving beginning loss of weight

2. Lengthening the duration of intervention of treatment

3. Focuses on the role of exercising

4. Merging ways of conducting with other therapies such as medication, surgical intervention, or strict diets

2.5 Environmental and resources factor

Rebuilding the environment that supports excess and inactivity might be an important aspect of weight loss and control. The house, the job, and the society are all part of the natural world (e.g., places of worship, eating places, stores, movie theaters). Environmental influences include the opportunities for low foods with highly nutritious, such as fruits, vegetables, nonfat dairy products, and other low-energy-density foods. Instead, of purchasing a piece of candy or packet of crisps and a Coke from a machine, environment rearrangement promotes known frequent dining options that create appetizing items with lower energy density and allow adequate time for eating a balanced diet. Modern lives and stressful work commitments can lead to obese habits that contribute to a less-than-ideal eating atmosphere, but modest modifications can help to break these patterns as shown in **Figure 5** [31].

New findings concepts imply that environmental variables (e.g., high-energy/high-fat meals, fast food intake, television viewing, etc.) instead of physiological factors are driving the present obesity pandemic. Images and offers of high fat, high calorie, extremely tasty, easy, and economical meals are constantly bombarding people. Such meals come in serving amounts that greatly surpass the regulatory guidelines [32]. In addition, our current societal physical needs have altered, culminating in a mismatch in energy imbalance. Hectic lives exacerbate the impact of environmental variables by obstructing weight reduction attempts and encouraging fat accumulation. Prevention and treatment necessitate changes in environmental and societal policies, particularly in the areas of serving sizes, accessibility of healthy foods, and physical exercise encouragement [33].

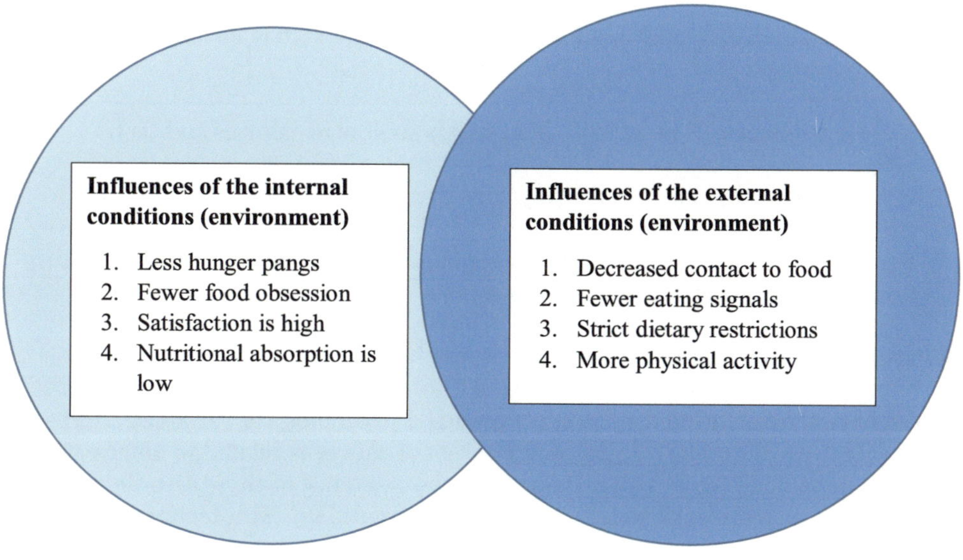

Figure 5.
Overweight prevention through environmental modulation.

2.6 Dietary counseling

Obesity and overweight management need the active engagement of the individual. Nutritionists can give clients a basis of education that will enable them to make informed dietary choices [9]. Nutrition education is separate from nutrition counseling, even though the two have a lot in common. The motivational, emotional, and psychological concerns related to the current job of weight reduction and weight maintenance are more directly addressed in health promotion and nutritional management. It discusses the how and why of dietary behavior adjustments [34]. Nutrition education, on the other hand, gives fundamental knowledge on the scientific foundations of nutrition, allowing individuals to make educated decisions regarding food, cooking techniques, dining out, and serving size. Nutrition curriculums may also cover topics such as the importance of nutrition in illness prevention, sports nutrition, and nutrition for pregnant and nursing women. Successful nutrition education provides nutrition knowledge and its application to healthy lifestyles [35].

2.7 Diet

There are two phases to weight-management initiatives: weight reduction and weight management. While exercise is the most essential component of a weight-loss scheme that impacts the pace of losing weight, it is apparent that food restriction is the most essential element of a weight-loss strategy that affects the rate of weight loss [36]. Food consumption contributes to 100% of daily intake, but movement contributes to just 15–30% of the energy requirement. As a result, limiting energy intake may have the greatest effect on the energy equation given. The number of diets recommended is nearly infinite, but regardless of the nomenclature, all diets should include an increase in protein, below in carbohydrates, low in fat amounts, and should be high in fiber diets [9].

Several low-fat foods are also rich in dietary fiber, and some researchers link low-fat diets' positive influences to their high proportion of dietary fiber-rich vegetables and fruits. High-fiber meals are recommended since they may lower calorie intake and affect metabolism. Nutritional fiber's positive benefits may be done through the following pathways: [37].

1. Caloric attenuation (most high-fiber meals are low in calories and fat).

2. Increased chewing and swallowing time decreases overall consumption.

3. Better stomach and intestinal movement and evacuation, with reduced absorption and reduced appetite and fullness.

2.8 Psychotherapist and consultation

Weight control is influenced by emotional and psychological variables. Counseling services are those that take into account emotional concerns related to binge eating and are designed to educate the patient about the existence of these disorders, their consequences, and the options for long-term treatment [38]. This technique is less complex, intensive, and long-lasting than counseling. Despite continuing counseling, it should be possible to assist patients to grasp the nature and extent of a destructive home or the phenomena of stress-related appetite. These services will be provided by a counselor or therapist in individual or group sessions. These counselors, on the other hand, should be well-versed in the challenges that come with weight-loss regimens, such as binge-eating disorders. Individual case management, as well as group sessions, can be useful in the short term since patients can hear the perspectives of others with good weight difficulties while tackling their problems [39].

2.9 Surgical procedure

Although it is unlikely that many members would be candidates for obesity surgery, a review of weight-loss regimens would be incomplete without including this possibility. The minor weight reduction via psychological treatment and/or medicines does not change the overweight status of enormously obese people (those with a body mass index (BMI) of 35 or 40). Obesity surgery may result in large, long-term weight loss for certain people. Numerous studies have indicated significant reductions in the incidence and death of patients who are morbidly obese, and surgery is being offered to these people more frequently [40].

3. An analysis of nutrient intervention for weight loss maintenance

Associated with weight gain are considered the world's largest fifth leading cause of mortality. In 2009, there were 2.5 billion obese persons worldwide, with 100 million overweight males and roughly 200 million overweight women. It is indeed common for eaters to return over 50% of their lost weight after a year, and also most eaters regain their original weight between 4 and 5 years. Researchers concur that maintaining even 10–15 percent of a person's losing weight is a major accomplishment [41]. Following weight reduction, weight stability is described as a bodyweight shift of up to 5% of the real body weight. Heat production decreases after fat burning, resulting in burning the fat barrier. The likelihood of increased energy consumption following weight reduction is caused by a decline in hormonal changes such as leptin and thyroid hormones. Adipocytes are subjected to cellular stress at this time, resulting in increased stored fat [42].

For work with various on weight control, with such a focus on dietary treatments such as meal replacement, diet component proportions, dietary habits, and special cuisines are the long-term maintaining of body weight which is considered a victory [43].

1. Meal replacement: Meal replacement is one of the most popular ways for avoiding excess weight. It is indeed secure, useful, and cost-effective, with no negative side effects. The degree of adherence is higher with this strategy, the nutritional intake is adequate, and the drop-out rate is low. Such dishes have a regulated calorie content and are also nutrient-dense. These nutritionally complete low-fat meals may be used to substitute major meals and snacks. While employing this strategy, there are many drawbacks. For starters, most study participants are volunteers, which means they are much more driven. Secondly, they might not be able to buy meal substitutes. Furthermore, if you eat the same meals every day, you may get nutritional tiredness [44].

2. Diet component proportions: Several studies tried many different macronutrient percentages to determine the best beneficial dietary combination for weight

management. Minimal carbohydrates, low glycemic index (LGI), low fat with strong Monounsaturated Fatty acids (MUFA), and protein-rich diets are examples of these types of diets. Nevertheless, there is indeed a lot of conflicting information in this field. In contrast to a reduced diet, a protein-rich Glycemic Index (GI) diet, increased Monounsaturated fatty acids diet (MUFA) and intensive support or nurse support, an increased carbohydrates/Protein diet, a limited carbohydrate diet, elevated monounsaturated fatty acids diet (MUFA), high carb glycemic index (GI) diet, increased carbohydrate with low glycemic index (GI) diet plus intensive support or nurse support, and fewer carbohydrates/Protein diet has no major effects on weight loss control [45].

3. Dietary habits: Individuals who have sustained their weight reduction longer than regainers stay up later less at night, engage in more physical activity following losing weight, consume fewer sweetener drinks, consume fewer calories through proteins, and receive more help and support. Dropping extra pounds during weight loss, keeping track of your weight, and eating nutritious meals are all thought to be essential elements in weight management. Those that do not acquire weight consume fewer calories than fat and obese persons. Other habits include eating more fiber, whole grains, veggies, and fruits while eating less fat and processed carbohydrates. When compared to others, weight regainers have distinct perceptions of hunger and cognitive processing. A higher level of adaptable eating regulation, as well as a lower level of uncontrolled eating and psychological discomfort, may have a role in weight management effectiveness [46].

4. Drawback of weight loss: reasons

Obesity is injurious to health, as we all understand. For a valid reason, healthful efforts have always highlighted the importance of weight management. Losing weight, on the other hand, is not a one-flavor recipe; there are numerous strategies to reach this aim. As a result, more is not necessarily better. Whenever it comes to diet reduction, getting too much go too soon might be dangerous to one's wellness [47].

It would be an exaggeration to suggest that excess weight reduction is not healthy. It is hazardous to your health! Excessive weight loss is described as a continuous loss of more than kg every week. Your system is doubtful to be capable of keeping up in such conditions, and indications are almost certain to arise. Just on appearance, certain symptoms, such as mild hair loss or feeling chilly more regularly, may appear to be innocuous. Certain adverse effects, on the other hand, might be extremely harmful to your biological and physiological health and quality of life [48].

The most serious side effects of excessive weight reduction are:

1. Muscle mass is lost—Not only do you lose fat whenever you lose weight, but you lose more muscle. A decrease in muscle mass is frequently accompanied by a decrease in metabolic rate, significantly unsettling the fat-to-muscle proportion. Poorer muscles make everyday chores like lifting heavy shopping or taking the stairs increasingly difficult. Although the number on the measure appears to be improving, your standard of living may not even be [49].

2. Electrolyte instability and nutritional inadequacies—Most of our body functions are controlled by materials found in nature. Anything mismatch in these compo-

nents' proportions might be harmful, resulting in diseases including strokes and arrhythmia. Electrolytes, for instance, are essential for cellular development and vitality. If either fails, the entire body will not take much time to comply. Excessive losing weight precludes your system of the nourishment it requires to operate normally. Deficits in some nutrients, such as vitamin D and calcium, might raise your risk of developing certain health problems or incline you to damage. Anemia, which is defined by sensations of tiredness and collapsing episodes and can develop when your iron intake is inadequate, is one instance of a condition linked to nutritional insufficiency [50].

3. Energy levels are declining dramatically—Inadequate calorie consumption or excessive calorie expenditure will have a negative impact on energy balance. Aside from feeling completely tired, your thought functions and creativity may suffer. Your mindset may be altered as well; extreme weight loss is usually followed by irritability. Even if you are not dieting, you may experience remarkable weight reduction. There is typically a more significant underlying condition that demands addressed in situations of persistent weight loss when more than 10 percent of a total of your body composition is dropped over 6 months [50].

5. Conclusion

Long-term management of body weight is considered successful. While meal replacement can help with weight loss, it cannot ensure that you will keep it off. Minimal carbohydrate, limited GI, and medium fat meals are recommended in balanced eating, although it is unclear if they are effective in avoiding excess weight. It appears that ingesting fewer calories aids weight loss maintenance. Several unique activities have also been linked to weight loss persistence. Eating less sugar-sweetened drinks, staying up later at night, and eating more nutritious foods are just a few instances of such habits. There is no unique meal that can guarantee weight control. As a result, additional study is needed to create techniques for weight management, with an emphasis on long-term weight reduction control.

Author details

Anvi Rana
Nutrition and Dietetics Department, Lovely Professional University, Punjab, India

*Address all correspondence to: anvirana001@gmail.com

References

[1] Phillips AC. Consultation and Development of Athlete Plans. NSCA's Guide to Sport and Exercise Nutrition. 2011. p. 223

[2] Magkos F, Fraterrigo G, Yoshino J, Luecking C, Kirbach K, Kelly SC, et al. Effects of moderate and subsequent progressive weight loss on metabolic function and adipose tissue biology in humans with obesity. Cell Metabolism. 2016;**23**(4):591-601

[3] Garcia Ulen C, Huizinga MM, Beech B, Elasy TA. Weight regain prevention. Clinical Diabetes. 2008;**26**(3):100-113

[4] Wing RR, Phelan S. Long-term weight loss maintenance. The American Journal of Clinical Nutrition. 2005;**82**(1):222S-225S

[5] Wing RR, Hill JO. Successful weight loss maintenance. Annual Review of Nutrition. 2001;**21**(1):323-341

[6] Gorin AA, Phelan S, Wing RR, Hill JO. Promoting long-term weight control: Does dieting consistency matter? International Journal of Obesity. 2004;**28**(2):278-281

[7] Dombrowski SU, Knittle K, Avenell A, Araújo-Soares V, Sniehotta FF. Long term maintenance of weight loss with non-surgical interventions in obese adults: Systematic review and meta-analyses of randomised controlled trials. BMJ. 2014;**348**:200-225

[8] Huang TT, Drewnowski A, Kumanyika SK, Glass TA. A systems-oriented multilevel framework for addressing obesity in the 21st century. Preventing Chronic Disease. 2009;**6**(3):360-379

[9] Varkevisser RDM, Van Stralen MM, Kroeze W, Ket JCF, Steenhuis IHM. Determinants of weight loss maintenance: A systematic review. Obesity Reviews. 2019;**20**(2):171-211

[10] Winter JE, MacInnis RJ, Wattanapenpaiboon N, Nowson CA. BMI and all-cause mortality in older adults: A meta-analysis. The American Journal of Clinical Nutrition. 2014;**99**(4):875-890

[11] Montesi L, El Ghoch M, Brodosi L, Calugi S, Marchesini G, Dalle Grave R. Long-term weight loss maintenance for obesity: A multidisciplinary approach. Diabetes, Metabolic Syndromc and Obesity: Targets and Therapy. 2016;**9**:37

[12] Sacks FM, Bray GA, Carey VJ, Smith SR, Ryan DH, Anton SD, et al. Comparison of weight-loss diets with different compositions of fat, protein, and carbohydrates. New England Journal of Medicine. 2009;**360**(9):859-873

[13] Waterlander WE, Steenhuis IH, de Boer MR, Schuit AJ, Seidell JC. Introducing taxes, subsidies or both: The effects of various food pricing strategies in a web-based supermarket randomized trial. Preventive Medicine. 2012;**54**(5):323-330

[14] Giel KE, Binkele M, Becker S, Stübler P, Zipfel S, Enck P. Weight reduction and maintenance in a specialized outpatient health care center. Obesity Research & Clinical Practice. 2008;**2**(3):143-150

[15] Bond MJ, McDowell AJ, Wilkinson JY. The measurement of dietary restraint, disinhibition and hunger: An examination of the factor structure of the Three Factor Eating Questionnaire

(TFEQ). International Journal of Obesity. 2001;**25**(6):900-906

[16] Mazzeo SE, Aggen SH, Anderson C, Tozzi F, Bulik CM. Investigating the structure of the eating inventory (three-factor eating questionnaire): A confirmatory approach. International Journal of Eating Disorders. 2003;**34**(2):255-264

[17] Karlsson J, Persson LO, Sjöström L, Sullivan M. Psychometric properties and factor structure of the Three-Factor Eating Questionnaire (TFEQ) in obese men and women. Results from the Swedish Obese Subjects (SOS) study. International Journal of Obesity. 2000;**24**(12):1715-1725

[18] Teixeira PJ, Going SB, Houtkooper LB, Cussler EC, Metcalfe LL, Blew RM, et al. Pretreatment predictors of attrition and successful weight management in women. International Journal of Obesity. 2004;**28**(9):1124-1133

[19] Cuntz U, Leibbrand R, Ehrig C, Shaw R, Fichter MM. Predictors of post-treatment weight reduction after in-patient behavioral therapy. International Journal of Obesity. 2001;**25**(1):S99-S101

[20] Newman E, O'Connor DB, Conner M. Daily hassles and eating behaviour: The role of cortisol reactivity status. Psychoneuroendocrinology. 2007;**32**(2):125-132

[21] Crowther JH, Sanftner J, Bonifazi DZ, Shepherd KL. The role of daily hassles in binge eating. International Journal of Eating Disorders. 2001;**29**(4):449-454

[22] Flora DB, Curran PJ. An empirical evaluation of alternative methods of estimation for confirmatory factor analysis with ordinal data. Psychological Methods. 2004;**9**(4):466

[23] Bischoff SC, Boirie Y, Cederholm T, Chourdakis M, Cuerda C, Delzenne NM, et al. Towards a multidisciplinary approach to understand and manage obesity and related diseases. Clinical Nutrition. 2017;**36**(4):917-938

[24] Nordmo M, Danielsen YS, Nordmo M. The challenge of keeping it off, a descriptive systematic review of high-quality, follow-up studies of obesity treatments. Obesity Reviews. 2020;**21**(1):e12949

[25] Cooper Z, Doll HA, Hawker DM, Byrne S, Bonner G, Eeley E, et al. Testing a new cognitive behavioural treatment for obesity: A randomized controlled trial with three-year follow-up. Behaviour Research and Therapy. 2010;**48**(8):706-713

[26] Kemp K, Griffiths J, Campbell S, Lovell K. An exploration of the follow-up up needs of patients with inflammatory bowel disease. Journal of Crohn's and Colitis. 2013;**7**(9):e386-e395

[27] Sumithran P, Proietto J. The defence of body weight: A physiological basis for weight regain after weight loss. Clinical Science. 2013;**124**(4):231-241

[28] Melby CL, Paris HL, Foright RM, Peth J. Attenuating the biologic drive for weight regain following weight loss: Must what goes down always go back up? Nutrients. 2017;**9**(5):468

[29] Camps SG, Verhoef SP, Westerterp KR. Weight loss, weight maintenance, and adaptive thermogenesis. The American of Clinical Nutrition. 2013;**97**(5):990-994

[30] Fothergill E, Juen Guo LH, Kerns JC, Robert Brychta KYC. Persistent metabolic adaptation six years after the biggest loser competition. Obesity. 2016;**24**(8):1612-1619

[31] MacLean PS, Wing RR, Davidson T, Epstein L, Goodpaster B, Hall KD, et al. NIH working group report: Innovative research to improve maintenance of weight loss. Obesity. 2015;**23**(1):7-15

[32] Kruseman M, Schmutz N, Carrard I. Long-term weight maintenance strategies are experienced as a burden by persons who have lost weight compared to persons with a lifetime normal, stable weight. Obesity Facts. 2017;**10**(4):373-385

[33] Elfhag K, Rössner S. Who succeeds in maintaining weight loss? A conceptual review of factors associated with weight loss maintenance and weight regain. Obesity Reviews. 2005;**6**(1):67-85

[34] Poulimeneas D, Yannakoulia M, Anastasiou CA, Scarmeas N. Weight loss maintenance: Have we missed the brain? Brain Sciences. 2018;**8**(9):174

[35] Johansson K, Neovius M, Hemmingsson E. Effects of anti-obesity drugs, diet, and exercise on weight-loss maintenance after a very-low-calorie diet or low-calorie diet: A systematic review and meta-analysis of randomized controlled trials. The American Journal of Clinical Nutrition. 2014;**99**(1):14-23

[36] Ross KM, Thomas JG, Wing RR. Successful weight loss maintenance associated with morning chronotype and better sleep quality. Journal of Behavioral Medicine. 2016;**39**(3):465-471

[37] Gettens KM, Gorin AA. Executive function in weight loss and weight loss maintenance: A conceptual review and novel neuropsychological model of weight control. Journal of Behavioral Medicine. 2017;**40**(5):687-701

[38] Hartmann-Boyce J, Aveyard P, Piernas C, Koshiaris C, Velardo C, Salvi D, et al. Cognitive and behavioural strategies for weight management in overweight adults: Results from the Oxford Food and Activity Behaviours (OxFAB) cohort study. Plos One. 2018;**13**(8):e0202072

[39] Greaves C, Poltawski L, Garside R, Briscoe S. Understanding the challenge of weight loss maintenance: A systematic review and synthesis of qualitative research on weight loss maintenance. Health Psychology Review. 2017;**11**(2):145-163

[40] Gupta H. Barriers to and facilitators of long term weight loss maintenance in adult UK people: A thematic analysis. International Journal of Preventive Medicine. 2014;**5**(12):1512

[41] Karfopoulou E, Mouliou K, Koutras Y, Yannakoulia M. Behaviours associated with weight loss maintenance and regaining in a Mediterranean population sample. A Qualitative Study. Clinical Obesity. 2013;**3**(5):141-149

[42] Kwasnicka D, Dombrowski SU, White M, Sniehotta FF. 'It's not a diet, it'sa lifestyle': A longitudinal, data-prompted interview study of weight loss maintenance. Psychology & Health. 2019;**34**(8):963-982

[43] Natvik E, Råheim M, Andersen JR, Moltu C. An experientially derived model of flexible and intentional actions for weight loss maintenance after severe obesity. Frontiers in Psychology. 2019;**10**:2503

[44] Coughlin JW, Brantley PJ, Champagne CM, Vollmer WM, Stevens VJ, Funk K, et al. The impact of continued intervention on weight: Five-year results from the weight loss maintenance trial obesity. Obesity (Silver Spring). 2016;**24**(5):1046-1053

[45] Phelan S, Hill JO, Lang W, Dibello JR, Wing RR. Recovery from relapse among

successful weight maintainers. The American Journal of Clinical Nutrition. 2003;**78**(6):1079-1084

[46] Tsai AG, Wadden TA. The evolution of very-low-calorie diets: An update and meta-analysis. Obesity. 2006;**14**(8):1283-1293

[47] Heshka S, Anderson JW, Atkinson RL, Greenway FL, Hill JO, Phinney SD, et al. Weight loss with self-help compared with a structured commercial program: A randomized trial. JAMA. 2003;**289**(14):1792-1798

[48] Latner JD. Self-help for obesity and binge eating. Nutrition Today. 2007;**42**(2):81-85

[49] Wadden TA, Berkowitz RI, Womble LG, Sarwer DB, Phelan S, Cato RK, et al. Randomized trial of lifestyle modification and pharmacotherapy for obesity. New England Journal of Medicine. 2005;**353**(20):2111-2120

[50] Wadden TA, Berkowitz RI, Sarwer DB, Prus-Wisniewski R, Steinberg C. Benefits of lifestyle modification in the pharmacologic treatment of obesity: A randomized trial. Archives of Internal Medicine. 2001;**161**(2):218-227

Section 3

Anorexia Nervosa Treatment

Chapter 11

Anorexia Nervosa: Opportunities and Challenges in Treatment

Kayode Olariike Oyindasola, Folake Funke Adedoyin and Adeoye Adeyemi Adedoyin

Abstract

Anorexia nervosa is an eating disorder condition characterized by an abnormal fear of gaining weight, driving people to starve themselves and become dangerously thin. It involves restricting food intake, which can lead to severe nutritional deficiencies. Anorexia nervosa can affect people of all ages, genders, races and ethnicities. The effects of anorexia nervosa can be life threatening, but counseling and treatment for underlying mental health issues can help people with this condition. Goals of treatment include restoring the person to a healthy weight, treating emotional issues such as low self-esteem, correcting distorted thinking patterns, and developing long-term behavioral changes. Early diagnosis and treatment are more likely to lead to a positive outcome. The physical signs and symptoms of anorexia nervosa are related to starvation. Anorexia also includes emotional and behavioral issues involving an unrealistic perception of body weight and an extremely strong fear of gaining weight or becoming fat. This chapter aimed to understand the opportunities embedded and challenges encountered in the treatment of anorexia nervosa. Information given will assist the patient and team of professionals (primary care physician, mental health professionals, nutritionist, counselors) in the treatment of this disorder to support recovery and prevent relapse.

Keywords: anorexia nervosa, eating disorder, opportunities and challenges

1. Introduction

Anorexia nervosa is an eating disorder condition portrayed by an abnormal fear of gaining weight this drives people to starve themselves and eventually become dangerously thin [1]. It is more prominent in females but can also be found in males, a life change or traumatic event may be associated with the development of the illness and a desire to excel in sports is a contributing factor [2].

Dieting behavior in anorexia nervosa is associated mostly by an intense fear becoming obese or gaining excess weight. Individuals with anorexia will say they want and are willing to gain weight; their behavior (action) is not in line with their intention. For instance, they consume minute amounts of low-energy giving foods and engaged in physical exercise beyond the usual. Also, persons with anorexia nervosa intermittently engage in binge eating and purge by vomiting or misuse of laxative. Anorexia nervosa is of two types:

- Restricting type, in this type individuals lose weight primarily by dieting, fasting or exercising excessively [3].

- Also, Binge – eating or purging type in which persons also engage in intermittent binge eating and purging behaviors.

The risk of evolving anorexia nervosa is greater in models, dancers, and athletes in sports where appearance and weight are important, especially among wrestlers, boxers, gymnast, and figure skaters.

People with anorexia tend to be very successful, they perform well in sports, school, work and other activities. They tend to be perfectionists with compulsive, anxious, and depressive symptoms. Most times it begins around the time of puberty, but can also develop at any time.

Over time, some of the following symptoms may develop related to starvation or purging behaviors:

- Menstrual periods cease

- Dizziness or fainting from dehydration

- Brittle hair/nails

Anorexia nervosa is characterized by the individuals' refusal to maintain adequate weight for their height, refusal to feed associated with distortion of the bodily image, and denial of their pathological condition [4].

People with anorexia find it difficult to recognize that they have a mental illness or psychiatric disorder. This is because it's hard for them to get out of the habits they have developed as a result of anorexia, to recover usually can take some time. Although people with anorexia respond to treatment, the earlier the treatment begins, the better the chances of a complete recovery. Treatment strategy usually involves talking therapies, which include cognitive behavioral therapy, the aim is to change the person's thoughts, feelings, and behavior around food. Nutritional support is essential and is offered to help gain weight properly.

2. Causes

The cause of anorexia is currently unknown [1]. Research suggests that a combination of certain personality traits, emotions, and thinking patterns, as well as biological and environmental factors might be responsible [5]. Cultural factors also play a role, where societies that value thinness have higher rates of the disease. Additionally, it can be found among those involved in activities that value thinness, such as high-level athletics, modeling, and dancing [6]. Diagnosis for the disease requires a significantly low weight and the severity of disease which is based on body mass index (BMI) in adults is classified as; mild disease having a body mass index of greater than 17, moderate a body mass index of 16 to

17, severe a body mass index of 15 to 16, and extreme a body mass index which is less than 15. For children, a body mass index for age percentile of less than the 5th percentile is often used [7].

3. Symptoms

The visible manifestation of anorexia nervosa is related to starvation. It includes emotional and behavioral issues encompassing an unrealistic perception of body weight and an extremely strong fear of gaining weight or becoming obese. Many atimes it is difficult to notice signs and symptoms because what is considered a low body weight is different from individual, while some individuals may not appear extremely thin. Also, people with eating disorder often conceal their thinness, eating habits or physical problems.

3.1 Symptoms/signs

Visible signs and symptoms of anorexia include:

- Insomnia
- Dizziness or fainting
- Hair that thins, breaks or falls out
- Thin appearance
- Abnormal blood counts
- Fatique
- Extreme weight loss or not making expected developmental weight gains
- Dizziness or fainting
- Bluish discoloration of the fingers
- Absence of menstruation
- Constipation and abdominal pain
- Intolerance of cold
- Irregular heart rhythms
- Low blood pressure
- Dehydration
- Swelling of arms or legs

4. Behavioral and emotional manifestation

Behavioral symptoms of anorexia include attempting to lose weight through:

- Exercising excessively
- Restricting food severely through skipping meals or fasting
- Binge eating and self-induced vomiting to get rid of food, this include the use of diet aids or herbal products and laxatives.

Emotional signs and symptoms are:

- Frequently skipping meals or refusing to eat
- Preoccupation with food, which sometimes includes cooking elaborate meals for others but not eating them
- Eating only a few certain "safe" foods, usually those low in fat and calories
- Denial of hunger or making excuses for not eating
- Not wanting to eat in public
- Lying about how much food has been eaten
- Fear of gaining weight that may include repeated weighing or measuring the body
- Frequent checking in the mirror for perceived flaws
- Social withdrawal
- Irritability

5. Treatment for anorexia nervosa

Goals of treatment include restoring the person to a healthy weight, treating emotional issues such as low self-esteem, correcting distorted thinking patterns, and developing long-term behavioral changes.

Treatment for anorexia recovery is paramount for person who is dealing with medical complications as a result starvation, such as gastrointestinal distress, cardio-vascular disorders such as low blood pressure, dehydration, and more. Psychological complications that would entail higher levels of care include urges to suicidal ideation or self-harm.

For a person recovering from anorexia nervosa and is medically stable, intensive medical intervention might not be necessary. Residential treatment for anorexia nervosa may be an appropriate level of care, this treatment may also be ideal for individual who is recuperating from anorexia nervosa but is mentally retarded and could not respond to partial hospitalization or outpatient treatment. The rehabilitation process for anorexia nervosa is a complex process, residential treatment can be a better choice for a person who is in need of multidisciplinary care for recovery. Treatment options will vary depending on the individual's needs, treatment most often involves a combination of the following treatment methods:

- *Psychotherapy*: This involves individual counseling that focuses on changing the thinking (cognitive therapy) and behavior (behavioral therapy). Treatment includes practical techniques for adopting healthy attitudes toward food and weight, as well as approaches for changing the way the person responds to difficult situations.

- *Medications*: Certain antidepressant medications can be used to help control anxiety and depression associated with eating disorder. Some antidepressants medications also help to improve sleep and stimulate appetite. Other forms medications can be given to help control anxiety and/or distorted attitudes toward eating and body perception.

- *Nutrition counseling*: This approach has been formulated to teach a healthy pattern to food and weight, to help restore ideal eating patterns, and to evaluate the importance of nutrition and following an adequate diet which is ideal for growth and well-being.

- *Group and/or family therapy*: Family support is very important for a treatment to be successful. It is important that family members understand the eating disorder and should be able to recognize its physical manifestation. Individuals with eating disorders might benefit from group therapy, where they can find support and care, discuss their feelings and concerns openly with others who also share common experiences and problems.

- *Hospitalization*: This is essential in order to treat severe weight loss that has resulted in malnutrition and other serious mental, psychological and physical health complications, such as depression, heart disorders, and risk of suicide. In some cases, the patient may need to be fed through intravenous feeding.

6. Anorexia Nervosa: Opportunities in Treatment

6.1 Levels of care

Majority of anorexia nervosa treatment centers provide multiple level of treatment to adequately support patients on the path to recovery. The outpatient or day treatment program is the least intensive level of care, this treatment type is formulated to help patients who are medically and psychiatrically stable, and can benefit from ongoing counseling. Most times, this level of care is endorsed to individuals who have undergone residential treatment as they integrate back into their daily lives.

In addition, majority of anorexia treatment centers render a more comprehensive residential treatment program. This type of treatment program is ideal for adolescents that may be experiencing both medical and psychological issues associated with eating disorder. Eating disorders such as anorexia nervosa requires medical supervision and guidance before or while a patient is working on the psychological aspects of the condition. With residential care, adolescents are able to get the treatment needed for any medical issues associated with the disorder and find comfort in a safe space where their thoughts and feelings can be fully utilized.

7. Engagement

Most people with anorexia nervosa find it difficult to admit that they have a problem and are undecided about change. This is a contributing factor to their reluctance to engage with treatment and services. Effective engagement of the patient in the treatment is a prerequisite for any successful treatment plan, health care workers who are involved in the treatment of anorexia nervosa should ensure to build an empathic, collaborative and supportive relationship with patients and, if possible, their careers. This should be paramount to the care given, motivation to change may go up and down over the course of treatment and the therapist must remain sensitive to this.

8. Comprehensive care offered within a controlled environment

One significant benefit of residential treatment is the comprehensive care which is being offered in a controlled environment, including medical, psychotherapy, and psychiatric supervision and treatment, medical nutrition therapy, support groups, and more. The kind of treatment provided is holistic, this can be advantageous for an individual who is in the early phases of recovery or needing constant supervision and monitoring.

Having the opportunity to establish recovery in a safe and supportive environment can be of added advantage for individual to heal and recover, particularly if their previous home condition or surroundings was not conducive to eating disorder recovery. There might be need for an individual to vacate temporarily from their environment or everyday demands in order to prioritize their healing and focus more on their recovery efforts.

9. Nutrition interventions help to normalize eating habits

Nutrition interventions and meal support can help an individual learn how to stabilize eating habits, restrict poor food behaviors, and learn to eat adequately for their own body needs. Therapy and nutrition interventions are implemented and monitored by specialized team members, which includes a psychotherapist and registered dietitian who specializes in eating disorders.

10. Challenges in Treating Anorexia Nervosa

From the Lancet, "Stephan Zipfel and colleagues present results of the Anorexia Nervosa Treatment of OutPatients (ANTOP) study, in which two manual-based outpatient treatments (focal psychodynamic therapy and enhanced cognitive behaviour therapy) were compared with optimised treatment as usual, which included careful and regular monitoring by family doctors linked to care at specialist treatment centres" [8]. The findings provide some rather sobering observations about treatment of anorexia nervosa, and highlight the difficulties of implementing clinical trials for this disorder. This include treatment for anorexia nervosa takes a long time, at an average of 10 months' duration. No brief interventions for the disorder have been judged effective. Also, response rate was low as almost a third of patients were lost to follow-up a year after the end of treatment (although, compared with other anorexia trials, this dropout rate is not bad). For many patients, psychotherapy alone did not suffice, and inpatient treatment was needed for some patients during the trial [8].

Challenges with residential treatment are of various dimensions and can include various factors, including intensity of treatment care and cost. If there is no insurance coverage, the cost of residential treatment can be difficult to afford, while some insurance companies will only cover a limited length of stay within residential care.

For some people, transiting from residential treatment to lower levels of treatment can be very difficult, as residents are not always prepared and equipped for the triggers of the outside world after their stay.

There should be allowances made for intermittent hospitalisations during anorexia outpatient trials because recovery from this disorder is rarely linear. Moreover, precipitous weight loss and other medical complications needing hospital treatment do not necessarily mean that outpatient care will ultimately fail.

Establishing a collaborative working relationship with families with a young person with anorexia nervosa presents a particular challenge that requires time and expertise to balance the competing needs of different family members.

A prominent challenge in treating anorexia is that people may not want treatment. Barriers to treatment include:

- Not seeing anorexia as an illness but rather a lifestyle choice
- Thinking you do not need treatment
- Fearing weight gain

People receiving inpatient treatment for anorexia nervosa have been found to be twice as likely to drop out of treatment compared to general psychiatric inpatients [9].

11. Conclusion

Anorexia nervosa is an eating disorder with short and long term physical consequences. Engagement of patient in treatment plan, getting support from family and friends are vital to successful treatment. Most patients with anorexia nervosa receive treatment solely on an outpatient basis. However, a substantial minority receive inpatient treatment. Hospital admission may be at ameliorating the effects of the illness on the patient's physical or at achieving progress toward full recovery.

12. Recommendations

- Patient and, where appropriate, careers preference, should be put into consideration in deciding which psychological treatment is to be offered.

- Majority of people with anorexia nervosa should be managed on an outpatient basis embedded with psychological treatment, this should be provided by a health care professional competent to give the treatment and also assess the physical risk of people with eating disorders.

- Treatment and physical monitoring for anorexia nervosa should not exceed six months' duration in psychological outpatient care.

- If outpatient psychological treatment does not lead to any significant improvement, inpatient care should be considered.

- Dietary counseling should be part of the treatment for anorexia nervosa

- Family members including siblings, should normally be included in the treatment of anorexia nervosa.

Author details

Kayode Olariike Oyindasola[1]*, Folake Funke Adedoyin[2]
and Adeoye Adeyemi Adedoyin[2]

1 Department of Human Nutrition and Dietetics, College of Health Sciences, Osun State University, Osogbo, Nigeria

2 Department of Nursing, All Saints University School of Medicine, Dominica

*Address all correspondence to: okeyoyinolariike@yahoo.com

References

[1] Attia E. Anorexia nervosa: Current status and future directions. Annual Review of Medicine. 2010;**61**(1):425-435. DOI: 10.1146/annurev.med.050208.20074

[2] Coelho GM, Soares EA, Ribeiro BG. Are female athletes at increased risk for disordered eating and its complications? Appetite. 2010;**55**(3):379-387

[3] Nattiv A, Loucks AB, Manore MM, Sanborn CF, Sundgot-Borgen J, Warren MP. American college of sports medicine position stand. The female athlete triad. Medicine and Science Sports and Exercise. 2007;**39**(10):1867-1882

[4] Borge NJB, Sicchieri JMF, Ribeiro RPP, Marchini JS, Santos JE. Eating disorders-clinical framework. Medicine USP Journals Portal. 2006;**39**(3):340-348. DOI: 10.11606/issn.2176-7262.v39i340-348

[5] Smitha B. Anorexia Nervosa. WebMD, LLC; 2020

[6] Arcelus J, Witcomb GL, Mitchell A. Prevalence of eating disorders amongst dancers: A systematic review and meta-analysis. European Eating Disorders Review. 2014;**22**(2):92-101. DOI: 10.1002erv.2271ee

[7] Diagnostic and Statistical Manual of mental disorders (DSM-5-TR) Washington. American Psychaitric Association. 2013:338-345

[8] Zipfel S, Wild B, Groß G, et al. Focal psychodynamic therapy, cognitive behaviour therapy, and optimised treatment as usual in outpatients with anorexia nervosa (ANTOP study): Randomised controlled trial. Lancet. 2014;**383**:127-137. DOI: 10.1016/S0140-6736(13)61746-8

[9] Kahn C, Pike KM. In search of predictors of dropout from inpatient treatment for anorexia nervosa. International Journal of Eating Disorders. 2001;**30**(3):237-244

Section 4

Miscellaneous

Chapter 12

Mechanism and Impact of Food Components in Burning Calories from White-to-Brown Adipose Tissue

Upasana

Abstract

Obesity is one of the nutritional public health concerns of today's world. It is defined as the abnormal accumulation of fat as a result of positive energy balance in the body. As the trend of overweight and obesity is increasing at the fastest pace affecting both children and adults; so, a search of new therapeutic guidelines is required to ameliorate the status of weight gain. Various researches are carried on regarding the activation of brown adipose tissue (BAT) for amplifying energy expenditure (EE) through heat production. Browning of white adipose tissue (WAT), now-a-days gained more attention and is considered as another tool for stimulating calorie burning. This chapter portrays the recent knowledge of some food ingredients that can enhance activation of BAT and browning of WAT with their beneficial health consequences.

Keywords: food components, burning, calories, adipose tissues, overweight, obesity

1. Introduction

Overweight and Obesity is considered as the main chauffeur for an umbrella of diseases like type 2 diabetes mellitus, insulin resistance (IR), non-alcoholic fatty liver, hypertension, dyslipidemia, heart diseases, orthopedic disorders, asthma, hormonal imbalances, several types of cancers, disability, and many other types of diseases. The fundamental causes of overweight and obesity are a result of positive energy balance between energy intake and its expenditure or a combination of both. The World Health Organization (WHO) has reported that obesity more than 1.9 billion adults were overweight; of these over 650 million were obese in the year 2016. It was also reported by WHO in the year 2019 that 38.3 million children under 5 were overweight or obese [1]. There are an array of factors that leads to overweight and obesity which include age, gender, genetic predisposition, sedentary lifestyle, socio-economic status, faulty eating habits (processed and energy-dense foods), and so on.

Generally, weight management is focused on two modifications i.e., lifestyle modification and improving eating habits. It is well known that the principal depot for energy storage is WAT and on the contrary basis, BAT is responsible for thermogenic energy expenditure. BAT had a significant capacity to dissipate energy and regulate triglycerides and glucose metabolism; act as a potential target for the treatment of overweight and obesity as well as metabolic disorders [2].

2. Adipose tissues: origin and development

Adipose tissue is fundamentally fabricated from adipocytes as well as pre-adipocytes, macrophages, endothelial cells, fibroblasts, and leucocytes that are considered as a major player of systemically metabolic regulation [3]. The adipose tissue acts as a central metabolic organ for systematic energy homeostasis by acting as a caloric reservoir [4]. It is characterized as an important endocrine organ that is responsible for the secretion of many molecules like proteins, lipids and, miRNA (microRNA) [5]. These elements act as paracrine and endocrine signals that are critical for the function of adipose tissue as well as for non-adipose tissues that are required for the regulation of the body's metabolism and insulin sensitivity [4, 5].

Broadly, adipocytes are classified into two main categories i.e., white or brown adipocytes depending upon their morphology and nature of work/function. Adipose tissues also act as endocrine organs that are responsible for the secretion of multiple hormones. WAT plays a role in fatty acid biosynthesis by storing lipids in form of triglycerides as its cell have large vacuoles and fewer mitochondria. Similarly, BAT plays a role in glucose uptake and fatty acid breakdown, leading to energy dissipation and heat production. Its cells are multilocular with central nuclei and mitochondria rich in the expression of uncoupling protein-1 (UCP-1) that mediates the uncoupling of electron transport that leads to a decrement in the generation of adenosine triphosphate (ATP) from adenosine diphosphate (ADP) with subsequent heat generation [5, 6]. The principal function of BAT is non-shivering thermogenesis; an energy-intensive process in which chemical energy is transformed into physical heat [5]. Further, the

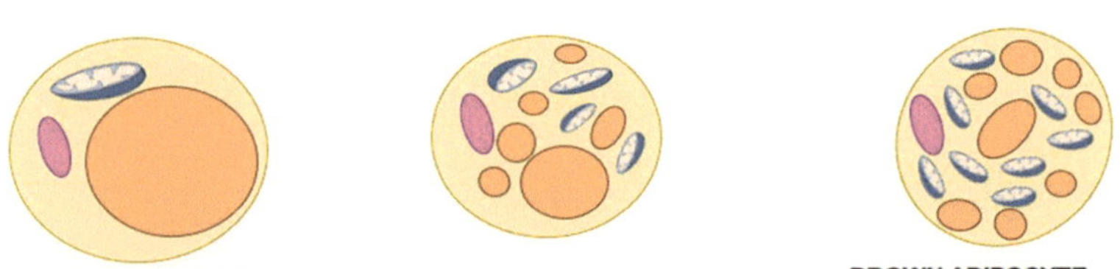

	WHITE ADIPOCYTE	BEIGE ADIPOCYTE	BROWN ADIPOCYTE
Localization	Subcutaneous, Intra-abdominal, Epicardial, Gonadal	Emerges in white tissue depots with appropriate stimuli	Interscapular, Paravertebral, Perirenal, Cervical, Supraclavicular
Morphology	Spherical	Spherical	Elliptical and Smaller than white
Cell Composition	Single lipid droplet, few mitochondria, flattened peripheral nucleus, little endoplasmic reticulum	Unilocular morphology but small lipid droplets after stimulation, mitochondria appear after stimulation	Multiple small lipid droplets, large number of mitochondria, oval central nucleus
Function	Storing energy	Thermogenic potential	Expending energy and heat production (non-shivering thermogenesis)
Uncoupling protein	Undetectable	Positive after stimulation	Thermogenic potential

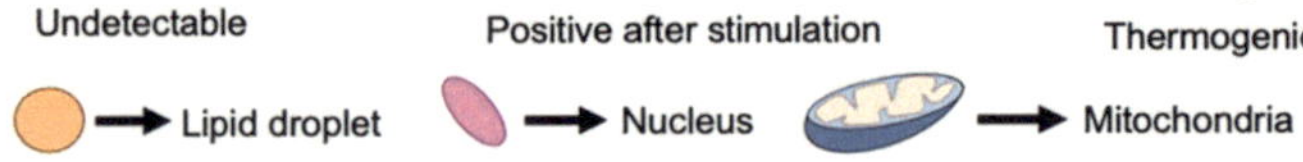

Figure 1.
Physiological, morphological, cell composition, and function of adipocytes. The figure was modified from the following research paper by El Hadi et al., 2019.

process of thermogenesis is also performed by the third type of adipose tissue cell known as beige adipocytes. Beige adipocytes have many properties similar to brown adipocytes i.e., the presence of multilocular lipid droplets and numerous mitochondria expressing UCP-1 [5]. However, the process of thermogenesis is not restricted to brown adipocytes but it may be done by beige adipocytes that may emerge within WAT depots in a process known as "WAT browning" [5–7]. The physiological, morphological, cell composition, and function of adipocytes are shown in **Figure 1**.

3. Food components involved in browning of WAT

Numerous dietary factors are involved in the activation of BAT or browning of WAT via the main physiologic mechanism well shown in **Figures 2** and **3**.

3.1 Polyunsaturated fatty acids (PUFAs)

The major sources of PUFAs, mostly Docosahexaenoic acid (DHA) and Eicosapentaenoic acid (EPA) are found in fatty fish such as salmon and anchovies as

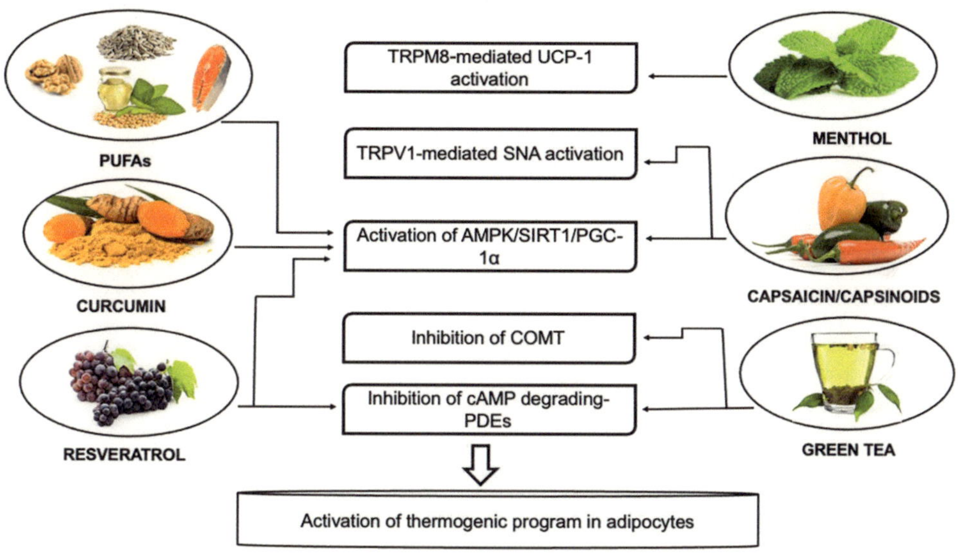

Figure 2.
Food components involved in the induction of WAT browning. Here, PUFAs- polyunsaturated fatty acids, WAT- white adipose tissue, TRPM8- transient receptor potential cation channel melastatin 8, UCP1- uncoupling protein 1, TRPV1-transient receptor potential vanilloid 1, SNA- sympathetic nerve activity; AMPK- adenosine monophosphate-activated protein kinase, SIRT1- sirtuin-1, PGC-1α-peroxisome proliferator-activated receptor gamma coactivator 1-alpha, COMT- catechol-O-methyl-transferase, cAMP- cyclic adenosine monophosphate, PDEs- phosphodiesterases. The figure was modified from the following research paper by El Hadi et al., 2019. The images used in drawing the figure were extracted from the following links as described below: 1. PUFAs- Walnut- https://5.imimg.com/data5/JR/AK/VJ/SELLER-2793878/walnut-500x500.jpg, fish- https://www.bigbasket.com/media/uploads/p/xxl/40186851_1-fresho-atlantic-salmon.jpg, soyabean oil- https://image.shutterstock.com/image-photo/soybean-oil-bottle-green-pods-260nw-310996568.jpg, sunflower seeds- https://zonefresh.com.au/wp-content/uploads/SUNFLOWER-KERNELS.jpg, 2. Curcumin- https://5.imimg.com/data5/SELLER/Default/2020/9/VE/PK/ZA/24380440/curcumin-extract-500x500.jpg, 3. Resveratrol- https://news.mit.edu/sites/default/files/styles/news_article__image_gallery/public/images/201303/20130307093438-0_0.jpg?itok=xnIFxN6G, 4. Menthol- https://smhttp-ssl-61936.nexcesscdn.net/media/catalog/product/optimized/7/5/75ea61bf1685045cff4a80f864b6472f/flavor-west-natural-menthol.jpg, 5. Capsaicin/capsinoids- https://article.innovadatabase.com/articleimgs/article_images/flavors8.jpg, 6. Green tea- https://femina.wwmindia.com/content/2018/nov/thumbnail1541742051.jpg.

well as fish oil supplements [6]. Previous studies reported that EPA activates white adipocytes to beige-like adipocytes in overweight human subjects by stimulating the activation of the adenosine monophosphate-activated protein kinase (AMPK)/ sirtuin-1 (SIRT1) /peroxisome proliferator-activated receptor gamma coactivator 1-alpha (PGC1- α axis) [6, 8]. Furthermore, many researchers also reported that fish oil contributes to brown adipogenesis by acting as a ligand of transient receptor potential vanilloid 1(TRPV1) in the digestive tract that triggers through the brain, a β 2-adrenergical sympathetic response in adipose depots [6].

3.2 Curcumin

Curcumin is the yellow-colored hydrophobic polyphenol that is available in extracts of turmeric roots belongs to the family of Zingiberaceae with genus

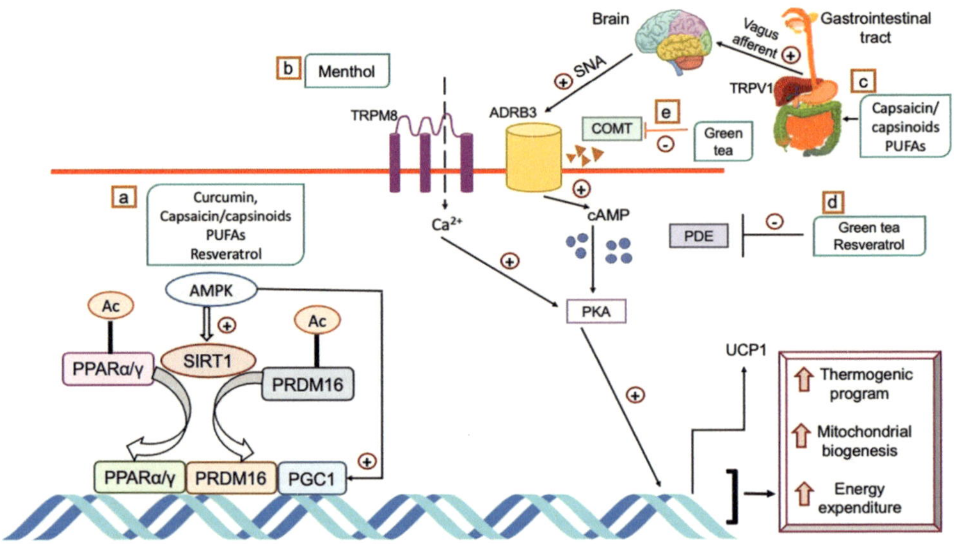

Figure 3.
Dietary components involved in the mechanism involved in brown adipogenesis, mitochondrial biogenesis, and energy expenditure. (a) Activation of SIRT1 either directly and/or indirectly through AMPK results in deacetylation and interaction of key transcription factors that induce brown and beige adipogenesis as PPAR α/γ and PRDM16. It was also found that PPAR/PRDM16 complex was able to bind and activate PGC1α, another co-factor expressed in brown and beige adipocytes that trigger the transcription of multiple genes engaged in thermogenesis and mitochondrial biogenesis. Likewise, AMPK may also directly magnify PGC1α activity by phosphorylation, which ultimately increases mitochondrial biogenesis. (b) The activation of TRPM8 in brown adipocytes increases the expression of thermogenic genes through the Ca2 + dependent PKA signaling pathway. (c) Due to the triggering of TRPV1 receptors in the gastrointestinal tract, and stimulation of the vagal afferent pathways, neurons within the ventromedial hypothalamus get activated. This leads to the induction of a cold-independent adrenergic response that intervenes brown adipogenesis. The adrenergic stimulation in brown adipocytes may also be promoted by decreasing the deterioration of (d) cAMP and (e) norepinephrine via direct inhibition of PDEs and COMT activity, respectively. Here, TRPM8-transient receptor potential cation channel melastatin 8, UCP1- uncoupling protein 1, TRPV1-transient receptor potential vanilloid 1, SNA- sympathetic nerve activity, AMPK- adenosine monophosphate-activated protein kinase, SIRT1- sirtuin-1, PGC-1α-peroxisome proliferator-activated receptor gamma coactivator 1-alpha, COMT- catechol-O-methyl-transferase, cAMP-cyclic adenosine monophosphate, PDEs- phosphodiesterases, PUFAs-polyunsaturated fatty acids, Ac-acetyl group, PPARα/γ peroxisome proliferator-activated receptor alpha/gamma, PKA- protein kinase A, PRDM16- PR-domain containing 16. (+) – stimulation, (-)- inhibition, increase. The figure was modified from the following research paper by El Hadi et al., 2019. The images used in drawing the figure were extracted from the following links as described below: 1. DNA- https:// images.freeimg.net/thumbs/dna-2316536_1280.png, 2. Brain- https://timvandevall.com/wp-content/uploads/ human-brain-parts-1.jpg, 3. Gastrointestinal tract- https://spng.subpng.com/20180425/fre/kisspng-gastrointestinal-tract-human-digestive-system-diag-abdominal-5ae0b2080064a3.8564190715246750800016.jpg.

Curcuma of the plant. It has numerous therapeutic potentials like anti-obesity, anti-diabetic, antioxidant, and anti-inflammatory; used as a spice in cooking generally in India. Akbari et al., 2019 stated that supplementation of curcumin decreases body mass index (BMI), percent body fat, leptin and increases adiponectin level in obese humans [9]. Earlier studies also reported that curcumin induces browning in WAT via adenosine monophosphate-activated protein kinase (AMPK) activation and inhibition of preadipocyte differentiation by downregulating the peroxisome proliferator-activated receptor gamma (PPAR γ) and CCCAAT/Enhancer Binding Protein α (C/EBP α) [5, 10–12].

3.3 Resveratrol

Resveratrol is a natural polyphenol that is mostly found in grapes (Vitaceae family with genus Vitis), blueberries (Ericaceae family with genus Vaccinium), cranberries (Ericaceae family with genus Vaccinium), red and white wines, peanuts (Fabaceae family with genus Arachis), cocoa and dark chocolates (Malvaceae family with genus Theobroma). It is well known that resveratrol plays numerous vital roles in the human body like anti-inflammatory as well as maintaining glucose metabolism and insulin sensitivity which are relevant to obesity [13]. It also possesses anti-lipolytic, cardio-protective, neuroprotective, and anti-cancerous effects [13]. Earlier studies revealed that resveratrol exerts thermogenic effects and contributes to increased respiration [14]. Another clinical study stated that resveratrol is considered a natural activator of the sirtuins family [15]. AMPK activation by resveratrol can stimulate mitochondrial biogenesis through SIRT1 [14]. Additionally, it also activates the deacetylation of PGC-1α, a regulator of energy metabolism that leads to ATP production by modulating mitochondrial function [13].

3.4 Menthol

Menthol is also called mint camphor that is produced from the plant peppermint (family Lamiaceae with genus Mentha) or maybe extracted synthetically. Menthol possesses various biological properties like anti-inflammatory, anti-bacterial, anti-pruritic, antitussive, and analgesic properties [6, 16]. Since menthol induces cooling sensation by activating the TRPM8 receptor, a $Ca2+-$ permeable non-selective channel that detects cold stimuli in the thermosensory system [6, 17, 18]. Several clinical studies also reported that menthol stimulates transient receptor potential cation channel melastatin 8 (TRPM8) expression on the white and brown adipocytes.

3.5 Capsaicin and Capsinoids

Capsaicin and capsinoids are the compounds that are generally found in red peppers belong to the family of Solanaceae with genus capsicum of the plant. Several studies reported that capsaicin and capsinoids have various properties like anti-obesity, anti-diabetic and anti-inflammatory. Earlier studies reported that capsaicin and capsinoids played a pivotal role in fat oxidation and EE [19]. Yoneshiro et al., 2013 reported that supplementation of capsinoids over 6 weeks decreases body weight in humans [20]. Despite the above, it was also reported that exposure of cold cumulative with ingestion of capsinoids results in activation of brown and beige adipose tissues [5, 20]. This activation happens as a result of activation of the transient receptor potential cation channel subfamily V member 1 (TRPV1) in the gastrointestinal tract which sends signals to the central nervous system (CNS) leading to 2-AR signaling activation in adipose tissue [5, 21]. It was also stated in earlier studies that capsaicin triggers browning of WAT by stimulating the expression of SIRT1, UCP1, bone morphogenetic protein 8B (BMP8B), and PPAR γ, PGC-1 α in white adipocytes.

3.6 Green tea

Green tea is considered a widely consumed beverage all over the world. It is extracted from fresh leaves of a green tea plant named Camellia sinensis belongs to the family of Theaceae. It contains huge amounts of polyphenols, mainly tea catechins like epicatechin, epicatechin gallate, and epigallocatechin that possesses properties like antioxidants, hypocholesterolemic, antihypertensive, and anticarcinogenic [14]. Various clinical studies also enumerated that consumption of green tea helps in weight management by modifying fat metabolism and calories expenditure. Earlier studies also reported that green tea contains a substantial amount of caffeine; which is known for its thermogenic properties [6, 22]. Dulloo et al., 1999 in human studies, also stated that green tea enhances fat oxidation and energy expenditure [23]. Nevertheless, catechins and caffeine may synergically mediate adrenergic-induced BAT thermogenesis by acting at different checkpoints of the norepinephrine-cyclic adenosine monophosphate (cAMP) axis. It was recommended that green tea catechins may promote sympathetic nerve activity (SNA) by decreasing the degradation of norepinephrine through direct inhibition of catechol-O-methyl-transferase (COMT) [6]. Furthermore, it was also reported that caffeine may synergically prolong the effects of norepinephrine by direct inhibition of phosphodiesterases (PDEs) activity [6, 23, 24].

4. Conclusion

Overweight and obesity are considered major risk factors for the number of non-communicable diseases like type 2 diabetes mellitus, non-alcoholic fatty liver, dyslipidemia, heart disease, some types of cancers, and many more. The main cause of overweight and obesity is increased fat mass; as all fat depots are not equally created. As we know that, adipocytes are present in WAT, contain large single fat droplets that act as a reservoir for energy storage. On the other hand, BAT play a specific role in thermoregulation. In this chapter, emphasis is given on some dietary components that have the potential to activate the regulation of BAT or beige fat development. Moreover, various clinical studies and trials showed that dietary components like PUFAs, curcumin, resveratrol, menthol, capsaicins/capsinoids, green tea, and many more when supplemented in adequate quantity show thermogenic effects. Therefore, further research is required to define and describe the methods by which these dietary components can be incorporated into the diet as well as about the bioavailability of these dietary components. Nevertheless, it can be stated that these dietary components may act as a boon in ameliorating the condition of overweight and obesity in the future.

Acknowledgements

A profound sense of gratitude to my beloved husband Mr. Nirmal Kumar for his love, understanding, opinion, encouragement, valuable suggestions, and useful comments throughout in writing this book chapter. I also apologize for not citing the research papers of all the authors that helped me in better understanding this topic.

Conflict of interest

The author declares no conflict of interest.

Author details

Upasana
Mahila College Dalmianagar, Dehri – on – Sone, Rohtas, Veer Kunwar Singh University, Ara, Bihar, India

*Address all correspondence to: me.upasana87@gmail.com

References

[1] World Health Organisation (WHO): Obesity. Available from: https://www.who.int/health-topics/obesity#tab=tab_1 [Accessed: October 18, 2021]

[2] Schulz TJ, Tseng Y. Brown adipose tissue: Development, metabolism and beyond. The Biochemical Journal. 2013;**453**(2):167-178. DOI: 10.1042/BJ20130457

[3] Luo L, Liu M. Adipose tissue in control of metabolism. The Journal of Endocrinology. 2016;**231**(3):R77-R99. DOI: 10.1530/JOE-16-0211

[4] Choe SS, Huh JY, Hwang IJ, Kim JI, Kim JB. Adipose tissue remodeling: Its role in energy metabolism and metabolic disorders. Frontiers in Endocrinology. 2016;**7**:30. DOI: 10.3389/fendo.2016.00030

[5] Brandao BB, Poojari A, Rabiee A. Thermogenic fat: Development, physiological function, and therapeutic potential. International Journal of Molecular Sciences. 2021;**22**:5906. DOI: 10.3390/ijms22115906

[6] El Hadi H, DI Vincenzo A, Vettor R, Rossato M. Food ingredients involved in white-to-Brown adipose tissue conversion and in calorie burning. Frontiers in Physiology. 2019;**9**:1954. DOI: 10.3389/fphys.2018.01954

[7] Kiefer FW. The significance of beige and brown fat in humans. Endocrine Connections. 2017;**6**(5):R70-R79. DOI: 10.1530/EC-17-0037

[8] Laiglesia LM, Lorente-Cebrian S, Prieto-Hontoria PL, Fernandez-Galilea M, Ribeiro SM, Sainz N, et al. Eicosapentaenoic acid promotes mitochondrial biogenesis and beige-like features in subcutaneous adipocytes from overweight subjects. The Journal of Nutritional Biochemistry. 2016;**37**:76-82. DOI: 10.1016/j.jnutbio.2016.07.019

[9] Akbari M, Lankarani KB, Tabrizi R, Ghayour-Mobarhan M, Peymani P, Ferns G, et al. The effects of curcumin on weight loss among patients with metabolic syndrome and related disorders: A systematic review and meta-analysis of randomized controlled trials. Frontiers in Pharmacology. 2019;**10**:649. DOI: 10.3389/fphar.2019.00649

[10] Lone J, Choi JH, Kim SW, Yun JW. Curcumin induces brown fat-like phenotype in 3T3-L1 and primary white adipocytes. The Journal of Nutritional Biochemistry. 2016;**27**:193-202. DOI: 10.1016/j.jnutbio.2015.09.006

[11] Wang S, Wang X, Ye Z, Xu C, Zhang M, Ruan B, et al. Curcumin promotes browning of white adipose tissue in a norepinephrine-dependent way. Biochemical and Biophysical Research Communications. 2015;**466**(2):247-253. DOI: 10.1016/j.bbrc.2015.09.018

[12] Ejaz A, Wu D, Kwan P, Meydani M. Curcumin inhibits adipogenesis in 3T3-L1 adipocytes and angiogenesis and obesity in C57/BL mice. The Journal of Nutrition. 2009;**139**(5):919-925. DOI: 10.3945/jn.108.100966

[13] Kim OY, Chung JY, Song J. Effect of resveratrol on adipokines and myokines involved in fat browning: Perspectives in healthy weight against obesity. Pharmacological Research. 2019;**148**:104411. DOI: 10.1016/j.phrs.2019.104411

[14] Okla M, Kim J, Koehler K, Chung S. Dietary factors promoting brown

and beige fat development and thermogenesis. Advances in Nutrition. 2017;**8**:473-483. DOI: 10.3945/an.116.014332

[15] Andrade JM, Frade AC, Guimaraes JB, Freitas KM, Lopes MT, Guimaraes AL, et al. Resveratrol increases brown adipose tissue thermogenesis markers by increasing SIRT1 and energy expenditure and decreasing fat accumulation in adipose tissue of mice fed a standard diet. European Journal of Nutrition. 2014;**53**(7):1503-1510. DOI: 10.1007/s00394-014-0655-6

[16] Patel T, Ishiuji Y, Yosipovitch G. Menthol: A refreshing look at this ancient compound. Journal of the American Academy of Dermatology. 2007;**57**(5):873-878. DOI: 10.1016/j.jaad.2007.04.008

[17] McKemy DD, Neuhausser WM, Julius D. Identification of a cold receptor reveals a general role for TRP channels in thermosensation. Nature. 2002;**416**(6876):52-58. DOI: 10.1038/nature719

[18] Bautista DM, Siemens J, Glazer JM, Tsuruda PR, Basbaum AI, Stucky CL, et al. The menthol receptor TRPM8 is the principal detector of environmental cold. Nature. 2007;**448**(7150):204-208. DOI: 10.1038/nature05910

[19] Ludy MJ, Moore GE, Mattes RD. The effects of capsaicin and capsiate on energy balance: Critical review and meta-analyses of studies in humans. Chemical Senses. 2012;**37**(3):103-121. DOI: 10.1093/chemse/bjr100

[20] Yoneshiro T, Aita S, Matsushita M, Kayahara T, Kameya T, Kawai Y, et al. Recruited brown adipose tissue as an antiobesity agent in humans. Journal of Clinical Investigation. 2013;**123**(8):3404-3408. DOI: 10.1172/JCI67803

[21] Ohyama K, Nogusa Y, Shinoda K, Suzuki K, Bannai M, Kajimura S. A synergistic antiobesity effect by a combination of capsinoids and cold temperature through promoting beige adipocyte biogenesis. Diabetes. 2016;**65**(5):1410-1423

[22] Westerterp-Plantenga M, Diepvens K, Joosen AM, Berube-Parent S, Tremblay A. Metabolic effects of spices, teas, and caffeine. Physiology & Behavior. 2006;**89**:85-91. DOI: 10.1016/j.physbeh.2006.01.027

[23] Dulloo AG, Duret C, Rohrer D, Girardier L, Mensi N, Fathi M, et al. Efficacy of a green tea extract rich in catechin polyphenols and caffeine in increasing 24-h energy expenditure and fat oxidation in humans. The American Journal of Clinical Nutrition. 1999;**70**(6):1040-1045. DOI: 10.1093/ajcn/70.6.1040

[24] Dulloo AG, Seydoux J, Girardier L, Chantre P, Vandermander J. Green tea and thermogenesis: Interactions between catechin-polyphenols, caffeine and sympathetic activity. International Journal of Obesity and Related Metabolic Disorders. 2000;**24**(2):252-258. DOI: 10.1038/sj.ijo.0801101

Chapter 13

Association of Fatness and Leg Power with Blood Pressure in Adolescents

Danladi Musa, Daniel Iornyior and Andrew Tyoakaa

Abstract

This cross-sectional study examined the independent and joint association of fatness and leg power (LP) with resting blood pressure (BP) in adolescents (12 to 15 years) in Benue state of Nigeria. The present study comprised 2047 adolescents, including 1087 girls. Participants were assessed for body mass index (BMI), LP, and resting BP. Multivariate regression models assessing the associations of the independent variables with BP were conducted. Fatness and LP were independent predictors of resting BP among participants and the relationship of LP with BP was more robust in girls than boys. Combined fatness and LP in predicting BP was modest (R^2 = 10.4–14.3%) after controlling for maturity status. Low LP was associated with systolic blood pressure (SBP) in both girls (R^2 = 9.0%, β = 0.260, p = 0.001) and boys (R^2 = 11.0%, β = 0.226, p = 0.001). In the model for diastolic blood pressure (DBP), only fatness was associated with BP in girls (p = 0.001). The odd of hypertension (HTN) risk among overweight girls was 2.6 times that compared to their healthy-weight peers. Girls with low LP were 0.40 times more likely to develop HTN risk compared to their counterparts with high LP. This study has demonstrated that lower body muscle power is more important than fatness in predicting HTN in adolescent boys and girls.

Keywords: adolescents, adiposity, hypertension, leg muscle power, ROC curves

1. Introduction

Hypertension (HTN) is a global health problem because of its high prevalence with concomitant risk of cardiovascular disease (CVD), kidney disease, and other co-morbidities [1]. Although HTN like many other CVD risk factors was previously considered an adult health problem, recent evidence has shown that it is increasingly becoming a pediatric health problem with its prevalence tracking into adulthood [2, 3]. Therefore, if youth at risk of this disorder are identified early, proactive steps can be initiated to enhance better health prospects in later life.

Previous studies in the pediatric population have identified HTN as a potent antecedent of CVD and its rising prevalence is noticeable not only in industrialized countries but more so in developing countries including those in Africa [3–5]. It has been documented that elevated blood pressure (BP) in adolescence can be associated with target organ damage, renal failure, and adverse changes in sympathetic nervous system, all of which can negatively impact cardiac output with resultant imbalance in cardiovascular homeostasis [2]. Although the specific etiology of HTN remains nebulous, high levels of body fat and low physical activity (PA) or fitness level have been found to be major predisposing factors [6]. Several studies in youth have demonstrated positive relationships between body fat and resting blood pressure [4, 7]. For instance, a cross-sectional study [7] found fatness as well as fitness to be independent predictors of resting blood pressure. There is increasing evidence linking muscle fitness including muscle power to cardiovascular health in youth [8, 9]. A population-based study of American adolescents [10] documented an independent association between lower body muscle strength and cardiometabolic risk including blood pressure.

Despite the emerging evidence linking muscle fitness to health outcomes in youth, studies examining the independent association of lower body muscle power (here-in referred to as LP or vertical jump power-VJP) and fatness with BP are exiguous. Further, the interactive effect of fatness and LP on BP needs to be explored. The present study aimed to examine the independent and combined associations of BMI and VJP with resting BP among in-school adolescents in Benue State, North central Nigeria. Specifically, the study determined the independent and joint associations of BMI and VJP with resting BP among adolescent girls and boys. The study further examined the relationships among BMI, VJP, and BP to determine population-specific thresholds for BMI and VJP for predicting risk of HTN among participants. The study also examined variations in fatness categories by VJP levels. A better understanding of these relationships will help inform more effective intervention programs that could lead to improved LP with a concomitant reduction in disease risk among youth including the overweight. Thus, it was hypothesized that LP would reduce BP values regardless of fatness levels.

2. Methods

2.1 Participants

This cross-sectional study included volunteer participants from selected secondary schools in Benue State, North Central Nigeria. Participants were eligible to participate in the study if they had no musculoskeletal problems, history of CVD, other reported health problems and sickness or had not participated in organized exercise programs at least 6 months before data collection. The study purpose and test procedures were fully explained to participants after permission was duly obtained from the heads of participating schools. The study protocol was approved by the health research ethics committee of Benue State University (Ref. No. BSUTHMKD/HREC/2013/017). Written informed consent of parents/guardians and assent of participants were sought before data collection. All tests were conducted in accordance with the ethical guidelines of the Helsinki declaration.

2.2 Study setting

The present study was conducted among adolescents aged 12–16 years in the three senatorial districts of Benue State, Nigeria (Benue North, Benue Central, and Benue South). Benue state with its capital at Makurdi is located in the North central geopolitical zone of Nigeria. The predominant tribes are Tivs, Idomas, Igedes and Etulos. The study covered 11 secondary schools comprising 2100 adolescent girls and boys. Like any typical state in Nigeria, secondary schools in Benue State are in two main categories: public and private. The public schools are owned by the government while private schools are owned by private individuals and Christian missionaries. The schools start lessons by 8:00 am and close by 2:00 pm with a 45 minutes break at 10 am.

2.3 Physical characteristics measurement

Participants' physical characteristic measurements were in accordance with the protocol of the International Society for the Advancement of Kinanthropometry (ISAK) [11]. Specifically, bare-foot body mass and stature were measured in light clothing without shoes and socks with the aid of a calibrated digital weighing scale (Model Sec-880, Seca Birmingham, UK) and wall-mounted stadiometer (Model Sec-206; Seca, Birmingham, UK) to the nearest 0.1 kg and 0.1 cm, respectively. BMI was computed by dividing body mass in kilograms by stature in meter-square (kg. m^{-2}). BMI was used to estimate body fatness. Body fat was estimated from triceps and medial calf skinfolds with the aid of Harpenden skinfold calipers (Creative Health Products, Ann Arbor, MI, USA). Measurements were taken three times on the right side of a participant's body and the median was recorded. The revised regression equations for black children were used to estimate percent body fat [12]. On the basis of their BMI values, participants were categorized into healthy weight (HW) and overweight (OW) according to FitnessGram revised data [12].

Waist circumference (WC) which estimates abdominal fat [13] was measured with a Lufkin non-extensible flexible anthropometric tape (W606PM Rosscraft, Canada) to the nearest 0.1 cm. Details of the measurement procedure have been previously described [7]. All physical characteristics measurements were conducted by an accredited ISAK-Certified level 2 Anthropometrist (Lead author).

2.4 Pilot test

Before data collection, a pilot test was conducted to refine test administration procedures and determine precision of the instruments for data collection. Forty adolescent girls and boys ranging in age from 12–15 years that did not form part of the sample were recruited for the pilot test. All measurements were made according to standard procedures and the Cronbach's Alpha coefficients were calculated to determine test reliability. In all cases, the alpha coefficients ranged from 0.820 to 0.896, indicating good internal consistency [14].

2.5 Leg power testing

Leg muscle power, a component of muscle fitness was assessed using a vertical jump (VJ) field test. The test was conducted indoors on a flat floor with a smooth wall using the countermovement jump (CMJ) protocol. Participants were instructed to rub chalk on the fingertips of the dominant hand and had a couple of practice sessions and then took their turns for the test. In the CMJ protocol, a participant stood with the dominant shoulder about 15 cm from the wall with both feet flat on the floor, reached as high as possible with the dominant hand, and made a chalk mark on the wall. He/she lowered the dominant hand, performed a countermovement by flexing the knees and hips, moving the trunk forward and downward and swinging the arms backward, and jumped with a swiping motion as high as possible making a second mark on the wall. The score was the vertical distance between the two chalk marks. Participants' scores were converted into VJP values using a regression equation [15]. Each participant was given two trials and the best recorded to the nearest centimeter. Detailed description of the protocol is available elsewhere [16]. Participants were categorized into high and low groups using their sex-specific VJP receiver operating characteristic (ROC) cut-off values.

2.6 Blood pressure measurement

Blood pressure of participants was assessed in the morning while they occupied a sitting position after 10 minutes of rest with an oscillometric device. (HEM-705 CP, Omron Tokyo, Japan). The resting systolic blood pressure (SBP) and diastolic blood pressure (DBP) were monitored on each participant's right arm using appropriate cuff sizes. Measurements were taken 3 times at 2-min intervals, and the average was recorded. Specific details of the BP protocol have been previously described [7]. The cut-off points for HTN (95th percentile for age and sex) in this study were based on the standards of the fourth report on the diagnosis, evaluation, and treatment of high blood pressure in children and adolescents 2004 [17].

2.7 Data analysis

Data were checked for normality before analyses with the Kolmogorov–Smirnov test. Complete data for all variables were available for 2047 out of 2100 adolescents, with a compliance rate of 97.5%. Descriptive statistics were presented as means ± SDs, frequencies, and percentage distributions. Student's t-test was used to compare the means of both genders on all study variables. Zero-order correlation coefficients were calculated to assess the relationships among BMI, VJP, and BP of participants. Multiple linear regression analyses were conducted to determine the independent and combined associations of BMI, VJP, and resting BP. All analyses were adjusted for biological maturation. Biological maturation was estimated from height and chronological age using the regression equation of Moore and Co-workers [18]. The equation estimates maturity offset (MO) directly. Then, age at peak height velocity (APHV) was estimated as the difference between chronological age and MO. The independent association of BMI and VJP with BP was further examined using binary logistics regression models. Separate analyses were conducted for girls and boys. Odd ratios (95%CI) of being hypertensive were calculated between BMI and VJP categories. The amount of variation in BP explained by the model was determined using the Cox and Snell R square and Nergelkerke R square [14]. Models were adjusted for MO as a potential confounding variable. The predictive capacities of the independent variables for the risk of BP were determined through the ROC analysis with 95% confidence intervals (95%CI). Threshold values for identifying risk of HTN were determined through area under curve (AUC) values, sensitivity, and specificity. A diagnostic test with AUC equal to 1 is perfectly accurate and another with a value of 0.5 has no discriminatory power. Tests with the AUC of 0.9–1.0 = highly accurate; 0.7–0.9 = moderate; and < 0.7 = less accurate [19]. All analyses were conducted using the statistical package for the social sciences (SPSS Version 20, IBM corporation, Armonk, NY, USA).

3. Results

3.1 Physical and performance characteristics

Participants' general characteristics are summarized in **Table 1**. Girls were taller (p = 0.032), heavier (p < 0.001), fatter (p < 0.001), had larger WC (p < 0.001), higher BMI (p = 0.021), and higher MO (p < 0.001) than boys. Boys had significantly higher lean body mass (LBM) (p = 0.003), greater vertical jump height (VJH) (p < 0.001), and APHV (p < 0.001) than girls. There were no gender differences in chronological age (p = 0.432) and VJP (p = 0.617). Prevalence of HTN among participants is presented in **Figure 1**. The average prevalence of HTN (combined) is 9.8% for systolic HTN and 8.9% for diastolic HTN. Details of the gender-specific prevalence are displayed in **Figure 1**. Prevalence of OW in the total sample is 4.7% (Girls = 5.0%; boys =4.7%). In the case of LP, the prevalence of low LP was 54.6% (girls = 54.4%; Boys =54.8%). Although, both genders had healthy BMI, the correlation coefficients between fatness and VJP were generally moderate.

3.2 Predicators of BP

As shown in **Table 2**, VJP had the strongest correlation with the dependent variables, especially SBP. Because MO also had strong relationship with the dependent variables, models were adjusted for MO in both genders. Multiple regression was conducted to determine independent association of fatness and LP with resting BP (**Table 3**). LP was the only independent predictor (p < 0.001) of SBP and DBP in both

Variable	Combined (n = 2047)	Girls (n = 1087)	Boys (n = 960)	t-value	p-value
Age (y)	13.6 ± 1.3	13.6 ± 1.3	13.6 ± 1.3	0.786	0.432
APHV (y)	13.4 ± 1.1	12.6 ± 0.7	14.2 ± 0.7	50.075	<0.001
Stature (cm)	150.3 ± 11.6	150.8 ± 11.0	149.7 ± 12.2	2.149	0.032
MO (y)	0.2 ± 1.4	1.0 ± 1.0	−0.6 ± 1.0	33.6	<0.001
Body mass (kg)	43.5 ± 9.0	44.2 ± 8.7	42.6 ± 9.3	3.931	<0.001
BMI (kg.m^{-2})	19.3 ± 3.8	19.5 ± 3.7	19.1 ± 3.9	2.319	0.021
Fat (%)	16.0 ± 6.5	18.4 ± 5.6	13.4 ± 6.4	18.597	<0.001
WC (cm)	66.2 ± 8.4	67.1 ± 8.2.	65.1 ± 8.5	5.460	<0.001
LBM (kg)	36.4 ± 7.4	35.9 ± 6.5	36.9 ± 8.3	2.935	0.003
VJH (cm)	23.8 ± 7.6	22.7 ± 7.1	25.0 ± 7.9	6.774	<0.001
VJP (w)	1397.9 ± 507.9	1392.6 ± 481.7	1403.9 ± 536.2	0.501	0.617
SBP (mmHg)	113.6 ± 17.4	115.5 ± 18.1	111.5 ± 16.4	5.174	<0.001
DBP (mmHg)	69.2 ± 13.7	68.8 ± 13.7	69.7 ± 13.7	1.465	0.143
r between BMI and VJP		0.504	0.517		

Table 1.
General characteristics of participants (n = 2047).

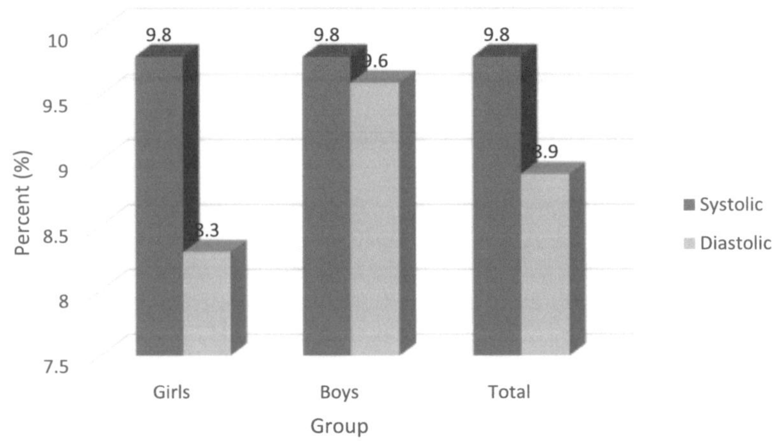

Figure 1.
Prevalence of hypertension in participants.

	SBP			DBP		
Group	**MO**	**BMI**	**VJP**	**MO**	**BMI**	**VJP**
Girls	0.207**	0.147**	0.314**	0.120**	0.110**	0.118**
Boys	0.298**	0.172**	0.334**	0.076*	0.072*	0.094*

$^*p < 0.05$ $^{**}p < 0.01$.

Table 2.
Correlation coefficients among BMI, VJP, and blood pressure.

Group	Dependent variable	Predictors	r^2	B	P
Girls	SBP	BMI	0.099	−0.016	0.662
		VJP		0.321	<0.001
	DBP	BMI	0.017	0.068	0.051
		VJP		0.084	0.016
Boys	SBP	BMI	0.111	−0.001	0.968
		VJP		0.335	<0.001
	DBP	BMI	0.010	0.032	0.398
		VJP		0.078	0.039

Table 3.
Fatness and leg power as predictors of SBP and DBP among participants.

genders, the association with the SBP being stronger. Fatness was not significantly associated ($p > 0.005$) with SBP and DBP in both genders.

3.3 Multivariate models for predicting BP

Hierarchical multiple regression analyses were conducted to determine the joint associations of fatness and LP with BP controlling for MO in both genders (**Table 4**).

For the girls' SBP model, the covariate explained only 4.3% of the variance in step 1. The addition of BMI and VJP in step 2 increased the total variance to 10.4% indicating that both the independent variables explained an additional variance of 6.1%. LP ($p < 0.001$) and MO ($p = 0.014$) were the significant predictors, with VJP presenting greater explanatory capacity. In the model for boys, fatness and LP explained 23.1% with only 8.9% contribution from MO. All variables made significant contributions, but MO presented the greatest explanatory power. In the model for DBP, only MO and BMI made significant ($p < 0.05$) contributions in girls, while in the boys' model, no independent variable made any statistically significant ($P > 0.005$) contribution. Details of the results can be found in **Table 4**.

Results of the logistic regression models (**Table 5**) indicated that in general only VJP and BMI made significant contributions, which were greater in girls. In the girls' model, both fatness (OR = 2.6, 95% CI = 1.29–5.35; $p = 0.008$) and LP (OR = 0.40, 95% CI = 0.25–0.64; $p < 0.001$) were associated with SBP. These results indicate that fat girls were 2.6 times likely to develop risk of HTN compared to their healthy weight peers. Further, the odd of HTN risk in girls with low LP was 0.40 times that of their counterparts with greater LP. As a whole, the model was able to explain between 4–9% of the variance in SBP and correctly classified 90.2% of the cases. In the Boys' model, no variable made any significant contribution. However, the model also explained between 4–9% of the variation in SBP and correctly classified 90.2% of the cases. For the DBP models, only MO (OR = 1.40, 95%CI = 1.15–1.62, $p < 0.001$) in girls made a significant contribution to the model. The model for boys was not significant ($p < 0.001$). Details of the results are in **Table 5**.

3.4 Threshold of independent variables for detecting HTN

The ROC curve analyses are presented in **Table 6**. In both genders, the AUCs were significantly greater than 0.5 for both VJP and BMI ($p < 0.05$). The optimal threshold

		Predictor	Model 1			Model 2		
Group	variable		r^2	B	P	r^2	B	p
Girls	SBP	MO	0.043	0.207	<0.001	0.104	0.087	0.014
		BMI	—	—	—	—	0.021	0.568
		VJP	—	—	—	—	0.263	<0.001
Boys		MO	0.089	0.298	<0.001	0.143	0.231	<0.001
		BMI	—	—	—	—	0.111	0.005
		VJP	—	—	—	—	0.165	<0.001
Girls	DBP	MO	0.014	0.120	<0.001	0.029	0.130	<0.001
		BMI	—	—	—	—	0.121	0.001
		VJP	—	—	—	—	−0.003	0.949
Boys		MO	0.006	0.076	0.019	0.013	0.071	0.091
		BMI	—	—	—	—	0.066	0.122
		VJP	—	—	—	—	0.026	0.592

Table 4.
Multiple regression analysis among Fatness, leg power, and BP among participants.

				SBP				DBP	
Group	**Pred**	**β**	**OR**	**95%CI**	*P*	**β**	**OR**	**95%CI**	*p*
Girls	MO	0.30	1.35	1.12–1.64	0.002	0.34	1.40	1.15–1.72	0.001
	BMI								
	HW OW	0.966	1 2.63	1.29–5.35	0.008	0.82	1 2.27	0.96– 5.34	0.061
	VJP								
	High Low	−0.923	1 0.40	0.25–0.64	<0.001	0.431	1 1.54	.96–2.48	0.076
Boys	MO	0.595	1.81	1.44–2.29	<0.001	0.194	1.20	0.96–1.53	0.103
	BMI								
	HW OW	0.920	1 2.51	0.96–6.56	0.060	−1.426	1 0.24	.032– 1.80	0.165
	VJP								
	High Low	−0.289	1 0.75	0.46–1.23	0.252	−0.312	1 0.73	0.45–1.19	0.208

Pred = predictor.

Table 5.
Odds of risk of HTN are stratified according to gender (n = 2047).

Group	Variable	AUC	95%CI	Cut-point	Se	Sp	*p*-value
Girls	BMI	0.573	.518–.627	18.9	0.575	0.516	0.014
	VJP	0.696	.649–.743	1501.5	0.698	0.373	<0.001
Boys	BMI	0.607	.547–.667	18.9	0.606	0.413	0.001
	VJP	0.667	.605–.729	1340.7	0.670	0.484	<0.001

Table 6.
Receiver operating characteristic analysis for risk of HTN (n = 2047).

in girls for VJP and BMI were 1501.5 W and 18.9 kg.m^{-2}, respectively. Corresponding values for boys were 1340.7 W and 18.9 kg.m^{-2}, respectively. Details of the results are shown in **Table 5**. The gender-specific ROC curves are presented in **Figures 2** and **3**.

In order to further evaluate the influence of fatness and LP on BP, participants were divided into four fat/power groups and the results are presented in **Table 7**. The proportion of girls within these categories was 42.1%, 53.0%, 3.6%, and 1.3% for low fat/high power, low fat/low power, high fat/high power, and high fat/low power, respectively. Corresponding values for boys were 42.2%, 53.3%, 3.0%, and 1.3%. There were significant group differences in SBP for both girls ($F_{(3,1083)} = 7.50$, $p < 0.001$) and boys ($F_{(3,956)} = 4.99, p < 0.002$). For both genders, the differences were between the fat/low power group and three other groups (low fat/high power, low fat/high power, and high fat/high power). The same group differences were documented for boys. For DBP in girls, there was a significant ($F_{(3,1083)} = 3.66, p = 0.012$) group difference, the difference was between the two extreme groups. In boys, there were no group differences ($p = 0.0165$).

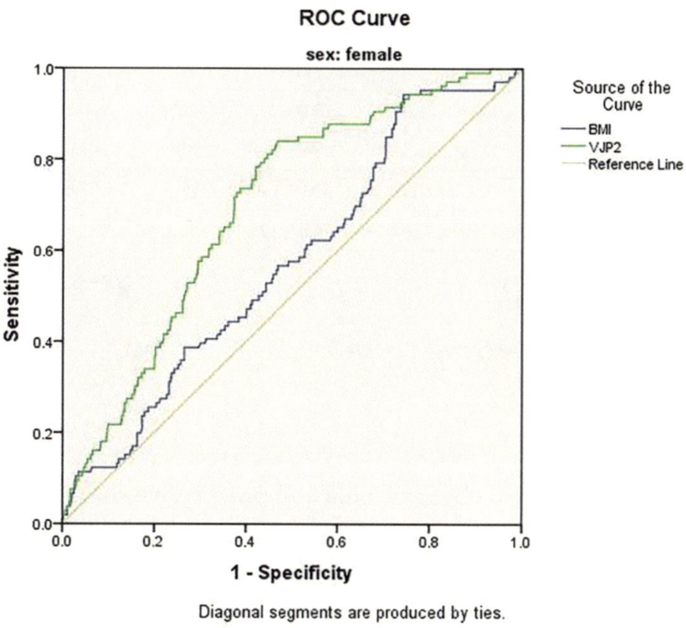

Figure 2.
Areas under the curve for BMI and VJP in girls.

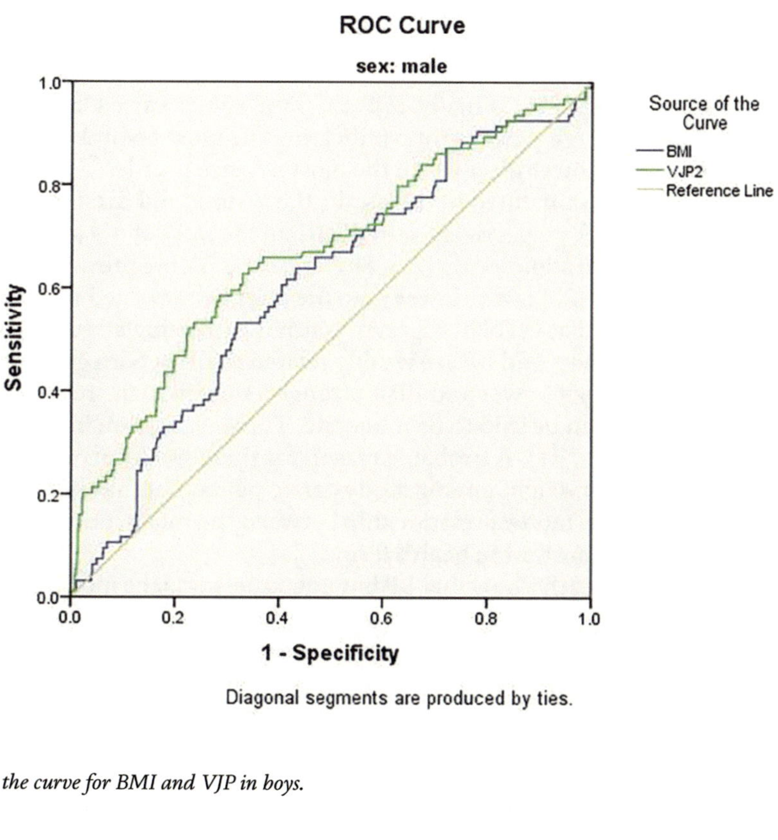

Figure 3.
Areas under the curve for BMI and VJP in boys.

	Girls (n = 1087)			Boys (n = 960)		
Group	**n**	**SBP**	**DBP**	**n**	**SBP**	**DBP**
Low fat/High power	458	108.6 ± 21.3	70.0 ± 13.5	407	106.2 ± 18.9	70.7 ± 13.7
Low fat/Low power	576	111.0 ± 16.3	67.6 ± 13.8	512	107.6 ± 15.2	68.8 ± 13.7
Fat/High power	39	108.3 ± 17.6	69.9 ± 12.3	29	102.8 ± 15.9	72.0 ± 13.1
Fat/Low power	14	128.0 ± 17.6	74.8 ± 19.6	12	123.4 ± 24.6	69.8 ± 12.2

HP=High power; LP = Low power.

Table 7.
Differences in BP according to fat/power groups (n = 2047).

4. Discussion

Recent evidence from both observational and prospective studies in high-and middle-income societies has shown overweight youth with low leg muscle power exhibit unfavorable cardiometabolic disease risk, including high BP [20, 21]. Although HTN, like in the developed world is becoming a health problem in sub-Saharan Africa, the significance of fatness and leg muscle power in the development of HTN remains to be fully investigated among Nigerian youth.

The main findings of this study include: First, the prevalence of HTN is comparable with prevalent rates documented in both industrialized and developing countries [22, 23] and it is higher in girls. Second, the relationships among the independent and dependent variables are generally weak to moderate. Third, Fatness and LP are independent predictors of BP, but LP demonstrated a greater explanatory capacity than fatness in girls. Fourth, the joint contribution of fatness and LP in predicting blood pressure is modest (10.4–14.3%). Finally, SBP and DBP values varied by fat-power groups, with the low fat-high power group indicating the most favorable BP profile compared to the fat-low power group with the most adverse profile.

For the total sample documented in this study, the systolic and diastolic HTN prevalence of 9.8% and 8.9, respectively, is higher than the rates of 4.9 and 6.5% reported for South African adolescents [22]. Similarly, the Global prevalence rate of 6.9% for African children [23] is also lower than the rates documented in the present study. This result implies that HTN in Nigerian youth is increasing at a disturbing rate.

In this study, both fatness and LP are weakly related to BP in both genders, though the relationship between leg power and BP is stronger. However, the relationship between fatness and LP can be said to be moderate. These results are in agreement with previous research [21, 24]. A probable reason for these weak correlations may be the low prevalence of overweight among study participants. This has been previously observed [25]. Despite the modest relationship between the independent variables and BP, the link is still important in health terms.

Results of this study clearly show that LP but not fatness was the independent predictor of SBP and DBP in both girls and boys. Our results are consistent with some previous reports [20, 25]. These results indicate that leg muscle power is a problem among the study participants. As indicated, large proportions of both girls (54.4%) and boys (54.8%) had low LP. This result highlights the need to focus on this aspect of fitness among this cohort of adolescents. Muscle power is now considered an important component of health-related physical fitness, which is associated with a positive health prognosis and a lower risk of developing CVD risk in the pediatric population [8].

The present study shows the joint contribution of fatness and LP in predicting resting SBP was moderate (Girls = 10.4%; Boys = 14.3%). But the major determinant of SBP in girls was LP while in boys, maturity status. The association of LP with SBP was stronger in girls than boys. A plausible reason for the result in girls may be early maturation (**Table 1**), they also often participate in less vigorous physical activities than boys, hence the higher BP levels. Our results are in agreement with those of several investigators [20, 21, 26]. But surprisingly, the relationship between LP and BP was positive, indicating that participants with greater leg power also had higher SBP. It has been observed that confounding variables such as excessive intake of salt, alcohol, and cigarette could lead to these results [20]. We are in agreement with these speculations as they appear plausible. Fatness was significantly associated with only SBP in boys and DBP in girls.

Findings from the present study clearly indicate that resting BP levels varied by cut-points of fatness and LP. The poorest BP profile was documented in adolescents who are overweight with low leg muscle power. Specifically, high levels of LP resulted in lower resting BP irrespective of fatness status. This result is supported by previous research in Norwegian adolescents [21]. This finding is of public health significance.

Based on our results and those of others, it may be realistic to believe that fatness and LP are important variables that contribute to the development of HTN in adolescents. Worthy of note is the importance of lower body muscle power in cardiovascular and musculoskeletal health. For instance, there is increasing evidence linking muscle fitness, including muscle power to cardiovascular and general health in youth [9, 26, 27]. Indeed, current physical activity guidelines for youth emphasize muscle-strengthening activities on a regular basis for improvement in muscle fitness [28, 29]. Based on empirical evidence, several authorities have emphasized the development of muscle fitness due to its overall health benefits [30–32]. Therefore, evidence from the present study and others should serve to stimulate effective public health strategies to minimize HTN in adolescents by improving leg muscle power and reducing fatness.

Findings from this study should be interpreted in the light of some limitations. The cross-sectional design precludes confirmation of cause-and-effect relationship. A major strength of this study was the use of valid field tests of health-related physical fitness. These tests use standards that discriminate well between children with more favorable cardiovascular health profiles from those with less favorable profiles. For instance, results from the logistic regression models showed a very high percentage accuracy classification (PAC) in both genders (Girls = 90.2%; Boys = 90.2%).

5. Conclusions

In conclusion, LP was independently associated with resting BP in Nigerian adolescents. The relationship of LP with BP was more robust in girls. Combination of fatness and LP in predicting BP was modest. Variation in BP for girls was best predicted by LP while that of boy was biological maturation. The combination of low LP and high fatness resulted in the most unfavorable BP profile. These results suggest that intervention targeting BP control in adolescents should focus more on leg muscle power with less emphasis on body composition, and this should be considered an important public health goal.

Acknowledgements

The authors gratefully acknowledge the cooperation of students, teachers, and head teachers of schools that participated in the project. The contribution of the research assistants who made data collection possible is gratefully acknowledged.

Conflict of interest

The authors declare no conflict of interest.

Author details

Danladi Musa[1*], Daniel Iornyior[2] and Andrew Tyoakaa[2]

1 Kogi State University, Anyigba, Nigeria

2 Benue State University, Makurdi, Nigeria

*Address all correspondence to: musa.d@ksu.edu.ng

References

[1] World Health Organisation. The world health report. In: Reducing Risk, Promoting Healthy Lifestyle. Vol. 2002. Geneva, Switzerland: World Health Organisation; 2002. pp. 101-146

[2] Chiolero A, Bovet P, Paradis G. Screening for evaluated blood pressure in children and adolescents: A critical appraisal. JAMA Pediatrics. 2013;**167**:266-273

[3] Ejike CE. Prevalence of HTN in Nigerian children and adolescents: A systematic review and trend analysis of data from the past four decades. Journal of Tropical Pediatrics. 2017;**63**:229-241

[4] Musa DI, Lawal B, Fawa MS. Body fat and blood pressure levels in school boys in Kano city, Nigeria. The African Symposium: An on-line Educational Research Journal. 2002;**2**:1-7

[5] Noubiap JJ, Essoumam BJJ, Jingi AM, Aminde LN, Nansseu JR. Prevalence of elevated blood pressure in children and adolescents in Africa: A systematic review and meta-analysis. Lancet Public Health. 2017;**2**:C375-C386

[6] Crump C, Sundquist J, winkleby MA, Sundquist K. Interactive effects of physical fitness and body mass index on risk of hypertension. JAMA Internal Medicine. 2016;**176**(2):210-216

[7] Musa DI, Williams CA. Cardiorespiratory fitness, fatness, and blood pressure associations in Nigerian youth. Medicine and Science in Sports and Exercise. 2012;**44**(10):1978-1985

[8] Smith JJ, Eather N, Morgan PJ, Plotnikoff RC, Figerbaum AD, Lubans DR. The health benefits of muscular fitness for children and adolescents: A systematic review and meta-analysis. Sports Medicine. 2014;**44**:1209-1223

[9] Janz KF, Baptista F, Ren S, Zhu W, Laurson KR, Mahar MT, et al. Associations among musculoskeletal fitness assessments and health outcomes: The Lisbon study for the development and evaluation of musculoskeletal fitness standards in youth. Measurement in Physical Education and Exercise Science. 2021;**25**(Suppl.):1-9. DOI: 10.1080/1091367x.2021.2000414

[10] Peterson MD, Zang P, Saltarelli WA, Visich PS, Gordon PM. Low muscle strength thresholds for the detection of cardiometabolic risk in adolescents. American Journal of Preventive Medicine. 2015;**50**(5):593-599. DOI: 10.1016/j.amepre.2015.09.019

[11] Mafell-Jones MJ, Stewart AD, de Ridder JH. International Standards for Anthropometric Assessment. Wellington, New Zealand: International Society for the Advancement of Kinanthropometry; 2012. pp. 32-89

[12] The Cooper Institute. Fitness Gram Test Administration Manual. 5th ed. Champaign, IL, USA: Human Kinetics; 2017. pp. 39-64

[13] Maffies C. Aetiology of overweight in children and adolescents. European Journal of Pediatrics. 2000;**159**:S35-S44

[14] Pallant J. SPPS Survival Manual: A Step-by-step Guide to Data Analysis Using SPSS. 5th ed. Berkshire, England: Open University Press; 2017

[15] Mahar MT, Welk GJ, Janz KF, Laurson K, Zhu W, Baptista F. Estimation of lower body muscle power from

vertical jump in youth. Measurement in Physical Education and Exercise Science. 2022;**26**(Suppl.):1-11. DOI: 10.1080/1091367x.2022.2041420

[16] Mcguigan M. Administration, scoring and interpretation of selected tests. In: Halt GG, Triplet NT, editors. (CDS). Essentials of strength training and conditioning. 4th ed. Champaign, IL: Human Kinetics; 2015

[17] National High Blood Pressure Education Working Group on High Blood Pressure in Children and Adolescents. The fourth report on the diagnosis, evaluation and treatment of high blood pressure in children and adolescents. Pediatrics. 2004;**114**:555-576

[18] Moore SA, McKay HA, Macdonald H, Nettlefold L, Baxter-Jones AD, Cameron N, et al. Enhancing somatic maturity prediction model. Medicine & Science in Sports & Exercise. 2015;**47**(8):1755-1764

[19] Swets JA. Measuring the accuracy of diagnostic systems. Science. 1988;**240**(4857):1285-1293

[20] Nunes HEG, Alves CAS Jr, Goncalves ECA, Silva DAS. What physical fitness component is most closely associated with adolescents' blood pressure? Perceptual and Motor Skills. 2017;**124**(6):1107-1120

[21] Steene-Johannessene J, Anderssen SA, Kolle E, Andesen LB. Low muscle fitness is associated with metabolic risk in youth. Medicine & Science in Sports & Exercise. 2009;**41**(7):1361-1367

[22] Awotidebe A, Monyeki MA, Moss SJ, Strydom GL, Amstrong M, Kemper HCG. Relationship of adiposity and cardiorespiratory fitness with resting blood pressure of South African adolescents: The PAHL study. Journal of Human Hypertension. 2015;**30**:245-251. DOI: 10.1038/jhh.2015.81

[23] Song P, Zhang Y, Yu J, Zha M, Zhu Y, Rahimi K, et al. Global prevalence of hypertension in children: A systematic review and meta-analysis. JAMA Pediatrics. 2019;**173**(12):1154-1163

[24] Buchan DS, Young JD, Boddy LM, Malina RM, Baker JS. Fitness and adiposity are independently associated with cardiometabolic risk in youth. BioMed Research International. 2013;**231**:1-6

[25] Eisenmann JC. Aerobic fitness, fatness and the metabolic syndrome in children and adolescents. Acta Pediatric. 2007;**96**:1723-1729

[26] Garcia-Artero E, Ortega FB, Ruiz R, et al. Lipid and metabolic profile in adolescents are affected more by physical fitness than physical activity (Avena Study). Revista Española de Cardiología. 2007;**60**(6):581-588

[27] Baptista F, Zymbal V, JanZ KF. Predictive validity of handgrip strength, vertical jump power and plank time in the identification of pediatric sarcopenia. Measurement in Physical Education and Exercise Science. 2021. DOI: 10.1080/1091307x.2021.1987242

[28] Welk G, Janz K, Laurson K, Mahar M, Zhu W, Paulovic A. Development of criterion- reference standards for musculoskeletal fitness in youth: Considerations and approaches by the fitnessgram scientific advisory board. Measurement in Physical Education and Exercise Science. 2022. DOI: 10.1080/1091367x.2021.2014331

[29] Weaver CM, Gordon CM, Janz KF, kalwarf HS, Lapped JM, Lewis R, et al. Peak bone mass development and

lifestyle factors: A systematic review and implementation recommendations. Osteoporosis International. 2016;**27**(4):1281-1386

[30] US Department of Health and Human Services. Physical Activity Guidelines for Americans. 2nd ed. Washington, DC, USA: US Department of Health and Human Services; 2018

[31] Corbin C, Jan KF, Baptista F. Good health: The power of power. Journal of Physical Education, Recreation & Dance. 2017;**88**(9):28-35

[32] Pate RR, Daniels S. Institute of Medicine report on fitness measures and health outcomes in youth. JAMA Pediatrics. 2013;**167**(3):221-222